JAY

D0943632

616 L85e
Long, James W.
The essential guide to
chronic illness

ESSENTIAL
GUIDE TO
CHRONIC
ILLNESS

FUNDS TO PURCHASE
THIS BOOK WERE
PROVIDED BY A
40TH ANNIVERSARY GRANT
FROM THE
FOELLINGER FOUNDATION.

THE ESSENTIAL GUIDE TO CHRONIC ILLNESS

The Active Patient's Handbook

James W. Long, M.D.

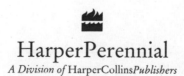

HarperPerennial
A Division of HarperCollinsPublishers

Allen County Public Library
900 Webster Street
PO Box 2270
Fort Wayne, IN 46801-2270

The author gratefully acknowledges permission to reprint the following excerpts:

From *Health Promotion and Disease Prevention in Clinical Practice*, by Steven H. Woolf, M.D., M.P.H., Williams and Wilkins, 1996, by permission of the author and publisher.

From *How We Die: Reflections on Life's Final Chapter*, by Sherwin B. Nuland, M.D., Knopf, 1994, by permission of the author and publisher.

From "Assisted Death: A Compassionate Response to a Medical Failure," originally published in the November 5, 1992 issue of the *New England Journal of Medicine*, Vol. 327, No. 19, by permission of the author, Howard Brody, M.D., Ph.D.

THE ESSENTIAL GUIDE TO CHRONIC ILLNESS. Copyright © 1997 by James W. Long, M.D. All rights reserved. Printed in the United States of America. No part of this book may be used or reproduced in any manner whatsoever without written permission except in the case of brief quotations embodied in critical articles and reviews. For information address HarperCollins Publishers Inc. 10 East 53rd Street, New York, NY 10022.

HarperCollins books may be purchased for educational, business, or sales promotional use. For information, please write to: Special Markets Department, HarperCollins Publishers Inc., 10 East 53rd Street, New York, NY 10022.

FIRST EDITION

Designed by Alma Hochhauser Orenstein

Library of Congress Cataloging-in-Publication Data
Long, James W.
    The essential guide to chronic illness: the active patient's handbook / James W. Long. — 1st ed.
        p.   cm.
    Includes bibliographical references and index.
    ISBN 0-06-271523-2 (hardcover). — ISBN 0-06-273137-8 (pbk.)
    1. Chronic diseases — Popular works. 2. Self-care, Health.
    I. Title.
    RC108.L66 1997
    616—dc21   96-47743

97 98 99 00 01 ❖/RRD 10 9 8 7 6 5 4 3 2 1
97 98 99 00 01 ❖/RRD 10 9 8 7 6 5 4 3 2 (pbk)

Contents

SECTION FOUR

SECTION FIVE

SECTION SIX

SECTION SEVEN

APPENDIXES

Author's Note

The unprecedented reformations currently taking place in America's health care system are causing considerable dismay among health care providers and consumers. Physicians and patients alike are finding it difficult to adjust to changes imposed by "managed care" philosophies and procedures. The crisis resulting from steady growth in demand for services and escalating costs of providing them is forcing us to seek better ways to meet the health care needs of the nation.

Although seemingly abrupt and somewhat disruptive, this evolution within our system of health care may well have some lasting beneficial effects. Quite recently, three new developments have emerged that express a common theme: the mutual sharing of knowledge, integrity, and responsibility by providers and consumers—physicians and patients—in the provision of health care on a national scale.

The first is a proposal by John Balint, M.D., and Wayne Shelton, Ph.D., of the Center for Medical Ethics, Education, and Research at Albany Medical College, New York. They propose a new model of the patient–physician relationship: "A patient–physician alliance based on mutual education of physician and patient about health and illness, values and persons, social responsibility, beneficence, trust, and a degree of paternalism."[1] This is a marked departure from the traditional paternalistic model in which the physician provides information and the patient makes unaided decisions. It also differs from the Libertarian model in which the patient's exaggerated autonomy tends to deter physician responsibility. The key element of this new patient–physician alliance is that the physician, as responsible teacher, must educate the patient regarding appropriate care so that the patient, as a fully informed recipient of care, can make rational and responsible decisions autonomously.

The second development is the rapid proliferation of "Mini-Med Schools" in numerous regions of the country.[2] Many prestigious medical institutions, including the University of Chicago Medical Center, the Uni-

[1]"A New Model of the Patient–Physician Relationship," J. Balint and W. Shelton, *JAMA*, March 20, 1996, Vol. 275, No. 11, pages 887–891.

[2]"'Mini-Med Schools' Offer Lay Public Lessons in the Science of Medicine," Joan Stephenson, Ph.D., *JAMA*, March 27, 1996, Vol. 275, No. 12, pages 897–899.

versity of Colorado Health Sciences Center, the National Institutes of
Health, and more than 20 others are offering local citizens the opportunity to attend formal classes in a diverse selection of basic and applied
medical sciences. The public response in each instance has been overwhelming, reflecting a genuine broad-based interest and hunger for
knowledge of the world of medicine.

The third development is the recently published *Guide to Clinical Preventive Services*, the second report of the U.S. Preventive Services Task
Force.[3] In a companion book written by members of the Task Force staff,[4]
the authors state:

> Discussions in this book about patient education and counseling empha-
> size a shared decision-making model and a respectful style of discourse
> between patients and clinicians. This approach differs from the old-fash-
> ioned paternalistic counseling style in which the doctor 'tells the patient
> what to do.' The philosophy espoused in this book is that patients are
> entitled to make informed decisions about how they live their lives and
> about their health care. Clinicians have a professional responsibility to
> ensure that patients' decisions are based on accurate and complete health
> information but do not have a right to force the outcome of decisions.
> [Again] this book encourages a collaborative model for decision-making,
> which permits the clinician and patient to work together to determine the
> best choice for that individual. The book speaks of choices, not 'orders';
> patient initiative, not 'compliance'; and partnership, not 'prescription.'

The idea for this book on chronic disorders was conceived several
years ago, before the welcome developments just described. However, it
was my affirmation of the same principles and practices discussed above
that prompted its creation. The aim of the book is to provide patients and
their families with information they can use to improve their interaction
with our health care community. It is in the patient's best interest to be as
fully informed as possible regarding his disorder and its management. All
health care providers should understand that a well-informed patient is
their best ally in achieving satisfactory treatment outcomes.

The information provided in this book is gleaned from the most recent
editions of well-established, authoritative medical textbooks; current
issues of leading medical journals; publications of federal government
agencies; and educational materials provided by disorder-oriented institutions and organizations. This broad spectrum of information reflects the
opinions and recommendations of individual authors and editors gener-

---

[3]*Guide to Clinical Preventive Services*, 2nd edition, Report of the U.S. Preventive
Services Task Force. Baltimore: Williams and Wilkins, 1996.

[4]*Health Promotion and Disease Prevention in Clinical Practice*, S.H. Woolf, S.
Jonas, and R.S. Lawrence. Baltimore: Williams and Wilkins, 1996.

ally recognized as experts in their respective fields. I fully acknowledge that this book is not all-inclusive; a book of this size and scope cannot provide coverage of all known diagnostic and therapeutic procedures for the disorders presented. As author-editor, I warrant only that the information has been carefully reviewed, thoughtfully selected, and accurately transcribed to the best of my ability. The inclusion of any management recommendations does not constitute endorsement or warranty of treatment outcomes by me, and I disclaim all responsibility for the consequences of selecting and utilizing any diagnostic or therapeutic procedure presented in this text. The author's intent is to provide information only, not to advise. The reader is urged to consult with personal medical advisers on all matters relating to disease prevention, diagnosis, and management.

This book is a medical reference volume intended primarily for the use of patients and their families. It is written solely to provide general information that the reader can use to facilitate communication with health care providers. It is not a source of medical advice to be used for self-diagnosis or self-treatment. Please read the detailed disclaimer statement above.

In accordance with the style used in Webster's New Collegiate Dictionary, the male pronouns *he*, *his*, and *him* are generally used throughout the text to represent humanity. The female pronouns *she* and *her* will be used when specific and appropriate.

Due to a lack of consensus in America's usage, the author has chosen to use the designation *black* to be synonymous with *Afro-American, colored*, and *negro*. This is in accord with the designation used in official government documents dealing with health statistics.

The disorders selected for inclusion in Section Three of this book meet three criteria: relative frequency in the United States; severity of impact on patient and family; and degree of difficulty in recognition or management.

Detailed drug information is not amenable to the size and scope of this book. Limited drug information is provided in Disorder Profiles when its significance justifies it. The reader is referred to Appendix 17 for authoritative sources of drug information in depth.

Many clinical trials involving serious medical disorders are being conducted in research centers throughout the United States. Because of the inherent uncertainty of when trials begin and end, firm dates are not published. However, information regarding current trials is available to those who need it. See Appendix 2 for a detailed discussion of clinical trials for malignant diseases.

Each physician develops his own favored pattern of diagnostic and therapeutic procedures, striving to establish a practice style that is comfortable, effective, and rewarding. The approach recommended by your physician to diagnose and treat your disorder may vary somewhat from the information provided in this book. It is important for you, the patient, to recognize and understand that many aspects of medical care are controversial. There can be marked variation in how any disorder manifests itself (symptoms and signs), and how each patient responds to treatment. If your physician's initial assessment and recommendations seem reasonable to you, follow his instructions as given. If your response is not what you expected, or you are uncertain about any aspect of your treatment, consult your physician before attempting any modification of therapy on your own. **Make a serious effort to learn as much as you can about your disorder—its diagnosis and treatment options. By doing so, you can acquire the knowledge and judgment needed to cooperate appropriately with your medical advisers and assure the best possible treatment outcome.**

JAMES W. LONG, M.D.
July 1996

Acknowledgments

The creation of a book of this nature is an arduous and sometimes oner-ous endeavor, but acknowledging the efforts of those who aided the undertaking is a genuine joy. Each of the following individuals has con-tributed in a unique and meaningful way. With sincere appreciation and gratitude, I respectfully acknowledge their collaboration.

To Dr. Jewell L. Osterholm, master neurosurgeon of Jefferson Medical College, Thomas Jefferson University, I owe a double measure of thanks. He astutely detected the cause of my six-year ordeal of pain and disabil-ity, skillfully corrected it, and made it possible for me to resume creative writing. In addition, the Profile of spinal stenosis in Section Three is the direct result of his tutelage and gracious review.

To Dr. Mary B. Burgoyne, rheumatologist, revered and respected by colleagues and patients alike, for her comprehensive review and insight-ful embellishment of Appendix 8, Nonsteroidal Anti-Inflammatory Drugs: A Guide to Selection for Therapy.

To Dr. James J. Rybacki, acclaimed specialist in pharmaceutical care and host of the popular radio program *The Pharmacist Minute*, my admi-ration and gratitude for his masterful assumption of sole editorship of *The Essential Guide to Prescription Drugs,* my major source of current drug information for the preparation of this book.

To Liz Freedlander, Executive Director, Talbot Hospice Foundation, for her time and generosity in providing me with the insight and operational philosophy of Hospice and graciously reviewing Section Four, Terminal Illness: The Dying Patient.

To Lois W. Sanger, M.L.S., Director of Library Services, Health Sciences Library, Easton Memorial Hospital, for making the world's medical litera-ture available to a retired physician living and writing in a small rural community. No matter the source of the book or the obscurity of the journal, Lois would obtain it—an indispensable health care professional.

To my wife, Alice R. Long, my editor/critic-in-residence, for reading the evolving manuscript from the patient's perspective and suggesting cogent revisions in both content and expression.

To Helen Moore, Publishing Manager and Senior Editor, HarperCollins Publishers, for providing that rare totality of superb editorial skills, intellectual support, and genuine personal concern that every author dreams of finding. Working with Helen is akin to the gratification felt by the sculptor's apprentice as he watches form and purpose emerge from rough-hewn stone.

To Elaine Verriest, Senior Production Editor, HarperCollins Publishers, for her most cordial accommodation and flawless efforts as she converted this unconventional manuscript to book form so effectively.

To John R. Day, Director, Electronic Publishing, HarperCollins Publishers, for his many years of invaluable guidance during my passage from typewriter to computer. John's consistent willingness to share his superlative expertise has contributed immeasurably to the accomplishment of this endeavor.

SECTION ONE

Introduction: Why This Book?

Our Evolving National Health Care System

Current revisions in traditional health services make it necessary to refocus our attention on how patients (health care consumers) go about obtaining the care they need and how the system (health care providers) responds to those needs. Although good communication between patient and physician has always been of fundamental importance, now, more than ever, it is the essential key to satisfactory medical encounters. The operational approach of many managed care organizations (MCOs) mandates that more patients be seen by fewer physicians, with added constraints of limited time and rationed services. As all physicians know and many patients understand, the circumspect evaluation and thoughtful diagnosis of many medical conditions are not amenable to assembly line conformity. Some disorders are relatively obvious, readily recognized, and easily managed. On the other hand, the true nature of numerous disorders is less apparent in early stages; careful, unhurried consideration is necessary to achieve a correct diagnosis. In using the managed-care settings evolving today, it is incumbent upon the patient to convey quickly and clearly his principal symptoms and concerns within the limited time made available. Because of the shortage of primary care physicians (only 20% of the physician workforce), MCOs may utilize physician assistants (PAs) and certified nurse practitioners (CNPs) to screen patients prior to seeing a physician. Although capable of providing an appropriate triage function, allied health professionals are not expected to possess the diagnostic acumen of fully trained and experienced physicians. This increases the risk of misinterpretation of the presentation made by an uninformed or inarticulate patient. It is increasingly apparent in today's health care settings that the well-informed patient can clearly influence the timely diagnosis of his illness and the outcome of its management. The advent of managed care has greatly accelerated the need for patient education and active participation in all aspects of health maintenance.

Using the "New and Improved" Health Care System

The principal goal of this book is to provide a useful source of information that will help patients and their families to participate beneficially in today's rapidly changing health care system. In a practical sense, this means addressing the concerns of the troubled patient with a medical problem. The basic concerns are two:

1. obtaining a correct diagnosis promptly
2. receiving timely, safe, and effective treatment

Attempts to achieve these goals involve the following procedures:

- selecting a Managed Care Organization (MCO)
- selecting a personal physician
- preparing for the initial and subsequent office visits
- presenting your case
- doing your homework

SELECTING A MANAGED CARE ORGANIZATION (MCO)

There is a growing variety of MCOs established throughout the country. The major ones include Health Maintenance Organizations (HMOs), Preferred Provider Organizations (PPOs), Independent Physician Associations (IPAs), and other similar groups. While all MCOs share the common goals of providing quality health care and cost containment, there are significant differences in management practices and services provided. If your MCO is selected for you (by your employer or insurance company), your situation may preclude alternate choices. However, if you are able to select from several MCOs available in your community, it is advisable to examine each one closely and choose the one that best fits your needs. In making your selection, consider the following features:

1. Can you continue to see the same personal physician that you have seen in the past? How much will you have to pay to see a physician who is not in the plan?
2. Does the plan cover preexisting medical conditions?
3. Which hospitals are in the plan? Does the plan cover outpatient surgery in a hospital or only in surgical centers?
4. What specific types of care are provided by the plan? What types of care are excluded from the plan?
5. Does the plan cover the costs of participating in clinical trials, such as those conducted by the NIH or other medical centers?
6. Do you need a referral each time you see a specialist? Who selects the specialist? Does the plan pay the specialist's fee? Is there a limit on the number of referrals to specialists?

7. How do you get a second opinion? Who chooses the consultant? Does the plan cover the consultant's fee?
8. What limits does the plan place on payments for medical care? Are you responsible for any co-payments?
9. If you need emergency care at any time, where do you go to obtain it? Is authorization required to go to an emergency room in a hospital? Does the plan cover services if you are taken by ambulance to a hospital that is not in the plan?
10. If you wish to withdraw from the plan, how do you accomplish this? Are there any penalties if you switch to another plan?

SELECTING A PERSONAL PHYSICIAN

Depending upon the MCO plan you choose, you may be free to select your primary care physician from all of those in your community who are taking new patients, or your choice may be limited to those on the staff of the plan. Finding the "right physician" for you is not an easy task. Begin your search by asking for recommendations from the following: a previous personal physician who has retired; a specialist physician in your community that you know and trust; a nurse (you know well) working in the community; your personal dentist; the director of the local hospice organization; your relatives, friends, and neighbors.

With the realization that your choices may be limited, look realistically for a physician that meets the following criteria (these are listed in the order of importance):

1. First and foremost—an attitude of *genuine caring*, honest interest in and concern for the patient's well-being.
2. Demonstrated *competence*—a wide reputation for diagnostic and therapeutic ability.
3. *Availability*—practical office hours and appointment scheduling; reasonable waiting periods to get an appointment and to be seen at time of appointment.
4. *Credentials*—fully licensed by appropriate state or municipal authority; has privileges to practice in accredited hospitals. Specialty board certification is a marker of superior training, but does not necessarily assure the first three attributes.

If you are fortunate enough to find a primary physician with these characteristics and he accepts you as a patient, respect his efforts and cooperate responsibly.

During the mythical "golden years" of medicine—before the juggernaut of managed care—thoughtful physicians and hopeful patients were well aware of the features that characterized the "ideal physician." It is unlikely that you will find such a person now. However, the list of features is presented here for those who wish to use a managed care organization in a spirit of benign assertiveness and find it appropriate to solicit any of the maxims that follow.

Characteristics of the ideal physician for managing chronic disorders:

1. His management overview is comprehensive; he attempts to provide
   - accurate diagnosis, as promptly and practically as possible;
   - intelligently conceived treatment plans, with realistic chances of benefit at acceptable risk and cost;
   - genuine concern for the patient's quality of life—as perceived by the patient.
2. He allows the patient to tell his story in his own words and in his own way, helping the patient as necessary to clarify the explanation. He does not interrupt needlessly or pressure the patient to "keep it short."
3. He actually *listens* to what the patient is saying; he tries to understand accurately what the patient is trying to tell him. He does not waste time talking about irrelevant matters.
4. His attitude clearly reflects genuine interest and concern for the patient's problems and respect for the patient's time. He prevents frequent and distracting interruptions during the consultation time reserved for the patient.
5. He recognizes that no two individuals are exactly alike—that any disorder can affect each patient differently. He acknowledges that subtle differences in chronic disease manifestations are frequent and expected. He explains that the "textbook picture" of many disorders is a convenient and necessary teaching tool, but is usually the exception in real life.
6. He does not "force fit" the patient's description of symptoms into a diagnostic pattern that he is familiar and comfortable with and can handle expeditiously. (This is a common cause of erroneous diagnosis.) He does not jump to conclusions and make "snap diagnoses" based on limited information.
7. When his diagnostic acumen fails to establish a plausible diagnosis promptly, he does not "cop out" with the terse conclusion that "it's all in your head."
8. He is circumspect. He plans short-term, intermediate-term, and long-term treatment goals intelligently and realistically, and discusses these with the patient.
9. He knows and explains that the best conceived treatment programs often do not produce the desired or predicted results. He monitors the patient's response to treatment at appropriate intervals and makes adjustments as necessary.
10. He does not practice "cookbook" medicine. He does not depend solely on laboratory tests and imaging techniques to make the diag-

nosis for him. He recognizes the variations and limitations inherent in many diagnostic procedures. He maintains an open-minded curiosity and diligence when the diagnosis is uncertain and elusive. He uses intuitive and probabilistic reasoning—the dying art of medicine.

11. He recognizes the value and wisdom of judicious "therapeutic trials" as an appropriate treatment in vague, borderline conditions, especially when diagnostic test results are inconclusive and the patient's condition warrants relief.

12. He is timely and forthright in seeking the opinions and suggestions of other physicians with pertinent expertise. He is not offended by a request for another opinion.

13. Knowing that the average patient remembers about 30% of what he is told during a medical encounter, the thoughtful physician provides written information (when appropriate) regarding the disorder and its management. This enhances the patient's understanding and compliance.

14. He asks if he has addressed the patient's concerns and answered his questions satisfactorily.

PREPARATION FOR SEEING THE PHYSICIAN

If you have just joined an MCO plan, the following procedures will help both you and your new physician significantly:

1. Call the receptionist and explain that you would like to schedule a "get-acquainted" appointment to meet with your new primary care physician and establish a patient–doctor relationship. It is advisable to do this while you are well—before you have a medical problem that requires prompt attention.

2. Assemble your medical records from previous physicians and take these with you on your first visit. These will be the first entries in your new file at the MCO, and will provide important medical history and background information for your new physician to use in evaluating future medical problems.

3. During your first visit, ask for available literature that the MCO provides describing their policies, practice procedures, and recommendations. Clarify any questions you may have regarding the medical services that are covered and those that are not covered by the plan.

4. When making all appointments, ask if you are to fast before reporting; if so, how many hours should you refrain from eating before your appointment time.

PRESENTING YOUR CASE

If you enjoy good health and have no ongoing medical conditions, your visits to the MCO will be primarily to utilize the preventive services offered by the plan. Occasional visits will be made to care for acute, self-limiting conditions; these usually require minimal preparation. When you experience a more persistent and possibly serious complaint, make an appointment for evaluation as soon as you can.

1. When you have an appointment to be seen for a significant medical problem, prepare for it properly *before you see the physician*. Clarify in your own thoughts exactly what you want to tell him. You may find it helpful to take a written list of points to be covered. Explain your symptoms and concerns clearly, concisely, and completely. Try to anticipate any questions you think he may ask, and have your answers ready. You may also consider taking a relative or close friend to help explain your symptoms clearly and to relieve anxiety.

2. Keep in mind that you and your physician are working together in a cooperative partnership; you both have active roles to play. Take your responsibility seriously; contribute to the success of the partnership in every way you can.

3. If you think you may have a particular disorder, read pertinent information about it before your appointment. Being familiar with the symptoms of a specific problem and other conditions that are similar, you will be able to communicate more effectively with the health care professional who sees you first. If you feel that your problem has not been evaluated adequately, insist on seeing your physician.

4. If you are advised to have diagnostic tests or procedures, ask your physician to describe the test, and to explain why the test in necessary, what is to be learned by doing the test, and any potential risks associated with the test. By providing answers to these questions, the MCO obtains your informed consent to perform the tests.

5. If you are given prescriptions for medications to treat your disorder, ask the physician to include in the labeling the name of the drug, the proper dosage, and the name of the disorder for which the drug is taken. If you prefer to keep the name of the condition private, that is your right, but make sure you have this information from the physician and consider adding it to the prescription label after it is filled. Many chronic conditions require the concurrent use of two or more drugs. Confusion regarding which drug is used to treat which condition is responsible for many medication errors.

6. If you have unanswered questions or need further explanation regarding your condition or its management, ask for clarification *before you leave the office*.

Doing Your Homework

After the diagnosis of your condition has been established, the next step is for you and your family to learn as much as you can about the nature of your disorder and its management. Providing such information is the principal purpose of this book. It will take several more years of evolution and refinement before our current MCOs achieve maximal efficiency and effectiveness. During this turbulent time, the patient and the family must learn to do all they can to maximize the benefits available from an imperfect system.

The following section explains how to use this book effectively. Each Disorder Profile (disorder review) in Section Three provides specific resources for increasing your knowledge and understanding. In addition, Appendixes 17 and 18 describe additional references for detailed information on medicinal drugs and general information on medical care.

How to Use This Book

A chronic disorder can be one of life's most difficult challenges. It can affect so many aspects of our lives—impairing the basic activities of daily living, compromising the pursuit of education and gainful employment, limiting social interaction, and seriously degrading the quality of life. For those among us who live with a chronic disorder, life is a continuous quest for help. News from the world of medicine is now a daily ritual. All major radio and television networks and many of our most popular publications regularly devote time and space to reporting the latest developments in health sciences. The last decade has seen a remarkable proliferation of fund-raising organizations that support education and research for specific chronic disorders. Our culture is embracing the concept that all of us—the ill and the well—should be active participants in the prevention and cure of disease.

Those who browse bookstores are aware of the ever-increasing number of lay publications in the health section that are devoted to specific disorders—single books on allergies, asthma, diabetes, heart disease, high blood pressure, menopause, prostate diseases, etc. These are useful sources of information for individuals with a specific disorder, and many of them are cited in respective Disorder Profiles found in Section Three of this book. However, many families, especially those spanning three generations, will experience a variety of disorders. The A-to-Z arrangement of the disorder profiles is designed to serve as a single source of information-in-depth on some of the chronic disorders that afflict Americans of all age groups today. The principal intent is to address those major concerns mentioned in Chapter 1: accurate diagnosis and effective treatment.

An Overview of This Book and Its Features

First, review the table of contents to get an idea of the scope and arrangement of the information provided. Then read the Author's Note and Chapter 1 of this section to understand the book's fundamental mission. Next, quickly read brief passages of each section, including the appendixes, to see how the information within each section relates to the others. Note the cross-references between sections that provide broader understanding.

The book consists of seven sections and 18 appendixes. Section One discusses the reformation of the nation's health care system now underway and considers the important role of information exchange as health care consumers and providers adjust to the changes imposed.

Section Two reviews the current status of preventive medicine and is provided as an incentive to increase public awareness of this important aspect of our health as individuals and our collective health as a nation. Managed care organizations are demonstrating that keeping healthy people well is cost-effective and does indeed prevent or delay the development of serious disorders in later life. This section summarizes practical steps that can be taken to prevent or modify the major causes of illness as we grow older.

Section Three is the heart of the book. It consists of Disorder Profiles—in-depth reviews of common and significant medical conditions that make it necessary for many of us to use the health care system. It is the information in the Profiles that enables the patient and the family to be active participants in the diagnosis and treatment of their chronic disorders. Each Profile contains 25 or more information categories, the aim of which is to provide the understanding and insight the patient needs to (1) communicate effectively with health care providers, and (2) collaborate responsibly to achieve satisfactory treatment outcomes. If time allows, select one Disorder Profile of interest to you and read it completely, noting the title of each information category. The "ALERT!" notices are designed to inform the reader of specific points that require emphasis. These may be useful in preventing misdiagnosis or misadventure in treatment.

Some information categories deserve special mention; these are the ones that deal with the principal concerns of accurate diagnosis and effective treatment:

- Principal Features and Natural History: A synopsis of the usual manifestations and course of the disorder.
- Diagnostic Symptoms and Signs: Those specific features that characterize the disorder and justify a "presumptive" diagnosis.
- Diagnostic Tests and Procedures: Those examinations that are usually done first to confirm the diagnosis.
- Diagnostic "Markers" for This Disorder: Very specific test findings that establish the diagnosis when other test results are inconclusive or present in similar disorders. Not all disorders have specific markers.
- Similar Conditions That May Confuse Diagnosis: A list of conditions that may resemble the Profile disorder in some respects. Consideration

of this group of similar disorders is referred to as the differential diagnosis. See the discussion below titled "A Correct Diagnosis: How Difficult Can It Be?"

- Goals of Treatment: Realistic expectations of desirable treatment outcomes.
- Currently Available Therapies for This Disorder: A list of drug and non-drug treatment procedures in general use at the time of publication.
- Management of Therapy: A discussion of some general principles that govern accepted therapy for the disorder.
- Resources: Specific citations to publications and organizations that provide additional information and services for patients with this disorder.

Section Four is a consideration of the ultimate chronic disorder—terminal illness and the end of life. It is not surprising that this has emerged as one of today's most pressing and controversial issues involving medical care. The remarkably rapid advances in medical technology that prolong our lives in unprecedented ways are also prolonging our deaths. The intensity of our focus on diagnosing and curing disease has deterred our responsible acknowledgment of reality: In spite of our medical brilliance, we all eventually die. While the experts debate the medical, legal, moral, and philosophical aspects of the dilemma we have compounded, each individual patient and family must confront the inevitable and find solutions that serve them best. This section is offered to help that process.

Section Five discusses the special considerations that are appropriate for managing chronic disorders in our elders. As we grow older, we all experience significant changes in body structures and functions. The processes of aging affect the course of disease and the response to medical management. This section provides guidelines for treating the older segments of our population.

Section Six consists of seven tables that summarize our present knowledge of disorders that are caused by medicinal drugs. Although drug-induced disease is not a common problem, it is a significant and important one. Because of its relative infrequency, the recognition of a causal relationship between a drug and a disorder is often delayed. The information provided in this section serves as a quick reference to ascertain if a newly diagnosed disorder could possibly be related to a recently used medicinal drug.

Section Seven is a glossary of terms that have no simple synonym and require clarification for understanding. Medical and related language is the essence of the information provided in a book of this nature. The author has tried to find a balance between the excessive use of medical jargon and the inadequate wording of superficial coverage. Throughout the text the reader is referred to this section for explanation of words that are likely to be unfamiliar. The more conversant the patient is regarding his condition, the more responsive the health care provider is likely to be.

An introductory list of Appendixes follows Section Seven. Each appendix provides a single source of expanded information that is relevant to several Disorder Profiles, thus avoiding needless repetition in each profile. The reader is referred to the pertinent appendix as appropriate.

A Correct Diagnosis: How Difficult Can It Be?

It is commonly said that a diagnosis can be made 90% of the time based upon the patient's symptoms. Stated more accurately, a "presumptive diagnosis" can be considered 90% of the time by an astute physician who knows how to elicit meaningful symptoms. Even in today's wonderful world of modern medical science, the good diagnostician must still practice the "art" of medicine. Many medical practitioners and the public alike have been deluded to think that accurate diagnosis of a medical condition is a relatively simple task. Unfortunately, the diagnostic tools provided by modern technology to serve as "diagnostic aids" are often used as "diagnosis makers." Advanced imaging procedures (CT scans, MRIs, sonograms, etc.) provide an expedient way to diagnose—often replacing (rather than augmenting) the careful evaluation of symptoms and the skillfully performed physical examination. Not infrequently, this leads to incomplete or erroneous diagnosis, followed by inappropriate therapy.

There are numerous factors that influence the accuracy of diagnosis. The major ones are the following:

PATIENT FACTORS
- The patient does not communicate well; he does not focus on the principal complaint at the beginning of the interview; he fails to give a clear and accurate description of his symptoms and concerns.
- He does not respond well to the physician's questions; he may omit important points, thinking them irrelevant; he cannot recall past events accurately.
- He allows the physician (or his surrogate) to "put words in his mouth"—to guide the patient's story into a pattern that is familiar to the questioner; the conclusions may be right or wrong.
- The patient or the family is unable to provide past medical records that may be relevant to the current problem.

PHYSICIAN FACTORS
- The physician does not listen to the patient attentively. (This is a universal complaint, the most common flaw cited in patient polls.) He interrupts inappropriately and hastens the interview; the patient's story is incomplete and inadequate.
- The physician's diagnostic acumen is limited; he ignores symptoms he does not understand and cannot explain; he "force fits" the

patient's symptoms into diagnostic patterns he knows and can manage comfortably.

- The physician's practice style is to "shoot from the hip" without taking careful aim; he makes snap judgments (and diagnoses) without circumspect consideration of differential diagnosis.
- The physician relies too heavily on diagnostic procedures. When these fail to make the diagnosis (as they often do), he lacks the intellectual capacity to pursue the problem and settles for treating the symptoms without identifying their cause.
- Unfortunately, medical knowledge is not shared uniformly throughout the profession, even within medical specialties. New diagnostic information of significance may or may not be published in scientific journals or presented at conferences, and is often available only to the limited number of practitioners who developed it. This contributes to erroneous diagnosis and ineffective treatment.

DISEASE FACTORS

- The early manifestations of many chronic disorders may be subtle and progress very slowly. They may raise suspicions in the minds of astute physicians, but they remain nonspecific and unreliable as diagnostic indicators. Such disorders require periodic evaluation over time, until a distinctive pattern emerges that supports a presumptive diagnosis.
- Many disorders reveal only some of their features and do not present the entire pattern. The "classical" or "textbook picture" of numerous conditions is actually uncommon. Marked variations among individuals can greatly influence the manifestations of disease states. It is often necessary to assume a tentative or "working diagnosis" based on incomplete information.
- Many disorders share features in common and resemble each other in various ways. In the absence of specific diagnostic markers or confirmatory tests, it may not be possible to establish a specific diagnosis with certainty.
- Relatively rare diseases—those not in the mainstream of medical practice—are usually the most difficult to diagnose. Over 30% of patients experiencing such disorders do not receive correct diagnoses for over five years. The "index of suspicion" for uncommon conditions is relatively low for the average physician.

DIAGNOSTIC TEST FACTORS

- Many diagnostic procedures are highly specific and readily confirm diagnosis: blood sugar measurements to diagnose and monitor the course of diabetes mellitus; electrocardiograms to identify heart rhythm disorders; tissue biopsies to determine cancer cell types, etc. On the other hand, some diagnostic tests are suggestive but not specifically diagnostic:

rheumatoid factor (a blood test) is present in several connective tissue disorders and infectious diseases, but is not specific for any one.

- The ability of a test to contribute to accurate diagnosis depends upon the *sensitivity* and the *specificity* of the test. *Sensitivity* is a measure of how many people with the disease will test positive; *specificity* is a measure of how many people without the disease will test negative. The effective diagnostician must know which tests are most sensitive and most specific for the disorder in question.
- Some tests yield false positive results: systemic lupus erythematosus (SLE) causing a false positive test for syphilis. Some tests yield false negative results: individuals with unmistakable Lyme disease testing negatively.
- Some test results have borderline significance—incapable of detecting mild or "subclinical" conditions with certainty. Diagnosis may require a therapeutic trial to clarify the true nature of the problem.
- Abnormal test results may be due to drugs as often as to diseases. The physician must be aware of all drugs taken by the patient in order to judge the validity of many abnormal test results.
- It is not unusual for imaging techniques (MRIs, CT scans) to disclose structural abnormalities that are later shown to have no causal relationship to the assumed diagnosis; this lack of correlation often applies to disorders of the lower spine.
- For many disorders there are no tests or procedures to confirm diagnosis. The "most probable" diagnosis is made by excluding the less probable.

SOME DISORDERS FREQUENTLY MISDIAGNOSED OR UNRECOGNIZED BY PHYSICIANS

The early symptoms experienced by the patient who is developing one of the following disorders are usually mild, vague, and nonspecific. During this period, accurate diagnosis is usually impossible. As the disorder progresses, a suggestive pattern emerges that justifies rational and "targeted" diagnostic procedures.

amyotrophic lateral sclerosis
brain tumors
carotid artery disease (transient ischemic attacks)
coronary artery disease (atypical angina patterns)
depressions
drug-induced Parkinson syndrome
fibromyalgia syndrome
hepatitis (chronic stage, without jaundice)
hyperthyroidism (in the elderly)
hypothyroidism (especially in the elderly)
Lyme disease (late stage manifestations)
multiple myeloma

multiple sclerosis
Paget's disease (early manifestations of advanced disease)
polymyalgia rheumatica
rheumatic fever (early stage without joint involvement)
sarcoidosis
schizophrenia (mild forms)
scleroderma
Sjögren's syndrome
spinal stenosis (especially cervical region)
systemic lupus erythematosus
temporal lobe epilepsy
Tourette syndrome

A Few Words About Treatment

As mentioned above, the Disorder Profiles in Section Three provide information on the types of therapy currently available for each disorder. When appropriate, some general principles of treatment management are discussed. On occasion, current controversies regarding therapy are explained so the reader will have some insight and understanding if the issues are pertinent to his condition and its management.

Specific recommendations regarding the details of treatment are beyond the scope of this book. Only the physicians who are actively caring for the patient are in a position to make rational judgments and recommendations regarding optimal therapy. In every instance, the selection and management of treatment must be highly individualized to ensure satisfactory results.

The reader is referred to Appendix 17 for sources of detailed drug information. The drugs listed in the Profiles are those currently recognized as relatively safe and effective for treating the disorder. However, the drug selection and the dosage schedule must be determined by the physician for each patient individually. Of the references cited in Appendix 17, you will find *The Essential Guide to Prescription Drugs* to be the most reader-friendly and patient-oriented; it provides the information needed to use drugs safely and effectively. Use the drug information provided to communicate with your physician—just as you use the disorder information found in this book.

Points for Consideration by the Patient

The individual who lives with a chronic disorder is faced with three realities:

coping with the health care system;
coping with the disorder;
coping with emotional adjustment.

Coping with the Health Care System

Just as you want your primary physician to be a "good doctor," it is appropriate that you give serious consideration to being a "good patient." If the doctor–patient relationship is to be a mutually beneficial partnership, both partners must behave responsibly. It is in your best interest to be the kind of patient that your physician will want to work with in providing the best possible care. The following patient characteristics are reasonable and appropriate:

- You request medical attention only when you truly need it; you do not abuse the system with trivial complaints that respond to self-care and time. You recognize the cost of modern health care and the need to use it judiciously.
- You keep your appointments and report at the designated time. You recognize that scheduling in a health care setting is done unavoidably by approximation and not with precision; a wait of 15 to 30 minutes is acceptable—if longer, discuss it with the office manager.
- You explain your symptoms and concerns clearly, concisely, and completely in as little time as possible.
- You answer questions truthfully and completely to best of your ability.
- If necessary, you ask for clarification of any explanations or instructions you are given before you leave the office.
- You request written information that describes your disorder and its management. You also request written information about any medications you are given.
- You comply with treatment recommendations to the best of your ability. If unable to comply fully, you consult your physician for guidance.
- You promptly report unfavorable reactions to medications and unexpected changes in your condition.
- You make a conscious effort to collaborate closely with your physician is all aspects of medical care—preventive and curative.
- You remember that the quality of the health care you receive depends upon the contributions made by both *you and your health care providers*.

Coping with the Disorder

As anyone living with a chronic disorder knows all too well, the "rules of the game" are written by the disorder itself. By their very nature, most chronic disorders do not have a true "fix"—a magic escape from all symptoms. Each disorder imposes its own burdens that must be dealt with one way or another. Understandably, available therapies vary greatly in their abilities to relieve or modify symptoms. The usual history of a chronic disorder is that the search for a diagnosis is then followed by a search for palliation. The following suggestions may be helpful in this search:

- If you have not already done so, begin a personal medical file that includes all pertinent records relating to the diagnosis and current management of your disorder. Keep this file up-to-date by adding notes, copies of reports, results of diagnostic procedures, etc., as they become available. This file will grow in value and importance for as long as your search continues. Make copies of it available to all health care professionals you consult for treatment.

- If you are still seeking a diagnosis, recognize that many chronic disorders need time to evolve before a diagnosis can be made. Discuss this openly with your physician so that impatience does not lead to ill-advised and fruitless searching for second opinions.

- Be reasonable in your requests for diagnostic tests and procedures. Understand the potential for conflict when you think a particular test is warranted and your physician disagrees. Managed care organizations have emerged because of the enormous abuse of medical technology. Ask your physician to explain the logic for selecting some tests and rejecting others. Be mindful of the cost vs. care dilemma.

- Recognize and understand that many aspects of medical diagnosis and treatment are controversial. The most well-informed authorities often disagree among themselves on the "best" test, the "interpretation" of test results, and the "preferred" method of treatment. The more informed you are, by doing your homework, the better prepared you are to make intelligent judgments and to actively participate in decision making.

- Once the diagnosis of your condition is established, educate yourself regarding the nature of the disorder and its management. Many sources of information are available: books such as this one; single-subject books devoted to the disorder; educational materials published by government agencies and national support groups; and your local library are all good starting places.

- Carefully explore the feasibility of the various treatment modalities currently used to treat the manifestations of your disorder. Ask your physician if any of them are appropriate for you and, if so, are they available to you.

- With the diagnosis of your disorder known and your treatment plan fully implemented, ask your physician to thoughtfully assess with you the "quality" of your life. Is there anything further that might be tried to make you more comfortable, improve your mobility, enable you to pursue your hobbies, enrich your life, and make it more meaningful?

Totally absorbed as they are in the limiting concerns of diagnosis and treatment, physicians can be forgiven for overlooking this aspect of patient care. But you are an active participant now, and you can raise the issue.

Coping with Emotional Adjustment

Many chronic disorders are so ever-present and intrusive that the patient's principal focus is often limited initially to getting through each day. During this struggle of endless coping, moments of introspection may come and go. At some point, these may expand and lead to a psychological burden as formidable as the physical one. If this development is not recognized and properly addressed, the suffering patient is further crippled and in need of additional medical care.

During the progression of your chronic illness, you may become aware of a spectrum of emotional responses: initially, denial that you have a serious problem; then anger, frustration, and irritability; if response to treatment is disappointing, despondency followed by depression. If you sense that you are experiencing any phase of emotional deterioration, consider the following suggestions.

SELF-DIRECTED PSYCHOTHERAPY

1. Try to develop a realistic overview and understanding of your total situation—the "big picture" of your disorder: its impact on you and your family; your resources for dealing with it (insurance, savings, etc.); your support systems (family, friends, medical care).
2. If you have not already done so, ask your physician to discuss the likely prognosis of your case. Explain why you are asking for this. Inform him of your current emotional state so he can judge your present and future needs.
3. Make a valiant effort to avoid an attitude of negative resignation: "the bottle is already half empty." Pessimism is self-defeating; it predisposes to reactive depression and weakens the body's defenses.
4. Make a genuine, all-out effort to adopt an attitude of *acceptance*: a realistic recognition and acknowledgment of the way things truly are—balanced with rational optimism of what is still possible and practical: "the bottle is still half full." It has been shown conclusively that a positive attitude has healing power and can favorably influence the course of disease.
5. Pursue practical hobbies that you genuinely enjoy. Mix active and passive entertainment as your condition allows.
6. Keep in touch with the world around you, even activities as seemingly simple as listening to the news on the radio or television or getting out to buy a newspaper are all positive accomplishments.

Professional Psychotherapy

If you (or your family) believe that you need professional help and guidance to stabilize your emotional health, ask your personal physician to evaluate your situation and advise you. He can make the judgment regarding the most appropriate therapist: pastoral counselor, clinical psychologist, or psychiatrist. Relieving depression and restoring normal mood will certainly improve your quality of life and ease the burden for all concerned.

Points for Consideration by Health Care Providers

Several recent discussions in the medical literature focus on significant shifts in physician attitudes regarding the doctor–patient relationship. Two such changes are noteworthy:

1. Health professionals should strive to provide "patient-centered" care in which the patient is seen as a person, an individual, a fellow human being—rather than as a brain tumor, a peptic ulcer, or a ruptured disc.
2. The patient is now an actively participating partner in a provider–consumer relationship in the business of health care provision.

These shifting perspectives suggest that physicians are evolving a new kind of respect for patients. If this is true and becomes a reality, it will certainly enhance the patient's respect for physicians—a needed and welcome improvement in the wake of managed care estrangements.

If the health care community is truly serious in its newfound respect for the patient's physical **and** psychological well-being, the patient–consumer community is most appreciative and offers the following points for consideration by all health care providers.

The Thoughtful Patient's Entreaty to His Physician

- Please respect my time as I respect yours. Do not schedule my appointment for 1 to 2 hours before you actually see me.
- When you are hearing my story, please also *listen* to what I am trying to tell you. If necessary, ask me questions to clarify my explanation; but please, accept my answers and do not substitute answers you want to hear.
- Please do not ignore my substantive input while you are trying to diagnose my disorder. Occasionally, an intelligent patient may know much about the subject.
- We are working together to solve my problems. Please do not resent my questions or construe them to be a challenge to your expertise. I respect you. I expect no less in return.
- Please honor my assessment of the pain and stress I live with. I do not ask you to empathize or sympathize; but I do ask you to provide

effective relief now—while diagnostic studies are underway.

- Please recognize when you are becoming a victim of the "interesting case" syndrome—mesmerized by the challenge of a chronic disorder of unknown cause and oblivious to my needs for symptom relief and emotional support.
- You are well aware of my disabilities and limitations; you know I do not malinger. If I tell you I need a handicapped parking permit, please provide it graciously for an appropriate period of time. Do not reduce me to a beggar.
- After the diagnosis of my disorder is known and treatment has begun, do what is possible to combat my *disease*, but please do not ignore my *illness*. If my disease is not curable, then it is irrelevant; the quality of my life is my major concern.
- If you are my surgeon, please do not resent or deny my request to have my personal primary physician attend me before and after surgery. He knows me as a patient and a person. Just as I need you to perform my surgery, I also need him to oversee my total care and well-being, and to provide professional and moral support.
- Please teach me how best to cope with my disorder, how best to care for myself. I prefer to call you only when I truly need your help or guidance.
- Please inform me if, in your judgment, the burden of any treatment may well outweigh the burden of my disorder. Please protect me from overly zealous consultants who propose risky therapies when a reasonable salvage is unlikely.
- Please strive for intellectual honesty and professional integrity as you struggle to balance the conflicting concerns of cost containment and quality care.
- If I am terminally ill, please honor my advance directives and my request for true hospice care. Please do nothing to prolong my life or my dying. And, especially, please provide effective relief from pain and suffering.

SECTION TWO

Health Promotion and Disease Prevention: Avoiding and Delaying Chronic Disorders

Preventive medicine has long been the stepchild of the medical establishment. There are valid explanations for this. Because of the long delay between a risky lifestyle and the manifestations of disease (smoking and lung cancer is a good example), the basic tenets of preventive medicine have not been convincing or compelling. Given the number and nature of chronic disorders that can afflict us, there is only a small amount of hard evidence that serious chronic diseases can be prevented. The formidable curricula of medical education provide little time or incentive for teaching clinical preventive practice. There is insufficient remuneration, and no glory, for preventing illness on a broad scale. The impact of modern medicine's technology—so totally focused on diagnosis and treatment—does not permit any substantive consideration of disease prevention as a practical, profitable matter. And lastly, individuals who find pleasure and gratification in risky lifestyles often rebel when advised to give them up, such as compulsive eaters with diabetes.

Given the volume and complexity of our collective diseases and disorders, and our insatiable drive for more sophisticated medical technology, it is not surprising that health care costs are outpacing our ability to pay for them. The forces that propel this trend are clearly evident, but opposing forces to reverse it are greatly outnumbered. A massive effort to undertake preventive measures on a large scale is long overdue. Only within the last 15 to 20 years have concerned segments of the medical community begun to create an appropriate body of knowledge that provides a framework for the clinical application of preventive procedures.

Good health and enjoyable longevity are everyone's earnest desire. Promoting health, maintaining wellness, and preventing illness are synonymous goals. At this time, what do we actually know and understand regarding the preservation of wellness and the prevention of illness? What can medical schools teach physicians? And what can physicians teach their patients?

Achieving Wellness and Deterring Illness

In the foreword to the recently published book *Health Promotion and Disease Prevention in Clinical Practice*[1], former U.S. Surgeon General C. Everett Koop, M.D., offers the following admonition to American physicians:

> If we are serious about promoting health and preventing disease, we must spend more of our time talking with patients about their health behaviors and less time subjecting them to tests and treatments. The time has come for a new approach to clinical practice in which the assessment and management of risk factors assumes as central a role in the doctor's office as the diagnosis and treatment of current complaints.

In terms of practical application, the concepts of disease prevention can be viewed within a framework of time—the span of a human life: primary, secondary, and tertiary prevention.

Primary Prevention

What is it? The use of procedures in healthy individuals which can prevent the initiation of disease.

When is it used? In childhood, adolescence, and early adult life.

How is it used? Routine immunizations. Early detection of incipient and reversible risk factors in healthy individuals. Examples: childhood obesity, teenage cigarette smoking, and excessive use of alcohol.

Secondary Prevention

What is it? The use of procedures in healthy individuals which can detect modifiable risk factors or early, asymptomatic disease.

When is it used? From early adult life into the eighth decade of life.

How is it used? Careful screening for risk factors that predispose to significant diseases or disorders; effective counseling to eliminate or modify potentially harmful risk factors. Example: total and permanent cessation of use of all forms of tobacco to reduce the risks of coronary artery disease, emphysema, and cancer of the mouth, throat, and lung. Careful screening

[1]Woolf, S.H., Jonas, S., Lawrence, R.S., eds., *Health Promotion and Disease Prevention in Clinical Practice*. Baltimore: Williams & Wilkins, 1996.

for early detection of asymptomatic disease; early therapeutic intervention to cure disease or arrest its progression. Example: Papanicolaou cervical smear (Pap test) reveals early cervical cancer, permitting surgical cure.

Tertiary Prevention

What is it? The use of procedures in symptomatic individuals (those with established disease) which serve to stabilize their condition, prevent complications, or arrest progression of disease. Tertiary prevention is largely an attempt to salvage an individual's quality of life in practical and meaningful ways.

When is it used? From infancy through senescence; most commonly from the fourth decade of life until death.

How is it used? Careful assessment of the status of the disease and the overall condition of the patient. Examples: performing an endarterectomy (removal of obstruction) in a carotid artery (in the neck) to prevent a stroke; determining the stage of a newly discovered breast cancer to select optimal treatment: type of surgery, adjuvant use of chemotherapy and/or radiation.

Strategies for Primary and Secondary Prevention

Immunizations

Active immunization (using vaccines) and passive immunization (using immune serums) are medicine's oldest tools of primary prevention. By providing control of many infectious diseases, vaccines have been a major contributor to the increased life expectancy in developed countries. The immunization schedules that follow are the current standards at the time of this writing. However, because live virus oral polio vaccine (OPV) is responsible for 8 to 10 cases of vaccine-associated paralysis in the United States each year, on June 20, 1996, the Advisory Committee on Immunization Practices of the Center for Disease Control and Prevention (CDC) recommended a change in polio immunization. The specific recommendation, to become effective in January 1997 if approved by the CDC, calls for giving enhanced inactivated polio vaccine (IPV) for the first two doses of the childhood schedule; oral vaccine (OPV) would be given for the remaining two doses of the schedule. It is probable that physicians and parents will have three options for polio immunization of children: all OPV, all IPV, or the two initial doses of IPV followed by two doses of OPV as recommended by the committee.

Note: Consult your physician regarding the advisability and scheduling of immunization procedures. Childhood vaccination schedules permit reasonable flexibility. There are significant contraindications to some adult immunizations that require consideration.

Many vaccines require multiple doses, generally given in a time-specific sequence. The number in parentheses following the vaccines below indicate the dosage in the sequence. When different schedule options are available, these are also noted.

Childhood Schedule: Beginning in Early Infancy

Age	Vaccines
Birth	Hepatitis B (1) (option 1)
2 Months	Hepatitis B (2) (option 1) or
	Hepatitis B (1) (option 2)
	Diphtheria-tetanus-pertussis (1)
	Oral polio vaccine (OPV) (1)
	Hemophilus influenzae B (1)
4 Months	Hepatitis B (2) (option 2)
	Diphtheria-tetanus-pertussis (2)
	Oral polio vaccine (OPV) (2)
	Hemophilus influenzae B (2)
6 Months	Diphtheria-tetanus-pertussis (3)
	Oral polio vaccine (3)
	Hemophilus influenae B (3)
12 Months	Hepatitis B (3)
	Diphtheria-tetanus-pertussis (4)
	Hemophilus influenzae B (4)
	Measles-mumps-rubella (1)
4–6 Years	Diphtheria-tetanus-pertussis (5)
	Oral polio vaccine (4)
	Measles-mumps-rubella (2) (option 1)
11–12 Years	Measles-mumps-rubella (2) (option 2)
11–16 Years	Tetanus-diphtheria booster

Childhood Schedule: Under Age 7, but Immunizations Not Started During First 2 Months of Infancy

Timing	Vaccines
FIRST VISIT	
2–11 Months of age	Diphtheria-tetanus-pertussis (1)
	Oral polio vaccine (1)
	Hemophilus influenzae B (1)
	Hepatitis B (1)
1 Year or older	Diphtheria-tetanus-pertussis (1)
	Oral polio vaccine (1)
	Measles-mumps-rubella (1)
	Hemophilus influenza B (1)
	Hepatitis B (1)
SECOND VISIT	
1 Month after first visit	Diphtheria-tetanus-pertussis (2)
	Hemophilus influenzae B (2)
	Hepatitis B (2)
THIRD VISIT	
1 Month after second visit	Diphtheria-tetanus-pertussis (3)
	Hemophilus influenzae B (3)

	Oral polio vaccine (2)
FOURTH VISIT	
6 Weeks after third visit	Oral polio vaccine (3)
FIFTH VISIT	
6 Months after third visit	Diphtheria-tetanus-pertussis (4)
	Hemophilus influenzae B (4)
	Hepatitis B (3)
4–6 Years	Diphtheria-tetanus-pertussis (5)
	Oral polio vaccine (4)
	Measles-mumps-rubella (2)
14–16 Years	Tetanus-diphtheria booster

Childhood Schedule: Beginning at Age 7 Years or Older

Timing	*Vaccines*
FIRST VISIT	
	Tetanus-diphtheria (1)
	Oral polio vaccine (1)
	Measles-mumps-rubella (1)
SECOND VISIT	
6–8 Weeks after first visit	Tetanus-diphtheria (2)
	Oral polio vaccine (2)
	Measles-mumps-rubella (2)
THIRD VISIT	
6 Months after second visit	Tetanus-diphtheria (3)
	Oral polio vaccine (3)
10 Years after Tetanus-Diphtheria (3)	Tetanus-diphtheria booster

Adult Immunization Schedule

Timing	*Vaccines*
Any age	Tetanus-diphtheria: without prior immunization, primary series: two doses, 1–2 months apart; third dose 6–12 months later. Booster every 10 years.
Any age	If HIV/AIDS infection or dysfunction of spleen: Hemophilus influenzae B, one dose.
Any age	If at high risk for hepatitis exposure: Hepatitis B vaccine: two doses, 1 month apart; third dose at 6 months after first dose.
Any age	Inactivated polio vaccine: without prior immunization, primary series: two doses, 4–8 weeks apart; third dose 6–12 months later.
Any age, without immunity	Measles vaccine, one dose.
Any age, without immunity	Mumps vaccine, one dose.
Any age, especially women of childbearing age without immunity	Rubella vaccine, one dose.
Age 65 and older	Influenza vaccine annually.
Age 65 and older	Pneumococcal vaccine, one dose.

Preventive Screening and Counseling

There is abundant evidence to document the claim that the majority of deaths among Americans below age 65 are preventable. The most valid approach to meaningful prevention is the evaluation of each individual for the presence of *known risk factors* and the attempt to favorably modify those that are amenable to change. To accomplish this effectively will require some interaction with health care providers. However, you—the most concerned participant—may find it necessary to take the initiative in determining your *personal risk profile* and (with your physician's help) to formulate an appropriate plan of preventive action. It is important to emphasize that the earlier in life you take such action, the greater the likelihood of preventing major disease.

In December 1995 the U.S. Preventive Services Task Force published the second edition of its *Guide to Clinical Preventive Services*. This monumental document represents a 5-year effort by over 650 scientific reviewers who evaluated more than 6,000 studies of screening tests, counseling topics, and interventions related to 70 specific diseases or conditions. Although some of the *Guide's* recommendations are at variance with prevention guidelines published by other professional organizations, it is generally thought to represent a state-of-the-art reference work for the clinical practice of health promotion and disease prevention. However, of the 70 final decisions made regarding routine screening tests, counseling, and interventions, 35 are recommendations for routine use, 12 withhold recommendation for routine use, and 23 are equivocal. In the words of the *Guide*, equivocal means: "There is insufficient evidence to recommend for or against the routine [use of a given procedure] in asymptomatic individuals." Among this group of noncommittal recommendations regarding routine screening are such conditions as asymptomatic coronary artery disease, skin cancer, oral cancer, diabetes, glaucoma, and osteoporosis. Among the group of diseases for which routine screening is not recommended are prostate cancer, lung cancer, thyroid cancer, and bladder cancer. The principal criteria used for reaching final recommendations for each procedure were (1) compelling evidence for effectiveness, and (2) evidence that benefits of the procedure outweigh risks. However, the clinical settings in which such recommendations may be applied are of paramount importance. After a review of the Task Force's recommendations, it is immediately apparent that if the practice of actual prevention is to be served, the highest priority should be *the identification of asymptomatic individuals who are at increased risk for the development of significant disease*. This should be the principal goal of screening—by history taking and clinical testing—so that timely counseling can facilitate prevention.

For a variety of reasons, you may not receive the help you need from your health care providers to assess your *personal risk profile*. In some managed care settings, sufficient time is not allotted for diagnosing and treating your current complaint *and* identifying your risks (if any) for the possible development of disease in the future. Also, some health care providers may elect to avoid procedures that, in their opinion, are not "cost-effective." In the short-term perspective, some preventive procedures may be viewed as not cost-effective and therefore wasteful of time and resources.

To assist you in determining your personal risk profile and devising a preventive health strategy (should one be advisable), the following guidelines are disorder-oriented rather than test-oriented. The disorders chosen are among the more common causes of serious chronic illness affecting Americans today. References to age, sex, and race are cited to indicate groups in which a disorder is more prevalent. By scanning the lists of risk factors, you can determine those of significance for you. The counseling recommendations that follow are the preventive procedures you should consider.

DISORDER, SCREENING, AND COUNSELING GUIDELINES

Bladder Cancer

Age Group
40 to 70 years
Sex
Male—75%, Female—25%
Risk Factors
Cigarette smoking
Occupational exposures: aniline dye industry; painting; hairdressing; drill press operators; agricultural workers; gardeners; workers in plastic, rubber, and leather industries
Use of cyclophosphamide medication
Screening
Periodic urine tests for blood
Counseling
Ask clinician for guidance

Breast Cancer

Age Group
25 to 90+ years
Sex
Male—1%, Female—99%
Risk Factors
Family history of breast cancer: mother or sister
Early onset of menstruation: age 11–12 years
Late menopause: age 55 years or older
First child after age 25 years
Oral contraceptive use: increased risk of premenopausal breast cancer if oral contraceptives were used for at least 4 years prior to the first pregnancy
Estrogen replacement therapy for menopause: increased risk if taken continuously for six years
High-fat and low-fiber diet during adolescence and early adulthood

Obesity: increased risk for postmenopausal breast cancer

Environmental exposures: increased risk with tobacco smoking and excessive use of alcohol or caffeine

Other cancers: the occurrence of salivary gland or uterine cancer increases the risk for developing breast cancer

Screening

Breast self-examination monthly, beginning at age 20 years

Clinical breast examination: every three years from age 20 to 39 years; annually for rest of life beginning at age 40 years

Mammogram: every two years from age 40 to 49 years; annually for rest of life beginning at age 50 years

If warranted by strong family history, genetic screening for BRCA-1 and BRCA-2

Counseling

Eat a low-fat and high-fiber diet.

Maintain normal weight for age and body build.

Limit alcohol to 2 ounces and caffeine to 2 servings daily.

Abstain totally from cigarette smoking; avoid secondhand smoke as much as possible.

Learn the proper technique for breast self-examination.

Avoid oral contraceptives if possible; consider other methods of contraception.

Consult your physician regarding the benefits and risks of estrogen replacement therapy during menopause.

Consult your physician regarding the advisability of using tamoxifen for prevention of breast cancer.

Cervical Cancer

Age Group

17 to 90+ years, mean age is 52 years

Race

Black-to-white ratio: 2 to 1

Risk Factors

Early onset of sexual activity, especially before age 16

Multiple sex partners before age 20

Continued multiple sex partners after age 20

Male partner at high risk for sexually transmitted diseases

Episodes of genital warts

Cigarette smoking, personal and secondhand

Renal transplantation (use of immunosuppressive drugs)

Screening

Papanicolaou cervical smear (Pap test) annually from age 18 to 20 years; then every three years for life

Counseling

Practice safe, protected sex; limit number of sexual partners.

Abstain totally from cigarette smoking; avoid secondhand smoke as much as possible.

Obtain prompt and adequate treatment of cervix if abnormal cells (dysplasia) are found by Pap test.

Cholesterol Abnormalities (Dyslipidemia)

Age Group

18 to 70 years

Sex

Male—total cholesterol over 200 mg/dl and LDL cholesterol over 130 mg/dl under age 55 years

Female—total cholesterol over 200 mg/dl and LDL cholesterol over 130 mg/dl over age 55 years

Risk Factors

Family history of high cholesterol in a parent or sibling

Family history of early heart attack, stroke, or peripheral vascular disease in a parent or sibling

High saturated-fat and high-cholesterol diet

Diabetes mellitus

Obesity

Screening

Blood tests for total cholesterol, HDL cholesterol, LDL cholesterol, and triglycerides every five years beginning at age 20 years

Counseling

Low-saturated fat, low-cholesterol, and high-fiber diet

Maintain normal weight for sex, age, and body build

Strict control of diabetes (if present)

Alcoholic beverage, 2 ounces daily to raise HDL cholesterol (if no history of alcohol abuse)

Note: The primary prevention of cholesterol disorders contributes significantly to the primary prevention of coronary artery disease, cerebrovascular disease (stroke), and peripheral vascular disease.

Chronic Bronchitis/Emphysema: Chronic Obstructive Pulmonary Diseases (COPD)

Age Group

45 to 75 years

Sex

Primarily male

Risk Factors

Cigarette smoking, personal and secondhand

Recurrent infections of the small and large bronchial tubes

Airborne allergens (chronic asthmatic bronchitis)

Screening

Lung function tests for early detection of airway obstruction

Allergy tests for causative allergens (if asthmatic bronchitis)

Counseling

Total abstention from all tobacco smoking

Prompt treatment of episodes of acute bronchitis

Appropriate desensitization therapy for allergic features of asthmatic bronchitis

Adequate control of recurrent asthma attacks

Colon/Rectal Cancer

Age Group

40 to 80 years

Sex

Male—50%, Female—50%

Risk Factors

Family history of colon or rectal cancer in parent or sibling

Family history of colon polyposis (numerous polyps)

Personal history of colon or rectal polyps

Personal history of ulcerative colitis or Crohn's disease of colon

For women: personal history of breast, ovarian, or uterine cancer

High-fat, low-fiber diet

High intake of salt-cured, salt-pickled, and smoked foods

Excessive alcohol consumption

Screening

Fecal test for occult (hidden) blood annually beginning at age 40 years

Digital rectal examination annually beginning at age 40 years

Sigmoidoscopy every three to five years beginning at age 50 years

Colonoscopy every three to five years beginning at age 18 years if there is a history of
    familial polyposis, or a personal history of adenomatous polyps or ulcerative colitis;
    beginning at age 40 years if there is a history of two or more first-degree relatives
    (parent or sibling) with colon cancer

Counseling

Eat a low-fat and high-fiber diet: fruits, vegetables, and whole grain cereals.

Avoid salt-cured, salt-pickled, and smoked foods.

Moderate alcohol consumption.

Maintain bowel regularity; avoid constipation.

Remove promptly all polyps when found.

Coronary Artery Disease (CAD)

Age Group

25 to 90+ years

Sex

Male—75%, Female—25%

Risk Factors

Family history of early CAD in first-degree relatives

Family history of cholesterol disorders

Personal cholesterol disorder: high LDL cholesterol and/or low HDL cholesterol; high
    triglycerides

Central obesity: 20% or more above normal weight

Cigarette smoking

Hypertension (uncontrolled)

Diabetes mellitus (uncontrolled)

Sedentary lifestyle: lack of regular exercise

Sustained psychological stress

Screening

Cholesterol fractions profile every five years beginning at age 20 years

Weight measurement monthly

Blood pressure measurement annually

Urine sugar test two hours after eating to detect latent diabetes (at physician's discretion)

Counseling

Eat a low-fat, low-cholesterol, high-fiber diet.

Maintain a normal weight for sex, age, and body build.

Abstain totally and permanently from cigarette smoking.

Monitor blood pressure; control hypertension.

Monitor blood sugar as needed; control diabetes.

Follow a program of regular, moderate exercise as prescribed by clinician.

Utilize stress management as required.

Chemoprophylaxis

Aspirin: antiplatelet effect may reduce risk of heart attack (acute myocardial infarction); consult your physician regarding the benefits and risks of daily aspirin for you.

Vitamin E: an effective antioxidant; studies suggest it may reduce the risk of developing CAD; consult your physician regarding use and dose.

Diabetes Mellitus

Age Group

Type I (insulin-dependent), under age 30 years, peak onset 11–14 years

Type II (noninsulin-dependent), over age 30 years

Sex

Type I—same incidence in males and females

Type II—greater incidence in females

Race

Higher incidence in blacks, American Indians, and Hispanics

Risk Factors

Predisposition to autoimmune disorders (see Appendix 5)

Family history of diabetes in parents or siblings

Obesity: 20% or more over ideal weight

Women: history of gestational diabetes (present only during pregnancy)

Evidence of early retinal vascular disease, coronary artery disease, cerebrovascular disease, or peripheral vascular disease

Screening

Annual urine sugar testing two hours after eating, beginning at age 18 years

Glucose tolerance test if urine sugar test is positive

If strong family history of diabetes, periodic eye examinations for retinal blood vessel changes; periodic complete urinalysis for evidence of kidney disease

Counseling

Maintain ideal weight for sex, age, and body build.

Eat a low-fat, low-cholesterol, high-fiber diet to deter development of vascular disease.

Avoid excessive intake of sugar.

Use alcohol moderately to avoid pancreatitis and associated diabetes.

Note: If diabetes develops, strict control of blood sugar levels is secondary prevention to deter the complications of retinal vascular disease, cardiovascular disease, kidney disease, and peripheral neuropathy.

Glaucoma

Age Group

Newborn to 75+ years; most common after age 45 years

Sex

Under 45 years—same incidence in males and females

45–64 years—more common in males

65 years and over—more common in females

Race

Blacks have a 4- to 5-times higher risk than whites for developing chronic open-angle glaucoma (the most common form).

Risk Factors
Family history of glaucoma
Nearsightedness (myopia)
Diabetes mellitus
Long-term use of cortisonelike (corticosteroid) drugs
Screening
Measurement of internal eye pressure every 2–4 years for ages 20–44 years
Measurement of internal eye pressure every 1–2 years for ages 45 years and older
Counseling
Recognize the early symptoms of glaucoma and request an eye examination:
- blurring of vision
- frequent need for change of glasses
- occasional headache
- colored halos seen around electric lights
- impaired visual adaptation to the dark (not due to aging)

if possible, avoid long-term use of cortisonelike drugs.
If you develop diabetes, request a thorough eye examination.

Hypertension (High Blood Pressure)

Age Group
13 to 80+ years
Sex
Under 45 years—same incidence in males and females
45–64 years—slightly more common in females
65 years and older—more common in females (2 to 1)
Risk Factors
Family history of hypertension
Obesity
Excessive salt intake (in salt-sensitive individuals)
Sedentary lifestyle
Sustained psychological stress
Screening
Measurement of blood pressure by clinician every 1–2 years beginning at age 18 years
If a strong family history of hypertension, self-monitoring of blood pressure (by automated instrument) at home and work site monthly
Counseling
Maintain a normal weight for sex, age, and body build.
Restrict use of salt: avoid salty foods, no added salt.
Maintain a program of regular, moderate exercise.
Follow programs for stress management as necessary.
Monitor blood pressure throughout life.

Lung Cancer

Age Group
45 to 70 years
Sex
Male—59%, Female—41%

Risk Factors

Exposure to tobacco smoke: primary smoking of cigarettes, cigars, and pipe
tobacco; secondary breathing of environmental tobacco smoke (secondhand
smoking)

Exposure to asbestos dust

Atmospheric pollution

Occupational exposure to radioactive ores: pitchblende (uranium) miners

Occupational exposures to metals: principally nickel and silver; also chromium, cadmium,
beryllium, cobalt, selenium, and steel

Occupational exposure to chemicals: chloromethyl ethers, mustard gas, and coke oven
emissions

Excessive exposure to diagnostic chest X-rays

Screening

Routine chest X-rays are not effective in detecting early disease in asymptomatic individuals. However, if a persistent cough develops, request evaluation by your physician.

Routine examination of sputum for cancer cells is not effective in detecting early disease
in asymptomatic individuals.

Counseling

Because early detection of this disease is unlikely and long-term survival depends upon
early detection, *the urgency of the need to abstain totally from tobacco smoking must
be emphasized!*

If any of the other risk factors listed above pertains to you, inform your primary physician.

Malignant Melanoma

Age Group

20 to 80+ years

Sex

Same incidence in males and females

Race

White-to-black ratio for melanoma is 25:1

Risk Factors

Family history of melanoma or multiple premalignant moles

Light skin color, red hair, blue eyes, freckles

Moles present at birth (congenital)

Residence in Hawaii, California, or southern U.S.

Episodes of severe sunburn in childhood

Intentional sunbathing to acquire skin tanning

Screening

Whites at risk should perform self-examination of entire body regularly to become
familiar with existing moles and thus prepared to recognize significant changes that
require evaluation.

Blacks at risk should perform self-examination of fingernails, palms of hands, toenails,
soles of feet, and lining of the mouth and throat for areas of suspicious color or texture change that require evaluation.

Counseling

Avoid intentional direct and excessive exposure to sun. There is no such thing as a
"healthy tan."

Avoid artificial sources of ultraviolet light, such as tanning beds.

Use sun-screening creams and lotions (sun protection factor of 15 or greater) when prolonged exposure to sun is unavoidable.

Wear sun-protective clothing.

Learn to recognize the changes in a mole that may indicate the development of melanoma:

- progressive changes in shape (asymmetry)
- borders that become notched and irregular
- color changes: development of red, white, gray, blue, or black areas
- sudden increases in size
- scaliness, erosion, or nodularity of surface

Report suspicious changes promptly for evaluation. *Early diagnosis and complete removal are mandatory for cure!*

Comply fully with instructions for long-term follow-up examinations.

Obesity

Age Group
Early childhood to senescence; greatest prevalence is between ages 20 and 55 years

Sex
Male—24%, Female—27%

Risk Factors
Family history of obesity; genetic predisposition

Sedentary lifestyle; decreased physical activity

Habitual and compulsive eating patterns

Lower socioeconomic class at birth

Childhood obesity is a risk factor for adult obesity

Screening
Classification of obesity: mild—20–40% overweight; moderate—41–100% overweight; severe—more than 100% overweight

Pattern of obesity: central—upper body or abdominal; peripheral—lower body or hip and thigh

Time of onset: adult-onset obesity is due to an increase in the *size* of fat cells (hypertrophic obesity); juvenile-onset obesity is mostly due to an increase in the *number* of fat cells (hyperplastic obesity).

Psychological factors: binge eating to relieve stress; habitual night-eating syndrome—little or no breakfast and lunch followed by high-caloric evening meal

Counseling
Nutrition education by a registered dietitian

Behavior modification by a psychotherapist

Graduated exercise instruction by a physical therapist

Note: The primary prevention of obesity contributes significantly to the primary prevention of the following:

- hypertension
- coronary artery disease
- cerebrovascular and peripheral vascular disease
- diabetes mellitus type II
- breast, ovarian, and uterine cancer
- gallstones
- osteoarthritis of weight-bearing joints

Oral Cancer

(Lips, tongue, mouth, and throat)

Age Group

Teens to 65 years

Sex

Male—80%, Female—20%

Risk Factors

Use of tobacco products: cigarettes, cigars, and pipe tobaccos, chewing tobaccos

Excessive consumption of alcoholic beverages

Regular use of mouthwashes with high alcohol content

Premalignant tissue changes: leukoplakia (white patches) and erythroplasia (red patches)

Poor oral hygiene; chronic irritation by broken teeth and poorly fitting dentures

Excessive exposure to sun (risk factor for lip cancer)

In middle-aged women: Plummer-Vinson syndrome—anemia, fissures in corners of the
    mouth, painful tongue, tissue webs in the esophagus

Cultural habits (southeast Asia): chewing betel leaves and nuts, reverse cigarette smoking

Screening

Periodic self-examination of lips, tongue, and mouth for abnormal tissue changes: white
    patches, red patches, ulcerations

Periodic examination of mouth and throat by dentist during routine prophylactic visits

Counseling

Abstain totally and permanently from use of all forms of tobacco.

Moderate intake of alcoholic beverages.

Use mouthwashes with low alcohol content.

Maintain good oral hygiene; regular prophylactic dental care.

Avoid excessive sun exposure.

Promptly consult with oral surgeon for evaluation of any persistent abnormal change in
    tissues of mouth or throat, or development of swollen glands in the neck.

Osteoporosis

Age Group

Type I (postmenopausal)—50 to 65 years

Type II (senile)—65 years and over

Sex

Male—10%, Female—90%

Risk Factors

Family history of osteoporosis (mother or sister)

Slender build, light-boned, white or Oriental race

Sedentary lifestyle or restricted physical activity

Low calcium intake

Cigarette smoking

Excessive consumption of alcoholic beverages

Habitual use of carbonated beverages

Excessive use of antacid drugs containing aluminum

Long-term use of cortisone-related drugs

Surgical or early natural menopause

Screening

Bone densitometry for those at high risk and considering use of estrogen replacement
    therapy.

Counseling

Perform regular weight-bearing activity such as walking 45–60 minutes 3–5 times per week.

Maintain ideal body weight.

Assure daily intake of calcium citrate 1500 mg and vitamin D 400 International Units.

Abstain from cigarette smoking.

Moderate intake of alcoholic and carbonated beverages.

Avoid aluminum/magnesium antacid preparations.

Consult your personal physician regarding the use of estrogen replacement therapy.

Chemoprophylaxis

For optimal benefit, estrogen replacement therapy should begin within three years following the cessation of menstruation. Consideration should be given to the following:

BENEFITS

Confirmed ability to prevent osteoporosis. Presumed ability to prevent or moderate coronary artery disease.

RISKS

Uterine cancer; this risk is eliminated by giving progesterone concurrently with estrogen.

Breast cancer; some studies support this risk if estrogen is taken continuously for six years.

Thrombophlebitis and embolism; this risk is minimal if natural estrogens are used.

Prostate Cancer

Age Group

40 to 90 years, median age at diagnosis is 72

Race

Lifetime risk for black males is 9.6%, for white males 5.2%

Risk Factors

Family history of prostate cancer in father or brother

High-fat diet

Occupational exposure in leather and cadmium industries

Sexual activity with many female partners

History of venereal disease

Benign prostatic hyperplasia (enlargement) is not a risk factor for prostate cancer.

Screening

Digital rectal examination of prostate gland annually beginning at age 40

Measurement of prostate-specific antigen (PSA) annually beginning at age 40

Counseling

Eat a low-fat, high-fiber diet.

Practice safe, protected sex with a limited number of female partners.

Men in the age group of 40 to 65 years should obtain regular screening tests annually.

Stroke

Age Group

30 to 90+ years

Sex

Male—54%, Female—46%

Risk Factors in Young Adults

Drug abuse

Uncontrolled hypertension

Blood disorders: sickle cell disease, leukemias, etc.
Heart disease
Concurrent cigarette smoking and use of oral contraceptives
Complications of migraine headache
Risk Factors in Older Adults
Hypertension
Atherosclerotic vascular diseases: cerebrovascular disease, carotid artery disease, coronary artery disease (secondary to chronic cholesterol disorders)
Diabetes mellitus
Tobacco smoking
Excessive use of alcoholic beverages
Central (abdominal) obesity
Atrial fibrillation (source of blood clots dispersed to brain—embolism).
Screening
Blood pressure monitoring of effectiveness of antihypertensive therapy
Periodic measurements of blood cholesterol fractions
Blood sugar monitoring of diabetes management
Periodic carotid artery examinations to detect narrowing
Periodic assessment of atrial fibrillation
Counseling
Maintain blood pressure in optimal range.
Learn to recognize transient ischemic attacks (TIAs) and understand their significance (see Disorder Profile of stroke in Section Three).
Comply fully with antianginal medication regimens.
Abstain totally and permanently from tobacco smoking.
Moderate use of alcoholic beverages.
Maintain normal weight for age, sex, and body build.
Chemoprophylaxis
Consult your physician regarding the use low-dose aspirin or warfarin (Coumadin) to prevent stroke.

Uterine Cancer

Age Group
35 to 80 years; median age of occurrence is 61 years
Risk Factors
Family history of uterine, breast, ovarian, or colon cancer in mother or sister
High-fat diet
Obesity increases risk tenfold
Early onset of menstruation; late menopause
History of infertility, irregular menstrual patterns, long periods of absent menstruation
Premenopausal use of sequential oral contraceptives
Postmenopausal use of estrogen without progesterone
Postmenopausal uterine bleeding
Screening
Endometrial (uterine lining) biopsy in high-risk individuals
Counseling
Eat a low-fat, high-fiber diet.
Maintain a normal body weight.
Avoid sequential oral contraceptives.

If using postmenopausal estrogen replacement therapy, take progesterone concurrently. Report promptly any occurrence of postmenopausal bleeding; immediate evaluation of the cause is mandatory.

Summary and Conclusions

Among the innovations proposed by managed care organizations as they strive to provide quality medical services and contain costs, the inclusion of preventive procedures is receiving increasing attention. However, it is unrealistic to expect a rapid quantum shift of focus from the traditional approach of "diagnose it and treat it" to one that also includes considerations of "how to prevent it." You, the individual patient, must assume personal responsibility for (1) self-education of preventive health procedures, and (2) self-discipline for practicing them in daily living. If you receive your medical care from an organization that claims to provide preventive services, take full advantage of all that is offered. If you are not informed that such services are available, ask to be scheduled to receive them. Refer to the guidelines outlined above to learn about risk factors and relevant modifications of lifestyle. In today's highly competitive health care world—cost- and profit-driven—you may come to realize that the one who is really most concerned about your future health is YOU.

The Health-Promoting, Disease-Preventing Lifestyle

- Obtain appropriate and timely immunizations for all members of the family.
- Maintain normal weight for sex, age, and body build. Avoid obesity throughout life.
- Assure sound nutrition: a balanced daily diet that includes fruits, vegetables, adequate fiber, and the full complement of recommended dietary allowances of vitamins and minerals; total fat limited to 30% of total calories, saturated fat limited to 10% of total calories, and dietary cholesterol limited to 300 mg daily. Avoid "megadoses" of vitamins and minerals.
- Establish a lifelong program of regular, moderate exercise: walking, bicycling, swimming, sports for 20 to 30 minutes three times per week.
- Abstain totally from the use of all forms of tobacco.
- Abstain totally from the use of all substances with potential for abuse or addiction.
- Limit the intake of alcohol to 3 or 4 ounces daily.
- Obtain adequate restful sleep on a regular basis, approximately 7 to 8 hours nightly.
- Maintain safe and prudent sexual behavior.

- Pursue meaningful and fulfilling activities. Maintain a positive, optimistic attitude. Use time wisely: allow time for work, time for play, and free time for relaxation.
- Perform periodic self-examinations of skin, mouth, breasts, and testicles for abnormalities that may require professional evaluation.
- Obtain prophylactic dental care every 6 months.
- Should a chronic disorder develop, comply fully with therapeutic recommendations to control it: hypertension, cholesterol disorders, diabetes, glaucoma, asthma, etc.

SECTION THREE

Disorder Profiles

ACNE ROSACEA
(AK nee ro ZAY sha)

Other Names Acne erythematosa, hypertrophic rosacea, rhinophyma, rosacea

Prevalence/Incidence in U.S. Current estimate is 13 million

Age Group Under 30: 13%; 30–39: 19%; 40–49: 25%; 50–59: 18%; over 60: 25%

Male-to-Female Ratio More common in females

Principal Features and Natural History
Rosacea is a chronic inflammatory skin disorder that usually affects the central area of the face in middle-aged people. Sometimes the skin of the forehead and chin may be affected. The pattern of development usually occurs in four stages. The first stage consists of frequent episodes of recurrent flushing of the nose and cheeks. The second stage includes persistent redness of the skin and the appearance of telangiectasia—spidery, dilated superficial veins on the cheeks and sides of the nose. In stage three, pimples, pustules, and nodules develop in the areas of inflamed skin. A small number of patients (mostly men) will experience progression to stage four. This involves more severe inflammatory changes in the skin structures of the nose that lead to marked swelling and permanent enlargement, a condition known as rhinophyma.

In addition to the involvement of facial skin, rosacea can also affect the eyes in up to 58% of cases. This can occur in several forms: inflammation and telangiectasia of eyelid margins, various kinds of conjunctivitis (red eye), and inflammation of the cornea (keratitis) with associated pain, burning, intolerance to light (photophobia), and the sensation of a foreign body in the eye. Eye symptoms can occur before, during, or following episodes of facial eruption.

Several known factors can provoke flare-ups of rosacea by causing an increase in flushing. These include exposure to sunlight, heat, or cold, and consumption of hot or spicy foods or alcoholic beverages. Some patients can identify specific foods, cosmetics, or household products that appear to trigger flare-ups.

Similar Conditions That May Confuse Diagnosis
Acne vulgaris
Cortisone-induced acne
Seborrheic dermatitis
Cutaneous lupus erythematosus
Cutaneous sarcoidosis

ALERT!
If the characteristic skin features of rosacea are mild or absent, many cases of ocular rosacea may be misdiagnosed. If the true nature of the eye manifestations are not recognized and properly treated, permanent scarring of the cornea and significant loss of vision can occur.

Causes

Established Causes
The primary cause of rosacea is not known.

Theoretical Causes
Rosacea is thought to be due to a combination of genetic and environmental factors. It occurs most frequently in fair-skinned individuals of northern European origin and is known as the "Celtic Curse." The mite *Demodex folliculorum* can be found in the facial hair follicles of rosacea patients and may possibly contribute to the inflammatory process that underlies the skin manifestations of rosacea.

Drugs That Can Cause This Disorder
There are no drugs that cause acne rosacea. However, the following drugs can cause acnelike eruptions:
bromides
disulfiram
iodides
isoniazid
lithium
phenobarbital

phenytoin
quinine
thiouracil
trimethadione

Goals of Treatment

Can This Disorder Be Cured?
There is no curative treatment available at this time.

Can This Disorder Be Treated Effectively?
Yes. The appropriate use of oral and topical medications can achieve improvement and symptom relief in 80% of cases. The appropriate use of surgical procedures can correct much of the disfigurement caused by advanced rosacea.

Specific Goals
- Initial suppression of inflammatory skin manifestations
- Long-term control of rosacea activity; prevention of flare-ups
- Prevention of permanent scarring, disfigurement, and loss of vision
- Correction of late-stage deformities: telangiectasia, rhinophyma

Health Professionals Who Participate in Managing This Disorder
Family physicians
General internists
Dermatologists
Ophthalmologists
Optometrists
Pharmacists
Plastic/Reconstructive surgeons

Currently Available Therapies for This Disorder

Drug Therapy
Oral antibiotics:
- tetracycline (the drug of choice)
- erythromycin
- minocycline
- doxycycline
- ampicillin
- metronidazole
Topical antibiotics (for local use):
- clindamycin
- erythromycin
- metronidazole (the drug of choice)

Retinoids:
- isotretinoin

Nondrug Treatment Methods
Surgical procedures:
- cryotherapy (freezing)
- dermabrasion
- electrosurgery
- excision and skin grafting
- tunable dye laser
- carbon dioxide laser

Management of Therapy
Oral antibiotics are used initially in high doses to reduce inflammation and eliminate pimples and pustules. Topical metronidazole gel is used concurrently with oral antibiotics.

When inflammation is adequately controlled, oral antibiotics are gradually withdrawn; topical metronidazole gel is continued to prevent recurrence of inflammation. Dosage schedules of both oral antibiotics and metronidazole gel must be adjusted as necessary to maintain optimal control of rosacea activity.

Isotretinoin should be used only for refractory cases that do not respond adequately to oral antibiotics and metronidazole gel.

Possible Drug Interactions of Significance
Erythromycin *taken concurrently* with
- astemizole (Hismanal) can cause serious heart rhythm abnormalities.
- terfenadine (Seldane) can cause serious heart rhythm abnormalities.

Special Considerations for Women
Observe the following precautions.

Pregnancy
See Appendix 15, FDA Pregnancy Categories.

Isotretinoin—Pregnancy Category X. Avoid completely during entire pregnancy.

Tetracycline—Pregnancy Category D. Avoid completely during entire pregnancy.

Breast-Feeding
Isotretinoin and tetracycline—avoid drugs or refrain from nursing.

Quality of Life Considerations
Rosacea is a chronic, recurrent disorder. It can have negative effects on self-image, self-esteem, and social interactions. Aggressive therapy can

yield significant improvement, bolster morale, and encourage adoption of a positive, optimistic attitude. Relief of symptoms is reported by 92% of patients who follow treatment instructions conscientiously.

The Role of Prevention in This Disorder

Primary Prevention

No practical means known at this time.

Secondary Prevention

This consists of (1) identifying and avoiding all factors that provoke flare-ups; and (2) complying fully with therapeutic programs that are designed to arrest progression of rosacea activity and minimize tissue damage.

Helpful Suggestions for Daily Living

Your Environment

Insofar as you can, minimize exposure to direct sunlight, wind, marked hot and cold weather.

Your Diet

- Keep a food diary for a while and try to discover specific foods or beverages that appear to trigger flare-ups within 24–48 hours after ingestion.
- Avoid hot, spicy, and highly seasoned foods; avoid alcoholic and caffeine-containing beverages.

Your Lifestyle

- Use cosmetics primarily to hide rosacea blemishes; minimize the use of cosmetics otherwise.
- Bathe in lukewarm water; avoid hot, steaming baths.
- Avoid strenuous exercising and prolonged physical activity.
- Maintain a calm, relaxed demeanor. Avoid situations that cause emotional stress of any kind.
- Obtain adequate sleep and rest on a regular basis.

Resource for Additional Information and Services

National Rosacea Society
800 South Northwest Highway, Suite 200
Barrington, IL 60010
Phone: (847) 382-8971

The Society publishes a quarterly newsletter and operates a physician referral service that provides the names and addresses of dermatologists throughout the country who treat rosacea. The Society also operates a telephone hotline on which patients can call to request information. The number is (847) 382-8971.

ACNE VULGARIS

Other Name Acne

Prevalence/Incidence in U.S.
Approximately 4.6 million cases: 2.4% of the population under 18 years of age; 3% of the population 18 to 44 years of age

Age Group
Most common in adolescents and young adults. Usually begins at puberty (9 to 12 years of age) and subsides at 18 to 20 years of age. A small percentage of cases will persist into the twenties and thirties.

Male-to-Female Ratio Slightly more common in women

Principal Features and Natural History
Common acne is a disorder of the hair follicles and sebaceous (oil-producing) glands of the skin. It is characterized by the formation of open comedones (blackheads), closed comedones (whiteheads), inflamed papules (pimples), and pustules in the superficial layers of the skin. The deep form of acne includes the formation of inflamed nodules and pus-filled cysts. These skin changes occur most commonly on the face, but are also found on the neck, chest, shoulders, and upper back. The degree of inflammation will vary from mild to severe throughout the course of the disorder. It is often worse in the winter and better during the summer, probably due to the beneficial effects of sun exposure.

Similar Conditions That May Confuse Diagnosis
Acne rosacea
Drug-induced acnelike skin eruptions (see below)
Seborrheic dermatitis

Causes
Acne is primarily due to overactivity of the oil-producing sebaceous glands. This usually begins with the changes of puberty when the associated increase in sex hormones (principally androgens) stimulates the growth and production of the glands. The opening of the gland becomes plugged with a mixture of dead skin cells, oils, and bacteria, resulting in a comedo; this progresses to the formation of fatty acids within the gland that causes inflammation, swelling, and eventual rupture into the skin. Contributing causes include familial predisposition, excessive heat and humidity, poor personal hygiene, the use of oil-based cosmetics, and exposure to industrial oils and tars.

Drugs That Can Cause This Disorder

The following drugs can initiate acne or aggravate existing acne:

androgens (male hormonelike drugs)

cortisonelike drugs

cytotoxic drugs (those used to treat various types of cancer)

methotrexate

oral contraceptives that contain norethindrone or norgestrel (Brevicon, Loestrin, Lo/Ovral, Micronor, Modicon, Norinyl, Norlestrin, Norlutin, Nor-Qd, Ortho-Novum, Ovcon, Ovral, Ovrette)

progesterone

The following drugs can cause acnelike eruptions but do not cause true comedo formation:

bromides

disulfiram

iodides

isoniazid

lithium

phenobarbital

phenytoin

quinine

thiouracil

trimethadione

vitamin B_{12}

Goals of Treatment

Can This Disorder Be Cured?

No curative treatment is known at this time.

Can This Disorder Be Treated Effectively?

Appropriate treatment, conscientiously followed, is beneficial in 95% of all cases.

Specific Goals

Improvement and control are the primary objectives.

• prevention of new blemishes
• prevention of scarring

Health Professionals Who Participate in Managing This Disorder

Family physicians

General internists

Dermatologists

Pharmacists

Plastic/Reconstructive surgeons

Currently Available Therapies for This Disorder

Drug Therapy
Locally (topically):
- benzoyl peroxide (Benzac-W Gel, Clearasil, Desquam-E Gel, Persa-Gel-W, etc.)
- adapalene (Differin)
- azelaic acid (Azelex)
- tretinoin (retinoic acid preparations, Retin-A)
- antibiotic lotions
- metronidazole gel (MetroGel)

Internally (systemically):
- tetracyclines (see Appendix 15, FDA Pregnancy Categories)
- erythromycin
- isotretinoin (see Appendix 15, FDA Pregnancy Categories)
- prednisone (see Appendix 6, Long-Term Corticosteroid Therapy)
- ibuprofen (see Appendix 15, FDA Pregnancy Categories)

Nondrug Treatment Methods
Cosmetic surgical procedures:
- dermabrasion for late scarring and pitting

Management of Therapy

Local (Topical) Drug Treatment
- Often sufficient to control superficial acne with mild to moderate inflammation
- May be used concurrently with internal (systemic) treatment for control of deep acne with severe inflammation, nodule and cyst formation
- Start treatment slowly; determine tolerance by applying small amounts of low-concentration products to small areas of skin.
- Limit applications to once or twice daily.
- Apply to *dry* skin, one-half hour after washing.
- Use soap and water to remove skin oils; wash skin no more than twice daily.
- Avoid abrasive preparations.
- Irritation from topical drugs is common; true allergy is uncommon

Use of Benzoyl Peroxide
- This is the single most effective drug for the topical treatment of acne. Many preparations are available without prescription. Its principal action is anti-infective; its primary use is treating superficial, inflammatory, papulopustular acne. This drug inactivates tretinoin (retinoic acid); do not apply these two drugs at the same time. This drug can bleach fabrics on contact; use with care.
- Start with a 5% preparation; apply once daily, in the morning.

Use of Tretinoin (Retinoic Acid)

- This is the only practical drug available for the topical management of comedones. It does require a prescription. It is used in all forms of acne to facilitate the removal of existing comedones and to prevent the formation of new ones. This drug may require continual use for up to 12 weeks to obtain initial benefit; continued control will require maintenance treatment for months or years. Drying and irritation of the skin are common. However, deliberate irritation and peeling are not necessary for benefit.
- Start with the 0.01% gel; increase the strength of the preparation as needed and tolerated. Apply once daily, in the evening or at bedtime.
- This drug may increase skin sensitivity to sunlight; use sunscreen preparations if necessary, but avoid them if possible.

Use of Topical Antibiotics

- Erythromycin is the drug of choice; tetracycline and clindamycin preparations are also used. These anti-infective drugs are used primarily to treat inflammatory acne; they do not clear existing lesions but do prevent the development of new ones. These drugs may require continual use for three to four weeks to obtain significant improvement.
- Apply twice daily, morning and evening.
- May be used concurrently with benzoyl peroxide or tretinoin.

Internal (Systemic) Drug Treatment

- Required for control of moderate to severe deep acne (inflammatory nodules, cysts, abscesses) and to reduce permanent scarring. A firm commitment to conscientious treatment for many months or years is often required to accomplish desired results.

Use of Tetracycline

- Generally considered to be the drug of choice for long-term use. Continual use for three months may be required to obtain optimal benefit. May be used alone or concurrently with benzoyl peroxide or tretinoin.
- Begin treatment with 500 mg to 1000 mg daily for four weeks or until a satisfactory result is obtained. Then reduce gradually to the smallest effective dose for long-term maintenance; this may be as low as 250 mg every one to three days.

  This is best taken on an empty stomach, one hour before or two hours after eating.
- If tetracycline is not effective or cannot be tolerated, erythromycin is the next drug of choice.

Use of Isotretinoin

- This drug is reserved for the treatment of severe acne that has not responded to conventional management. Continual use for 20 or more weeks is usually required to produce significant benefit. Within one to six weeks after starting treatment, severe flares of acne may occur. Reduced dosage for the first month may be necessary.

Its primary action is to inhibit the production of sebum (a mix of sebaceous oils and skin cell debris). This reduces the source of fatty acids that cause inflammatory reaction.

Do not use this drug during pregnancy. Use effective birth control measures while taking it.

- Monitor triglyceride blood levels during use; if level exceeds 400 mg, reduce the dose; if level exceeds 600 mg, discontinue this drug.
- Use this drug with caution in those with type I diabetes or inflammatory bowel disease (Crohn's disease, ulcerative colitis).

Use of Prednisone

- Cortisonelike drugs may induce acne in some individuals. However, it may be useful for some with extensive, severe inflammatory acne that is unresponsive to other treatments. Initiate treatment with 30 mg to 45 mg of prednisone daily, gradually reducing this dose within one month. Low-dose maintenance using 2.5 mg each evening may extend control.

Use of Ibuprofen

- This anti-inflammatory drug may enhance the beneficial effects of systemic tetracycline. A trial of 600 mg four times per day is warranted for those with severe inflammatory acne that has shown limited benefit from standard drug therapy.

Use of Oral Contraceptives

- High-estrogen birth control pills that contain a nonandrogenic progestin (ethynodrel, norethisterone, norethynodrel) are sometimes used to treat severe acne.
- The beneficial action of these preparations is the reduction of sebum formation.
- Because of the inherent risks, this use of oral contraceptives as therapy is generally not recommended.

Ancillary Drug Treatment (as required)

For candidiasis (yeast infection of genital or anal region, a complication of long-term antibiotic or oral contraceptive use):

- clotrimazole (Lotrimin)
- nystatin (Mycostatin)

Note: Drug selection, dosage, and administration schedule must be determined by the physician for each patient individually.

Possible Drug Interactions of Significance

Tetracyclines *taken concurrently* with isotretinoin may cause pseudotumor cerebri (swelling of the brain). Avoid this combination completely.

Special Considerations for Women

For those who choose to use oral contraceptives to prevent pregnancy, the following preparations are recommended because the progestin component has a very low androgen (male hormone) effect and therefore less likely to aggravate existing acne:

- desogestrel (Desogen, Ortho-Cept)
- norgestinate (Ortho-Cyclen, Ortho Tri-Cyclen)

ALERT!

Women with acne who also have excessive growth of body hair (hirsutism) and a history of irregular menstrual periods may have an abnormally high production of androgens (male sex hormones). Consult your physician regarding the need to evaluate this.

Pregnancy

Isotretinoin (Accutane) has an FDA Pregnancy Category rating of X (see Appendix 15). Follow the guidelines provided by the manufacturer precisely. Comply fully with your physician's instructions regarding the prevention of pregnancy.

Resources

Recommended Reading

Treating Acne: A Guide for Teens and Adults, Richard A. Walzer, Consumer Reports Books, 1992.

Additional Information and Services

Acne Research Institute
1236 Somerset Lane
Newport Beach, CA 92260
Phone: (714) 722-1805
Telecommunications services: 1-800-235-2263 (outside CA); 1-800-225-2263 (within CA); Fax: (714) 722-6828

Publications available.

AIDS

Other Names Acquired immune deficiency syndrome, AIDS-related complex, ARC, HIV infection

Prevalence/Incidence in U.S.

Current estimate of HIV-infected Americans—1 to 1.5 million; 1 in 250 persons.

Total through June 30, 1996—548,102 cases; 343,000 deaths (63%).

Persons living with HIV infection, not AIDS—73,217.

Persons living with AIDS—195,720.

Prevalence of HIV infection (with and without AIDS) in June 1996—268,937, with 75% of the cases occurring between the ages of 25 and 44

Racial proportions of cases: Whites—47%; Blacks—34%; Hispanics—18%; Asians—0.7%; Am. Indians/Alaskans—0.3%

Male-to-Female Ratio Male cases—81%; female cases—19%

Principal Features and Natural History

The term "AIDS," as loosely used prior to 1987, encompassed all stages and manifestations of infection with the human immunodeficiency virus (HIV). Strictly speaking, AIDS refers to the later stages of the infection when failure of the immune system results in the development of serious and life-threatening infections and malignancies. The span of this illness extends from the onset of infection (when the HIV virus first enters the body) through the terminal manifestations that cause death. This period of time varies from several months to as long as 15 years. The course of the illness in adults is usually a slow progression through the following stages.

1. *Early HIV Infection with Transient Symptoms*:

   The number of contacts with the virus that is required to cause infection is not known. The incubation period for the infecting virus to result in mild, transient flu-like symptoms is usually two to six weeks. The interval between infection and the onset of significant, chronic symptoms varies from one to seven years, with an average of two to four years. A negative blood test does not exclude the possibility of contact with the virus. Anyone at risk for AIDS should have periodic blood tests to monitor his/her status. There is a time lag between actual infection by the virus and the conversion of appropriate blood tests from negative to positive. This is the time required for the immune system to develop specific antibodies to the infecting virus; antibodies can usually be detected within three months after infection, but time lags of more than six months have been reported.

2. *HIV Infection with Early Symptoms*:

   The earliest manifestations of HIV infection are not specific. Because they are common to many types of virus infection, they usually do not arouse suspicion of HIV infection. Symptoms may include fatigue, loss of appetite, mild weight loss, diarrhea, low-grade fever, night sweats, and swollen lymph glands. The initial pattern may suggest infectious mononucleosis. This phase of infection may be transient or intermittent, followed by a period of variable length during which there are few or no significant symptoms.

3. *HIV Infection with Later Symptoms—AIDS-Related Complex*:

   During the period of no symptoms or relatively mild illness, the immune system is undergoing continuous challenge and stress. A specific class of white blood cells (CD4 lymphocytes), an essential component of the immune system, is being infected and slowly destroyed by HIV. The speed and intensity of this process are quite variable. The progressive destruction can run its course in several months or persist for several years. A common group of symptoms are characteristic of this AIDS-related complex or ARC (also referred to as suspected AIDS, pre-AIDS, and lymphadenopathy syndrome). These include fever, night sweats, swollen lymph glands, persistent diarrhea (three or more months), and loss of weight (15 or more pounds). Although not included in the original pattern of ARC, other significant disorders resulting from HIV infection (but not AIDS-defining) are now recognized. These include severe dermatitis, personality changes, intellectual impairment, peripheral neuritis, yeast infections of the mouth, pneumonias, myocarditis, nephritis, and arthritis. Approximately 40% of patients in this group will progress to AIDS within three years. The usual interval from the development of a positive blood test to the onset of AIDS is 8 to 11 years.

4. *HIV Infection with Associated Indicator Diseases—AIDS*:

AIDS is now defined as a specific group of diseases or conditions which are indicative of severe immunosuppression related to infection with the human immunodeficiency virus (HIV). As chronic HIV infection progresses, the immune system undergoes increasing impairment until it is no longer able to prevent the development of "opportunistic" infections and/or malignancies. These so-called "indicator diseases" include the following, listed in the order of decreasing frequency:

Pneumocystis carinii pneumonia
HIV wasting syndrome (chronically active HIV infection)
candida (yeast) infection of the mouth and esophagus
Kaposi's sarcoma (a form of cancer)
tuberculosis and related infections
HIV infection of the brain (encephalitis with dementia)
toxoplasmosis of the brain (a protozoan infection)
cryptococcosis infection (a yeastlike infection)
herpes simplex virus infections of mouth, esophagus, lung
lymphoma, several forms (types of cancer)
cytomegalovirus infections of retina and other organs
candida (yeast) infection of the trachea, bronchial tubes, or lung
cryptosporidiosis infection of the intestine (a protozoan infection)

It is estimated that this stage of infection, what can be thought of as full-blown AIDS is reached after 7 years of infection in 50% of cases and by 15 years in 78% to 100%. At this time, there is no curative treatment for AIDS. Available drugs can only retard the activity of the HIV virus for a limited time; they cannot eliminate it. When the immune system is depleted, anti-infective drugs alone are unable to control intercurrent infections. Annual case-fatality rates have averaged 62.4 for adults and adolescents, and 56.4 for children since 1981.

Diagnostic Symptoms and Signs

Early
A transient flu-like illness with no specific diagnostic features. This may indicate initial infection.

Intermediate
Persistent, generalized swelling of lymph glands, with or without symptoms of low-grade infection (fever, fatigue, loss of appetite, aching)

Late
Progressive pattern of systemic disease: fever, weakness, loss of weight, skin rashes, yeast infections in mouth, cough, diarrhea, headaches, dementia, leg pains

Specific opportunistic infections and cancers: see "Indicator Diseases" above

Diagnostic Tests and Procedures
"OraSure" oral specimen collection device for detecting HIV antibodies in oral fluids.

Standard blood screening test: ELISA (enzyme-linked immunosorbent assay) for HIV antibody. If positive, ELISA testing is repeated and a confirmatory Western blot test is mandatory.

Complete blood cell counts, including CD4 cell counts

Routine blood chemistry panel to establish baseline values for future comparison

Routine blood test for syphilis

Chest X-ray

Tuberculin skin test

Cervical Pap smear

Blood tests for hepatitis viral infections

Blood tests for toxoplasmosis

Measurement of G-6-PD (glucose-6-phosphate dehydrogenase) levels in red blood cells

Measurement of HIV viral load or burden (viral particles in a sample of blood)

Causes
The primary cause of AIDS is the severe and protracted suppression of the immune system resulting from infection with the human immunodeficiency virus (HIV-1 or HIV-2).

HIV infection can be acquired in several ways. The virus has been found in semen, vaginal secretions, blood, saliva, human breast milk, and certain body tissues (including those used for organ donation). It has not been found in sweat or tears. Exposures to possible infection and their relative frequency in established cases are illustrated in the following categories:

Adult Exposure Category	1995 Cases
Men who have sex with men	51%
Men and women who inject drugs	26%
Men who have sex with men and inject drugs	6%
Men who have heterosexual contact	5%
Women who have heterosexual contact	38%
Transfusion of infected blood	1%

Child Exposure Category	
HIV-infected mother	91%
Transfusion of infected blood	3%

Frequently Asked Questions Regarding the Transmission of HIV Infection

Q. Can transmission occur during ordinary, daily activities involving contact with others in customary social settings: home, workplace, school, shopping areas, restaurants, theaters, etc.?

A. There is no evidence to indicate that the virus is airborne, waterborne, or foodborne; no evidence of infection by insect bites; no evidence of infection by nonsexual personal contact.

Q. Are any precautions necessary among household contacts?

A. Yes. The HIV-infected person should not share razors, toothbrushes, or any other items that could carry blood residues. If an HIV-infected person experiences a wound that bleeds, any surface that is contaminated by infected blood should be cleaned thoroughly and disinfected. Household bleach (diluted with water, 1 part to 10) is recommended for disinfection.

Q. Is there risk of transmission while participating in sports or sharing athletic facilities with infected individuals?

A. Ordinarily, no. The HIV is not found in sweat. However, an infected individual who sustains a wound that bleeds could be a potential source of transmission. Contamination of any part of the body with infected blood must be avoided. If contamination occurs, thoroughly wash and disinfect the area of contact immediately.

Q. Should an HIV-infected individual inform health care workers of his/her status?

A. Yes. Although the risk of transmission is small, all HIV-positive patients should inform physicians, dentists, nurses, and other health care workers that they are infected. Infected individuals should not donate blood, semen, body organs, or other tissues.

Q. Can HIV infection be transmitted by kissing?

A. HIV has been found in saliva. Studies to date indicate that casual, closed-mouth kissing does not transmit infection. However, open-mouth, passionate kissing is thought to be a possible means of transmission.

Q. What forms of sex are "safe?"

A. Only one: mutually monogamous sexual intercourse between uninfected individuals carries no risk of HIV infection. All forms of sexual contact—genital, oral–genital, rectal—with an HIV-infected individual carry risk of transmission. An HIV-infected partner can transmit the virus even though he or she is free of symptoms, appears to be completely healthy, and still has a negative blood test for HIV infection. Infection can occur after a single exposure.

Q. What precautions can be taken to permit "safer" sex?

A. It is important to know that available measures to use for "safer" sex can reduce the risk of HIV transmission but not eliminate the risk completely. The following are recommended: (1) The regular use of latex condoms; nonlatex condoms are less effective. Reported rates of condom failure are 5% during vaginal intercourse and 8% during rectal intercourse. (2) The use of spermicidal jelly. Preparations containing nonoxynol 9 (Ortho-Gynol, others) may inactivate HIV. It is thought that the combined use of a latex condom and spermicidal jelly should provide the greatest reduction of risk.

Q. Are home test kits available for detection of HIV infection?

A. Yes. The FDA-approved HIV home testing and counseling service, called Confide, became available on a limited basis in Florida and Texas in June, 1996. It will be available nationwide in early 1997. The test and accompanying service include:

- an information booklet and pretest counseling
- a test kit with instructions and materials for obtaining a blood sample (by finger prick and special paper)
- a prepaid, preaddressed mailer for mailing the sample to a national clinical reference laboratory. The special sample paper contains a unique identification number; the test subject does not include his/her name or other identifying information.
- a toll-free 800 telephone number for the user to call after seven days to obtain test results and further counseling

Q. Can an HIV-infected person transmit the virus while taking an antiviral drug such as AZT?

A. Yes. The use of any drug currently available does not prevent the transmission of infection by established routes: sexual contact, sharing infected needles, receiving transfusion of infected blood or donation of infected tissue, pregnancy transmission by mother to child.

Drugs That Can Cause This Disorder

There are no drugs that can cause AIDS. This group of life-threatening conditions is the direct result of irreversible suppression of the immune system caused by HIV infection.

Theoretically, the following immunosuppressive drugs could impair the user's immune system and thereby increase susceptibility to HIV infection:

azathioprine (Imuran)
chlorambucil (Leukeran)
corticosteroid drugs (prednisone, etc.)
cyclophosphamide (Cytoxan, Neosar)
cyclosporine (Sandimmune)
methotrexate (Folex, Mexate)

Goals of Treatment

Although prevention and cure of HIV infection are the ultimate goals, there are no drugs or vaccines now available that are capable of this.

Using the drugs listed below to optimal advantage, present treatment goals include the following:

* to initiate treatment with antiviral drugs at the earliest appropriate time to retard the destruction of CD4 lymphocytes and thus delay the onset of symptoms related to HIV infection.
* to determine the lowest effective dose of antiviral drugs that will achieve the best possible benefit-to-risk outcome.
* to initiate treatment with selected drugs at the appropriate time to prevent the development of opportunistic infections.
* to initiate treatment with appropriate drugs as soon as possible to cure, control, or suppress intercurrent infections.
* to relieve symptoms and suffering to the greatest extent possible.

Health Professionals Who Participate in Managing This Disorder

Family physicians
General internists
Pediatricians
Infectious disease physicians
Infectious disease nurses
Neurologists
Ophthalmologists
Optometrists
Dentists
Pulmonologists
Gynecologists
Obstetricians

Dermatologists
Rheumatologists
Psychiatrists
Pharmacists
Physician assistants
Nurse practitioners
Nutritionists
Medical social workers
Pastoral counselors

Currently Available Therapies for This Disorder

Drug Therapy

Antiviral drugs specifically for HIV infection:

- didanosine (DDI, Videx)—nucleoside analog
- lamivudine (Epivir)—nucleoside analog
- stavudine (d4T, Zerit)—nucleoside analog
- zalcitabine (DDC, Hivid)—nucleoside analog
- zidovudine (AZT, ZDV, Retrovir)—nucleoside analog
- indinavir (Crixivan)—protease inhibitor
- ritonavir (Norvir)—protease inhibitor
- saquinavir (Invirase)—protease inhibitor
- nevirapine (Viramune)—reverse transcriptase inhibitor

Drugs used to treat the "indicator diseases" of AIDS:

- acyclovir for herpes simplex and varicella-zoster virus infections
- amphotericin B for cryptococcosis
- atovaquone for *Pneumocystis carinii* pneumonia and toxoplasmosis
- azithromycin for cryptosporidiosis and *Mycobacterium avium* infections
- ciprofloxacin for *Mycobacterium avium* infections
- clarithromycin for *Mycobacterium avium* infections
- clindamycin for *Pneumocystis carinii* pneumonia and toxoplasmosis
- clofazimine for *Mycobacterium avium* infections
- clotrimazole for candidiasis (yeast infections)
- dapsone for *Pneumocystis carinii* pneumonia
- ethambutol for tuberculosis
- fluconazole for treatment of candidiasis and suppression of cryptococcal infections
- flucytosine for cryptococcal meningitis
- foscarnet for cytomegalovirus retinitis and herpes virus infections
- ganciclovir for cytomegalovirus infections
- isoniazid for tuberculosis
- itraconazole for histoplasmosis, cryptococcosis, aspergillosis, and candidiasis

- ketoconazole for treatment of candidiasis and suppression of histoplasmosis
- nystatin for candidiasis (yeast infections)
- paromomycin for cryptosporidiosis
- pentamidine for *Pneumocystis carinii* pneumonia
- primaquine for *Pneumocystis carinii* pneumonia
- pyrazinamide for tuberculosis
- pyrimethamine for toxoplasmosis
- rifabutin for *Mycobacterium avium* infections
- rifampin for tuberculosis
- sulfadiazine for toxoplasmosis
- sulfamethoxazole for *Pneumocystis carinii* pneumonia, isosporiasis, and salmonellosis
- trimethoprim for *Pneumocystis carinii* pneumonia, isosporiasis, and salmoncllosis
- trimetrexate for *Pneumocystis carinii* pneumonia

New Drugs in Development for Treating This Disorder

Current research on the development of new therapeutic agents for use against HIV infection includes the following:

- vaccines
- passive hyperimmune globulin (now in phase III trials)
- gene therapy engineered to destroy the HIV genome in HIV-infected patients (see Appendix 11)

For further information call the AIDS Clinical Trials Information Service, 1-800-TRIALS-A.

Management of Therapy

The natural history of HIV infection and the spectrum of illness that it causes permits a division of its progression into observable stages. Experience of attempts to manage the various manifestations of this chronic infection has taught that careful evaluation of the patient's status at the time of diagnosis provides a basis for determining specific treatment. By "staging" the individual's status of disease, the best drug(s) and method(s) of use can be initiated. Knowledge of typical disease progression provides a basis for (1) interpreting the significance of the patient's symptoms, and (2) assessing the patient's prognosis.

The manifestations of ARC and AIDS vary greatly from person to person and from stage to stage. All aspects of treatment must be carefully individualized. Drug selection and administration require meticulous consideration of benefits versus risks in each case.

The CD4 lymphocyte count is used to assess the state of immune suppression. Periodic counts serve decision making regarding the stage of the disease and the selection of drug therapies. The normal range of the

CD4 count is 500 to 1,400 cells per cubic millimeter of blood. If the count is over 600, testing should be done every 6 months; if the count is between 200 and 600, testing should be repeated every 3 months. CD4 counts under 200 require closer monitoring on an individual basis.

Measurement of the viral burden (or load) is now regarded as the best indicator of the status of infection. The CD4 lymphocyte count and the viral burden value, used together, provide the best estimate of disease status and prognosis.

Use of Antiviral Drugs

The use of the nucleoside analog drugs (didanosine, stavudine, zalcitabine, and zidovudine) has been the principal therapy for HIV infection since 1987. Used singly and in various combinations, they provided variable results in delaying progression of disease and the onset of late symptoms, and in extending life. However, these drugs are not curative.

The recently approved protease inhibitor drugs (indinavir, ritonavir, and saquinavir) appear to be ten times more effective against HIV infection than the nucleoside analog drugs. By inhibiting the enzyme protease in the HIV, these drugs impair the development of functional (infectious) viruses and cause the production of immature, noninfectious HIV particles. In addition, protease inhibitor drugs are effective against HIV strains that have developed resistance to nucleoside analog drugs. To date, protease inhibitors are significantly less toxic than nucleoside analogs.

Current studies are under way to determine the optimal use of these two classes of drugs in combination. Early trials have demonstrated that certain combinations can significantly reduce viral blood levels, increase CD4 cell counts, and decrease death rates. For current information regarding the most effective drug therapies available at this time, call 1-800-TRIALS-A, the National Institute of Allergy and Infectious Diseases.

Drug Treatment of Common HIV-Related Infections

Pneumocystis carinii pneumonia: This is the initial opportunistic infection in 60% of AIDS cases, and eventually occurs in 70% of all cases. The drugs of choice are combined trimethoprim and sulfamethoxazole; these are given in full dosage for 21 days. Alternate drugs include atovaquone, pentamidine; combined dapsone and trimethoprim; combined clindamycin and primaquine.

Toxoplasmosis: This protozoan infection of the brain is the initial manifestation of AIDS in 2% of cases. The drugs of choice are combined sulfadiazine and pyrimethamine; these are given for a prolonged period of time to prevent relapse.

Cryptococcosis: This yeastlike infection is the initial opportunistic disease in 7% of AIDS cases. It usually causes meningitis or infections in the respiratory tract. The drug of choice is amphotericin B (given intravenously). The antifungal drug fluconazole (given by mouth) is under study for effectiveness in treating this infection.

Mycobacterium Avium-Intracellulare (MAI) infections: This tuberculo-sislike infection occurs in 60% of AIDS cases. Unlike typical tuberculosis, it usually causes infection in the gastrointestinal tract, liver, and bone marrow rather than the lung. There are no established drugs of choice for treatment. Drugs commonly tried are combinations of amikacin (given intravenously), clarithromycin, azithromycin, ciprofoxacin, ethambutol, rifampin, or rifabutin, given orally.

Isosporiasis: This protozoan infection of the intestine is a common cause of chronic diarrhea in AIDS cases; its exact incidence is not known. The drugs of choice are combined trimethoprim and sulfamethoxazole given for several weeks. An alternate drug, equally effective, is pyrimethamine.

Herpes simplex infection: This viral infection occurs in 20% of patients with ARC or AIDS. The drug of choice is acyclovir given by mouth in doses of 200 to 400 mg five times daily for acute infections and 400 mg twice daily to prevent recurrence. The long-term suppressive dose has not been established.

Candidiasis: This very common yeast infection causes thrush (infection of the mouth and throat) in 90% of AIDS patients, and infection of the esophagus in 50% of cases. The drugs of choice for treatment are keto-conazole by mouth (200 to 400 mg daily) or fluconazole by mouth (200 mg as initial dose, then 100 mg daily).

Tuberculosis: Now considered to be an AIDS-defining illness, the inci-dence of active tuberculous infection of the lungs has increased significantly in HIV-infected individuals. The following drug regimen is the current treat-ment of choice: (1) isoniazid (300 mg), rifampin (600 mg), and pyrazi-namide (15 to 30 mg/kg to a maximum dose of 2 grams) for two months; then (2) isoniazid and rifampin (in the above doses) for four more months. Selected cases may require treatment for 9 to 12 months.

Ancillary Drug Treatment (as required)

For yeast infection of mouth and throat:
- nystatin oral suspension
- clotrimazole troches

For seborrheic dermatitis:
- 1% hydrocortisone cream
- ketoconazole by mouth

For fungal skin infections:
- clotrimazole skin preparations
- miconazole skin preparations
- griseofulvin by mouth

For peripheral neuropathy:
- amitriptyline

For chronic nonspecific diarrhea:
- loperamide

For impaired attention and response:
- methylphenidate

Note: Drug selection, dosage, and administration schedule must be determined by the physician for each patient individually.

Possible Drug Interactions of Significance

The following drugs should not be used concurrently with indinavir (Crixivan):

astemizole (Hismanal)
cisapride (Propulsid)
didanosine (ddI, Videx)—use separate dosing
midazolam (Versed)
rifampin (Rifadin, Rimactane)
terfenadine (Seldane)
triazolam (Halcion)

The following drugs should not be used concurrently with ritonavir (Norvir):

alprazolam (Xanax)
amiodarone (Cordarone)
astemizole (Hismanal)
bepridil (Vascor)
bupropion (Wellbutrin)
cisapride (Propulsid)
clorazepate (Tranxene)
clozapine (Clozaril)
diazepam (Valium)
disulfiram (Antabuse)—disulfiram reaction (see Glossary)
encainide (Enkaid)
estazolam (ProSom)
flecainide (Tambocor)
flurazepam (Dalmane)
meperidine (Demerol)
metronidazole (Flagyl)—disulfiramlike reaction (see Glossary)
midazolam (Versed)
oral contraceptives—possible reduced effectiveness
piroxicam (Feldene)
propafenone (Rythmol)
propoxyphene (Darvon)
quinidine (Quinora)
rifabutin (Mycobutin)
saquinavir (Invirase)—safety not established
terfenadine (Seldane)

triazolam (Halcion)

zolpidem (Ambien)

Monitor closely if the following drugs are used concurrently with saquinavir (Invirase):

astemizole (Hismanal)

calcium-channel blockers—monitor for toxicity

carbamazepine (Tegretol)—decreased saquinavir levels

clindamycin (Cleocin)—monitor for toxicity

dapsone—monitor for toxicity

dexamethasone (Decadron)—decreased saquinavir levels

phenobarbital—decreased saquinavir levels

phenytoin (Dilantin)—decreased saquinavir levels

rifabutin (Mycobutin)—saquinavir levels decreased 40%

rifampin (Rifadin, Rimactane)—saquinavir levels decreased 80%

terfenadine (Seldane)

triazolam (Halcion)—monitor for toxicity

Special Considerations for Women

- HIV infection is often associated with other sexually transmitted diseases. Appropriate tests for chlamydial infection, gonorrhea, and syphilis are advisable.
- HIV-infected women should have Pap smears of the cervix soon after diagnosis and annually thereafter. Accumulated data shows that HIV infection predisposes to precancerous changes in the cervix that progress rapidly to invasive cancer if not treated promptly.
- HIV-infected women are at increased risk for pelvic inflammatory disease (PID). Abscesses of the ovaries and fallopian tubes often require prolonged antibiotic therapy and surgery.

Pregnancy

The following points deserve consideration by the HIV-infected woman:

- If she is interested in contraception, the effective use of condoms has three important advantages: prevention of pregnancy; prevention of HIV transmission to uninfected partners; and prevention of infection by another sexually transmitted disease.
- There is no evidence that pregnancy or childbirth has deleterious effects on the progression of HIV infection.
- The risk of transmission of HIV infection from mother to infant ranges from 13–39%. Recent trials have shown that treatment with zidovudine (AZT) reduces the rate of transmission during pregnancy.
- Pregnancy outcomes of HIV infected mothers are at increased risk for stillbirth and low-birth-weight infants.

Breast-Feeding

The HIV has been found in human breast milk. Viral transmission can occur with breast-feeding. This practice is not recommended for HIV-infected mothers.

The Role of Prevention in This Disorder

Primary Prevention

Measures taken to avoid HIV infection are obvious:

- Practice "safe sex." Refrain from sexual activities with high-risk partners. Use latex condoms and spermicidal jelly as appropriate.
- Refrain from intravenous drug use.
- Refrain from sharing razors, toothbrushes, or other items with blood residues that are used by HIV-infected persons.
- Promptly disinfect skin exposed to HIV-contaminated blood.
- Assure that all blood and blood products that you are to receive have been properly screened for HIV.

Secondary Prevention

It is advisable to provide the following vaccinations to HIV-infected persons as early as possible, preferably when the CD4 count is above 200:

- pneumococcal vaccine
- influenza vaccine
- hepatitis B vaccine
- hemophilus influenza Type B vaccine
- measles, mumps, and rubella vaccines for susceptible persons
- inactivated polio vaccine (IPV). *Do not give oral polio vaccine (OPV)!*
- tetanus-diphtheria vaccine, with booster doses every 10 years

Resources

Recommended Reading

Evaluation and Management of Early HIV Infection, Clinical Practice Guideline Number 7, Agency for Health Care Policy and Research, Public Health Service, U.S. Department of Health and Human Services, AHCPR Publication No. 94-0572, January 1994. Source: CDC National AIDS Hotline, 1-800-342-AIDS.

The Guide to Living with HIV Infection, John G. Bartlett, M.D., and Ann K. Finkbeiner. Baltimore: Johns Hopkins AIDS Clinic.

No Time to Wait: A Complete Guide to Treating, Managing, and Living with HIV Infection, Nick Siano and Suzanne Lipsett. New York: Bantam Books, 1993.

AIDS Care at Home: A Guide for Caregivers, Loved Ones, and People with AIDS, Judith Greif and Beth Ann Golden. New York: Wiley, 1994.

Additional Information and Services

National AIDS Hotline

Phone: 1-800-342-2437 (7 days/week, 24 hours/day)
Spanish access: 1-800-344-7432 (7 days/week, 8 A.M.–2 A.M. EST)
TDD deaf access: 1-800-243-7889 (M–F, 10 A.M.–10 P.M. EST)

Provides confidential information, referrals, and educational material on AIDS.

CDC National AIDS Clearing House
P.O. Box 6003
Rockville, MD 20849-6003
Phone: 1-800-458-5231; (301) 217-0023
TDD deaf access: 1-800-243-7012
Telecommunications services: Fax: (301) 738-6616

Provides information on AIDS, AIDS-related services, and educational resources. Offers referral service. Publications available.

American Foundation for AIDS Research (AmFAR)
5900 Wilshire Blvd, 2nd Floor
E. Satellite
Los Angeles, CA 90036
Phone: 1-800-39-AMFAR; (213) 857-5900

Publishes the *AIDS/HIV Treatment Directory.*

National Library of Medicine: AID TO AIDS INQUIRERS
Phone: 1-800-HIV-0440

Health information experts provide answers regarding up-to-date treatments for AIDS.

Monday–Friday, 9 A.M.–7 P.M. EDT. All calls are completely confidential.

Disease Management Expertise

National Institute of Allergy and Infectious Diseases
AIDS Clinical Trials Group
Dr. Maureen Myers
6003 Executive Blvd., Room 200P
Rockville, MD 20852
Phone: 1-800-TRIALS-A; (301) 496-8210˙

Provides information on current treatment trials using new drugs for AIDS. Explains access to individuals who may wish to participate.

ALZHEIMER'S DISEASE

Other Names AD, Alzheimer's presenile dementia, Alzheimer's senile dementia, senile dementia (Alzheimer type)

Prevalence/Incidence in U.S.

Approximately 4 million; 7% of the American population aged over 65 years; 10% of those 75 to 85 years old; 47% of those over 85 years old. Alzheimer's disease causes 60% of all progressive dementias.

Estimated deaths annually: 100,000

Age Group

Occurs occasionally under 50 years of age; uncommon before 65 years; the majority occurs over 65 years: mild dementia in 5% and moderate to severe in 10–20%. Moderate to severe dementia occurs in 20% of all cases over 80. AD now affects 47% of all people over 85 years old.

Male-to-Female Ratio More common in women

Principal Features and Natural History

Insidious onset leading to progressive and permanent decline of all intellectual functions

Mood changes: apathy, depression, irritability, anxiety, paranoia

Loss of recent memory, inability to recall facts of common knowledge, disorientation, confusion, delusions, hallucinations, all worse at night

Impaired attention, understanding, judgment. Loss of ability to think abstractly, to use language correctly, to calculate

Eventual gait disturbances, incoordination of movements

Social skills may be retained until late in course of disease

Course is from 3 to 20 years, with mean duration of 7 years

Diagnostic Symptoms and Signs

Criteria for the diagnosis of "clinically probable" Alzheimer's disease:

dementia (see Glossary) established by clinical examination and confirmed by neuropsychological testing

deficits in more than one cognitive area: memory, attention, language, personality, visual–spatial functions, mental calculation

mental deterioration is progressive

normal function of all senses; no delirium

onset between 40 and 90 years of age, usually after 65 years of age

absence of other illness or disorder that could affect the brain or produce dementia

Diagnostic Tests and Procedures

At this time, there are no definitive tests for Alzheimer's disease. Basic laboratory tests and imaging procedures of the brain may be done to exclude other causes of dementia.

In November 1994, an article published in the journal *Science* reported that individuals who have AD are unusually sensitive to the action of tropicamide, a drug used by ophthalmologists to dilate the pupils during eye examinations. The pupils of healthy patients and those with other dementias dilate only 5% following the instillation of tropicamide eye-drops; the pupils of patients with AD dilate from 13–23%. Confirmatory studies are now underway to determine if this procedure can be utilized as a definitive test to establish the presence of Alzheimer's disease.

Diagnostic "Markers" for This Disorder

Excessive numbers of neurofibrillar tangles and neuritic plaques in the outer layer (cortex) of the brain. These are microscopic tissue changes (degenerated nerve cells) found at postmortem examination (autopsy), confirming the diagnosis of Alzheimer's disease.

Similar Conditions That May Confuse Diagnosis

Age-associated memory impairment
Mini-strokes due to cerebral vascular disease
Psychiatric depression and "pseudodementias"
Unrecognized and untreated hypothyroidism in the elderly
Undiagnosed late-stage Lyme disease with dementia
Pick's disease: a rare degenerative disorder of the frontal and temporal
    lobes of the brain
AIDS-associated dementia
Syphilis-associated dementia
Drug-induced dementia
Alcoholic dementia syndrome
Vitamin B_{12} deficiency

ALERT!

Neurologists estimate that at least 25% of patients who are diagnosed as having Alzheimer's disease actually have another disorder that is readily treatable. An initial diagnosis of AD is clearly one that warrants a second opinion.

Causes

Degeneration of nerve cells in the areas of the brain that control intellectual functions. The actual cause of degeneration is unknown. Genetic predisposition appears probable; Alzheimer-type dementia is four times more frequent among family members than in the general population. There is a history of previous head injury in 15–20% of cases. One common feature is a marked deficiency of the nerve transmitter acetylcholine in critical brain tissues.

There is no scientific consensus that aluminum deposits in brain tissue are causally related to Alzheimer's disease.

Drugs That Can Cause This Disorder

No drugs cause true Alzheimer's dementia. However, 3% of all dementias

are drug-induced. The following drugs can cause symptoms in the elderly that resemble Alzheimer's disease (see Appendix 16: Drug Classes):
    antidepressants
    atropinelike drugs
    barbiturates
    benzodiazepines
    butyrophenones
    cortisonelike drugs
    digitalis preparations
    MAO inhibitors

Goals of Treatment
- Temporary improvement of alertness and memory
- Relief of confusion, depression, and behavioral disturbances

Health Professionals Who Participate in Managing This Disorder
Family physicians
General internists
Geriatricians
Neurologists
Psychiatrists
Registered nurses
Nurse technicians
Nurses' aides
Behavioral therapists
Medical social workers

Currently Available Therapies for This Disorder

Drug Therapy
No specific or truly effective drug treatment is available at this time. Treatment is symptomatic.
- Ergoloid mesylates (Deapril-ST, Hydergine) are tried during the early stages to relieve symptoms; benefits are infrequent, negligible, and fleeting.
- Tacrine (THA, Cognex) appears to improve mental function in a minority of patients with mild to moderate Alzheimer's disease (see below).

New Drugs in Development for Treating This Disorder
- Experimental drugs: choline, physostigmine (none are curative or significantly beneficial). Nimodipine, a calcium-channel-blocking drug, is currently under study for human use. It has been shown to accelerate learning in aged rabbits.

- Huperzine A, an extract of club moss, appears to be "more effective and more specific" than tacrine in raising acetylcholine levels in brain tissue. Testing in humans is planned pending FDA approval.

Management of Therapy

- Keep all medications to a minimum.
- If any drug is used, start treatment with small doses, increase the dosage cautiously and monitor the response very closely.
- Avoid drugs with strong atropinelike effects and strong sedative effects.
- Ergoloid mesylates may act as a mild antidepressant and may improve mood. If it is tolerated well, a trial of six months is justified.
- Lecithin may increase the acetylcholine content of brain tissue and temporarily improve memory in some individuals. It is available in health food stores without prescription. It is safe to try. Ask your physician for guidance.
- Use antipsychotics (Haldol, Mellaril, etc.) and sedatives (chloral hydrate, Benadryl, etc.) only when clearly needed. Use the smallest dose that proves to be effective.
- The appropriate use of electroconvulsive therapy (ECT) may provide safe and effective treatment for severe depression that is unresponsive to antidepressant drugs.

Use of Tacrine (Cognex)

This drug is not a cure and does not alter the progression of Alzheimer's disease. It may improve memory by raising the level of acetylcholine in brain tissues. Studies to date indicate that tacrine produces a modest, temporary improvement in a minority of patients with mild to moderate Alzheimer's disease when treated for 12 to 30 weeks. Common side effects include loss of appetite, indigestion, nausea, vomiting, diarrhea, rash, muscle aches, and unsteady gait.

The dose ranges from 10 to 40 mg four times daily. The maximal daily dose should not exceed 160 mg.

Studies have shown that tacrine can cause liver toxicity in more than a quarter of the people who take it. Liver function tests must be done weekly for the first 18 weeks of treatment. If no liver reactions are found, testing can be reduced to every three months for the duration of treatment.

Ancillary Drug Treatment (as required)

For anxiety:
- buspirone (BuSpar)
- lorazepam (Ativan)

For agitation, confusion:
- haloperidol (Haldol)
- thioridazine (Mellaril)
- thiothixene (Navane)

For delusions:
- molindone (Moban)
- clozapine (Clozaril)
- risperidone (Risperdal)

For insomnia:
- lorazepam (Ativan)
- chloral hydrate (capsules, syrup, suppositories)
- diphenhydramine (Benadryl)

For depression:
- fluoxetine (Prozac)
- sertraline (Zoloft)
- venlafaxine (Effexor)

For constipation:
- docusate (Colace, Doxinate, Surfak, etc.)

Note: Drug selection, dosage, and administration schedule must be determined by the physician for each patient individually.

Special Considerations for Women

The results of a study performed at the University of Southern California School of Medicine (reported in February 1995) indicate that women who used estrogen replacement therapy (ERT) following menopause showed a 30% lower risk of developing Alzheimer's disease than women who did not use estrogen. Women taking the highest doses of estrogen had the lowest risk of developing AD. Consult your physician for guidance. The benefits and risks of long-term estrogen therapy must be considered for each woman individually.

Quality of Life Considerations

Regarding the Patient

To the observer of a person with advancing AD, the quality of the patient's life would appear to be pitiful and dismal. However, the patient's perception and understanding of what is happening are progressively blunted. Emotional suffering becomes shallow and fleeting. Periods of agitation, confusion, and depression can be managed reasonably well with appropriate medications. Good custodial care will help greatly to stabilize the patient's behavior.

Regarding the Caregivers

Of greater concern is the quality of the caregiver's life. During the period of the patient's progressive decline, care is often provided in the home. Those providing the care must cope with the continuous physical, emotional, and financial stresses involved. Sources of help must be sought and utilized as appropriate. These include local support groups sponsored by the Alzheimer's Association, home health care agencies, local day care centers, respite care services, and community hospice organizations. Health care professionals should simultaneously monitor the status of the AD patient and those providing the care. For more information and appropriate help for caregivers, contact the Well Spouse Foundation, 610 Lexington Avenue, Suite 814, New York, NY 10022. Phone: 1-800-838-0879, (212) 644-1241.

Resources

Recommended Reading

The Alzheimer's Cope Book: The Complete Care Manual for Patients and Their Families, R.E. Markin. New York: Carol Publishing Group, 1992.

When Memory Fails: Helping the Alzheimer's and Dementia Patient, Allen J. Edwards. New York: Plenum Press, 1994.

The 36-Hour Day: A Family Guide to Caring for Persons with Alzheimer's Disease, Related Dementing Diseases, and Memory Loss in Later Life, N.L. Mace and P.V. Rabins. Baltimore: Johns Hopkins University Press, 1981.

Understanding Alzheimer's Disease: What It Is; How to Cope with It; Future Directions, M.K. Aronson, ed. New York: Charles Scribner's Sons, 1988.

Additional Information and Services

Alzheimer's Association
919 North Michigan Avenue, Suite 1000
Chicago, IL 60611-1676
Phone: (312) 335-8700, 1-800-272 3900
TDD: (312) 335-8882; Fax: (312) 335-1110

Toll-free information and referral service. Sends packet of information; offers information by phone. National network of 220 chapters and 2,000 support groups. Publishes a free quarterly newsletter.

Disease Management Expertise

National Institutes of Health
National Institute of Neurological Disorders and Stroke
Medical Neurology Branch
Building 10, Room 5N236
Bethesda, MD 20892
Phone: (301) 496-9526

ASTHMA

Other Names Bronchial asthma, reversible airway disease, reversible obstructive airway disease

Prevalence/Incidence in U.S.

Current estimate: 14 to 15 million, 5.7% of the population
Estimated deaths annually: 5,000 fatal attacks

Age Group

Under 18 years—4.8 million; 18 to 44 years—5.4 million; 45 to 64 years—3.1 million; 65 to 74 years—1.2 million; 75 years and over—500,000

Male-to-Female Ratio Male—46%, Female—54%

Principal Features and Natural History

Recurring acute attacks of shortness of breath, wheezing (labored breathing), a sensation of tightness in the chest and cough, with symptom-free intervals between attacks. Episodes of active asthma may last an hour to several days. The acute attack begins with tightening of muscles in the walls of bronchial tubes (airways), which causes constriction and reduced air flow. This is followed by swelling of the lining of bronchial tubes and the excessive production of mucus, both of which cause additional narrowing of the airways, forced breathing, and coughing. Severe asthma may be accompanied by sweating, insomnia, and bluish discoloration of the face and extremities (cyanosis). Asthma that begins in infancy (under 2 years of age) may persist into adulthood. With onset after 2 years, 50% of asthma cases will "outgrow" the disorder by 16 years. Asthma with onset in adulthood is often severe and persistent.

Diagnostic Symptoms and Signs

During an attack of acute asthma, the breathing pattern is characterized by a distinct difficulty in exhaling, as though something is obstructing the outflow of air. Inhaling is unimpaired. Narrowed airways (constricted bronchial tubes) produces a whistlelike effect with characteristic "wheezing" as air is forced out of the lungs. Coughing may or may not occur during the asthmatic episode.

Diagnostic Tests and Procedures

Skin testing by an allergist to identify possible causes (allergens) that may
   provoke acute attacks of asthma
Pulmonary function studies to measure lung capacity and rates of airflow
   during forced breathing
Tests to demonstrate (1) the degree of sensitivity of bronchial tubes to
   agents that provoke constriction; (2) the degree of reversibility of constricted bronchial tubes

Possible Effects of Drugs on Test Results

Antihistamines and cortisonelike (corticosteroid) drugs taken prior to skin testing can suppress an allergic response and cause false negative test results.

Bronchodilator drugs taken prior to pulmonary function testing can affect test results.

Consult your physician regarding proper preparation for diagnostic procedures.

Similar Conditions That May Confuse Diagnosis

Episodes of acute infectious bronchitis: bacterial or viral

Other chronic obstructive pulmonary disorders (COPD): chronic bronchitis, emphysema

Causes

Extrinsic (Allergic) Asthma

Due to a true allergy (allergen–antibody reaction); hereditary susceptibility to the development of allergies. Common allergens are house dust (and mites in house dust), pollens, animal danders, feathers, wool, molds.

Intrinsic (Idiosyncratic) Asthma

Due to an unusual individual sensitivity (not a true allergy). Onset usually 35 to 45 years of age; 10–15% are sensitive to aspirin and have nasal polyps.

Occupational Asthma

An important type of asthma that is often unrecognized. It can be due to a wide variety of allergens that are peculiar to certain occupations. Common examples are the following:

Allergen	Occupation
Cat, mouse, guinea pig	Laboratory staff, veterinarians
Flour	Bakers, food workers
Acacia	Printers
Metals	Nickel, platinum, etc., workers
Toluene	Auto, paint, plastic workers
Hair bleach and dyes	Beauticians
Western red cedar	Wood workers

Exercise-Induced Asthma

Usually in children and young adults; occurs alone or with other types of asthma; often worse 15 minutes after exercise.

Asthma "Triggers"

Cold air; smoke; cooking odors; perfumes; respiratory infections; emotional stress; food additives: monosodium glutamate (MSG), sulfites, tartrazine (yellow dye No. 5), yeast (see Appendix 14)

Drugs That Can Cause This Disorder

acetaminophen
aspirin (and substitutes)
beta-blocker drugs
erythromycin
griseofulvin
hydralazine
ibuprofen
indomethacin
ketoprofen
mefenamic acid
monoamine oxidase inhibitors
naproxen
nitrofurantoin
oral contraceptives
penicillin
pentazocine
phenothiazines
phenylbutazone
procainamide
propoxyphene
reserpine
tartrazine dye

Goals of Treatment

Can This Disorder Be Cured?

Episodes of extrinsic asthma can be eliminated if all responsible allergens and "triggers" are avoided. Some states of allergy (hypersensitivity) can be modified by hyposensitization therapy.

Nonallergic forms of asthma are not amenable to cure.

Can This Disorder Be Treated Effectively?

The majority of cases respond well to appropriate therapy. Satisfactory control requires close monitoring and timely use of effective medications.

Specific Goals

- Prompt relief of acute asthmatic attacks
- Prevention of recurrent acute attacks; maintenance of normal activities
- Stabilization of lung function: freedom from asthma to the greatest degree possible, with a minimal use of drugs
- Prevention of later complications: bronchiectasis, emphysema, heart disease (cor pulmonale)

Health Professionals Who Participate in Managing This Disorder
Family physicians
General internists
Pediatricians
Geriatricians
Allergists
Pulmonologists
Occupational medicine physicians
Psychiatrists
Clinical psychologists
Sports medicine physicians
Pharmacists

Currently Available Therapies for This Disorder

Drug Therapy
XANTHINE PREPARATIONS
- aminophylline (Aminophyllin, Aminodur, etc.)
- oxtriphylline (Brondecon, Choledyl)
- theophylline (Bronkodyl, Slo-bid, Theo-Dur, etc.)

BETA-ADRENERGIC DRUGS
"Selective" beta$_2$ stimulants:
- albuterol (Proventil, Ventolin)
- bitolterol (Tornalate)
- isoetharine (Bronkometer, Bronkosol)
- metaproterenol (Alupent, Metaprel)
- pirbuterol (Maxair)
- salmeterol (Serevent)
- terbutaline (Brethine, Bricanyl)
  Nonselective beta$_1$ and beta$_2$ stimulants:
- ephedrine
- epinephrine
- isoproterenol (Isuprel, Medihaler-Iso, etc.)

CORTISONELIKE STEROIDS
- beclomethasone aerosol (Beclovent, Vanceril)
- budesonide (Pulmicort)
- dexamethasone aerosol (Decadron Respihaler)
- flunisolide aerosol (AeroBid)
- fluticasone aerosol (Flovent)
- prednisolone (Delta-Cortef, Sterane, etc.)
- prednisone (Deltasone, Meticorten, etc.)
- triamcinolone aerosol (Azmacort)

OTHERS
- cromolyn (Intal)
- ipratropium (Atrovent)
- nedocromil (Tilade)
- oxygen
- zafirlukast (Accolate)

Nondrug Treatment Methods
- Hyposensitization therapies to reduce sensitivity to specific allergens ("allergy shots")
- Removal of dust (and dust mites) from residence
- Air filters in residential heating and cooling systems
- Avoidance of primary and secondary cigarette smoke
- Avoidance of occupational irritants and dusts

Management of Therapy

For Extrinsic (Allergic) Asthma
- For occasional and predictable acute attacks, start treatment with a "selective" $beta_2$-adrenergic inhaler.
- For attacks of increasing frequency and duration, add $beta_2$-adrenergic tablets or a long-acting oral theophylline preparation.
- For severe acute attacks or aggravation of chronic asthma, add beclomethasone, budesonide, flunisolide, or triamcinolone aerosol inhaler.
- If control is not adequate, use $beta_2$-adrenergic tablets and a theophylline preparation concurrently.
- If control is still inadequate, add cromolyn on a regular basis.
- If an adequate trial of all of the above fails to produce satisfactory relief and control, add cortisonelike steroids (tablets by mouth).

For Intrinsic (Idiosyncratic, Late-Onset) Asthma
- Attacks may be less responsive to the use of the bronchodilators (beta-adrenergics and theophylline) as outlined above.
- Earlier control may require the use of cromolyn or nedocromil and cortisonelike preparations on a regular schedule.

For Exercise-Induced Asthma
- Preferred first step: Use a "selective" beta-adrenergic inhalant (albuterol, terbutaline, etc.) 15 to 20 minutes before exercise for prevention.
- If control is not adequate, add cromolyn inhalant 15 minutes before exercise.
- If control is still inadequate, add ipratropium inhalant to the above.

For Nocturnal Asthma
Asthma is often most severe at night; 75% of asthmatics experience episodes of varying severity during the night.

- As a first step, ensure that the daytime program of asthma management is optimal, with emphasis on adequate doses of inhalant cortisonelike (steroid) preparations and "selective" beta-adrenergic bronchodilators.
- If conventional daytime therapy does not prevent nocturnal episodes, the following medications may be tried at bedtime: ipratropium inhalant, salmeterol inhalant (a longer-acting "selective" beta-adrenergic bronchodilator), longer-acting oral beta-adrenergics, and long-acting forms of theophylline.

Use of Theophylline Preparations

Theophylline elixir and uncoated tablets are used for prompt relief of acute asthma. The sustained-release forms (Slo-bid, Slo-phyllin, Theo-Dur) are used for smooth maintenance therapy of chronic asthma. Theophylline blood levels are helpful in determining optimal dosage schedules.

Theophylline potentiates beta-adrenergic bronchodilators and increases their effectiveness. See the Drug Profile of theophylline in Section Two of *The Essential Guide to Prescription Drugs* by J.J. Rybacki, for a complete listing of drug interactions.

Use of Beta-Adrenergic Bronchodilators

- "Selective" beta$_2$-adrenergics are the drugs of choice for asthma management (see above listing). These pressurized inhalers are potent drugs that must be used cautiously. Avoid excessive use; follow dosage schedules precisely. Current recommendations favor their use on an "as needed" basis. They are most effective at the beginning of an asthmatic attack and before exercise that induces asthma.
- For the most effective use of aerosol bronchodilators, learn the correct procedure: exhale through the mouth to empty lungs; squirt and inhale the first dose at the same time; hold your breath and count to 10, then exhale. If necessary, use a second inhalation in 10 to 15 minutes. Limit inhalations to one or two at a time, and at least three to four hours apart.
- Do not use isoproterenol (Isuprel) aerosol and epinephrine (Adrenalin) aerosol concurrently.
- Salmeterol is a long-acting "selective" beta$_2$-adrenergic bronchodilator for inhalation. Because of its delayed onset of action (10 to 20 minutes), it should not be used to treat acute episodes of asthma. However, its duration of action (up to 12 hours) makes it ideal for maintenance treatment of chronic asthma with twice-a-day dosing. It is not a substitute for short-acting beta-adrenergic inhalants.

Use of Cortisonelike Steroids

- Steroids are not bronchodilators; they will not relieve acute asthma. This includes all of the steroid aerosols listed above. In the past, the use of these drugs was restricted to the treatment of severe acute and chronic asthma that was not controlled by conventional drugs. This recommendation is now under revision. Many authorities now consider asthma to be a chronic inflammatory disorder of the airways, and they recommend the use of steroid inhalants as first-line drugs for the management of chronic asthma (see "Current Controversies in Drug Management" below). Steroids should never be used as the sole drug for managing asthma.

- When asthma becomes severe and continuous and cannot be controlled by conventional drug regimens, a trial period of two to four weeks of steroids by mouth is justified. The optimal long-term use consists of a relatively large single dose of prednisone (or prednisolone) every other morning (alternate-day schedule). This provides adequate asthma control with minimal adverse effects of long-term steroid use.
- The steroids beclomethasone, flunisolide, or triamcinolone, inhaled in aerosol form, are used to control asthma as steroid tablets are withdrawn.

Use of Cromolyn

- Cromolyn is not a bronchodilator; it will not relieve acute asthma. Its action is anti-inflammatory, an essential element in the management of chronic asthma. It is used only by inhalation; powder and liquid aerosol forms are available.
- A trial of cromolyn (as an asthma preventive) should begin while you are free of asthma, before acute attacks occur.
- When used on a regular schedule, cromolyn is 70–75% effective in preventing recurrences of acute asthma.
- Cromolyn is most effective in preventing extrinsic (allergic) asthma, and least effective in preventing intrinsic (idiosyncratic) asthma. It may or may not prevent exercise-induced asthma but is worth a trial.
- Cromolyn should be used on a regular basis for 8 to 10 weeks to evaluate its protective benefit. For best results, a beta-adrenergic aerosol should be used 10 minutes before inhaling cromolyn.
- Nedocromil (Tilade), a similar drug of greater potency, is well tolerated and useful as a preventive for maintenance treatment of chronic asthma.

Use of Ipratropium

This atropinelike drug has bronchodilator action, but no undesirable systemic side effects. Its action is slower and weaker than beta-adrenergic bronchodilators, but it may be useful for those with asthma who are unable to tolerate the side-effects of adrenergic drugs.

It is used adjunctively with cortisonelike steroid inhalants and cromolyn or nedocromil. It is not effective in all asthmatic patients.

Therapeutic Drug Monitoring (Blood Levels)

If it is necessary to use theophylline in high doses or for extended periods of time, it is advisable to monitor blood levels.

Sampling times: two hours after regular dosage forms; five hours after sustained-release dosage forms

Recommended therapeutic range: 10 to 20 mcg/ml

Ancillary Drug Treatment (as required)

For anxiety:
- promethazine (Phenergan)

Note: Avoid *all* sedatives during active asthma.

For pain, mild to moderate:
- acetaminophen (Tylenol, etc.)

For pain, severe:
- methotrimeprazine (Levoprome). This does not depress respiration.

For bacterial infection of respiratory tract (complicating asthma):
- ampicillin
- amoxicillin
- trimethoprim and sulfamethoxazole
- tetracycline (avoid during pregnancy and under 8 years of age)

For viral infection of respiratory tract (triggering asthma):
- steroids: prednisone and methylprednisolone

Note: Drug selection, dosage, and administration schedule must be determined by the physician for each patient individually.

Current Controversies in Drug Management

The beta-adrenergic aerosols for inhalation (see above) are the most effective bronchodilators in current use. However, it is now thought by many that the increased use of these drugs has contributed to the growing prevalence of severe asthmatic illness and rising death rates, especially in the elderly. It appears that their effectiveness has led to excessive use—large doses and unwarranted frequency. Several studies have shown that the regular use of these aerosols appears to *increase* the sensitivity and reactivity of bronchial tissues in those with asthma; periods of initial relief are followed by greater bronchoconstriction, leading to more frequent use of the drugs and higher doses. A major factor responsible for chronic asthma (with recurrent acute attacks) is persistent inflammation of bronchial tissues. Beta-adrenergic aerosols have little or no effect on chronic bronchial inflammation. By contrast, steroid (cortisonelike) aerosols (see above) are potent anti-inflammatory drugs that have proven to be quite effective in the management of chronic asthma. A consensus is emerging that favors the use of steroid aerosols as primary drugs for the routine treatment of chronic severe asthma, supplemented by beta-adrenergic aerosols "on demand" (only as needed) to control acute episodes of asthma.

Possible Drug Interactions of Significance

Theophylline may *decrease* the effects of
- lithium (Lithane, Lithobid, etc.), and reduce its effectiveness.

Theophylline *taken concurrently* with
- phenytoin (Dilantin) may cause *decreased* effects of both drugs. Monitor blood levels and adjust dosages as appropriate.

The following drugs may *increase* the effects of theophylline:
- disulfiram (Antabuse)
- influenza vaccine
- oral contraceptives
- tacrine (Cognex)

The following drugs may *decrease* the effects of theophylline:
- beta-blocker drugs (see Appendix 16, Drug Classes)
- primidone (Mysoline)

Special Considerations for Women

Oral contraceptives may increase the effects of theophylline. Observe for any effects of theophylline overdosage: nausea, vomiting, restlessness, irritability.

Pregnancy

Theophylline is designated FDA Pregnancy Category C (see Appendix 15). Significant birth defects were reported in mice. It is advisable to avoid this drug during the first three months of pregnancy.

Breast-Feeding

If taken in prescribed dosage, theophylline is found in breast milk. Avoid theophylline or refrain from nursing.

Special Considerations for the Elderly

Asthma in older individuals is often associated with other forms of chronic obstructive pulmonary disease (COPD)—chronic bronchitis and emphysema. Some degree of each of these three conditions usually coexist. Treatment goals include control of asthma and cough, reduction of mucus formation in the bronchial tubes, and the prevention of lung infections (pneumonia).

Older persons are more sensitive to the effects of theophylline; small doses are advised until full effects are known. It is also advisable to refrain from using coffee and other sources of caffeine while taking theophylline; the combined effects may cause excessive stimulation and hyperactivity.

Resources

Recommended Reading

The Asthma Sourcebook, Francis V. Adams, M.D. Lowell House, 1995.

Living Well with Chronic Asthma, Bronchitis, and Emphysema, M.B. Shayevitz, M.D., and B.R. Shayevitz, M.D. Consumer Reports Books, 1991.

Additional Information and Services
Asthma and Allergy Foundation of America
1125 15th Street NW, Suite 502
Washington, DC 20005
Phone: (202) 466-7643, 1-800-7-ASTHMA; Fax: (202) 466-8940
  Publications available.

National Jewish Center for Immunology and Respiratory Medicine
1400 Jackson Street
Denver, CO 80206
Phone: 1-800-222-LUNG, (303) 388-4461
  Publications available: *Lung Line Letter.*

National Allergy and Asthma Network
3554 Chain Bridge Road, Suite 200
Fairfax, VA 22030-2709
Phone: (703) 385-4403, 1-800-878-4403; Fax: (703) 352-4354
  Publications, resource booklet, videotapes available.

ATTENTION DEFICIT/HYPERACTIVITY DISORDER

Other Names AD/HD, attention deficit disorder, ADD, hyperactivity, hyperkinetic syndrome

Prevalence/Incidence in U.S. Approximately 3% to 5% of school-aged children; 1% to 2% of adults

Age Group Early childhood through adulthood

Male-to-Female Ratio In childhood: 4 to 1; in adulthood: 1 to 1

Principal Features and Natural History
Formerly referred to as "minimal brain dysfunction" and "hyperactivity," attention deficit/hyperactivity disorder now refers to a spectrum of difficulties in sustaining attention and controlling activity. While behavior patterns of individuals with this disorder differ somewhat in children and adults, the dominant features are the same: distractibility, impulsivity, and hyperactivity.

In childhood, AD/HD is usually observed before the child reaches 4 years of age. In many instances it is not recognized and diagnosed until he starts school and sustained attention is required. The behavior of the child with AD/HD is clearly inappropriate and disruptive. Typical features in young children include excessive running, jumping, and climbing; in older children and adolescents, there is restlessness, fidgeting, interrupting, and antisocial behavior. Children of all ages display impatience, frustration, outbursts of ill temper, low self-esteem, and poor academic achievement.

About 25% of children who have AD/HD continue to experience it as adults. While the outward manifestations are somewhat less obvious in adults, the principal features are still apparent. Some appear calm and controlled on the surface but can be seen nervously tapping their fingers or jiggling a foot. Many cannot concentrate long enough to finish reading a paragraph or follow a list of instructions. Others go on irrational buying sprees or engage in risky and hazardous activities. The pattern is chronic and pervasive—a way of life.

Diagnostic Symptoms and Signs
Short attention span, distractibility
Excessive and accelerated activity
Restlessness
Impatience
Impulsiveness
Antisocial behavior
Learning disabilities
Poor academic performance

Diagnostic Tests and Procedures
There are no specific diagnostic tests for AD/HD.
Diagnosis is based on observation of behavioral patterns.

Similar Conditions That May Confuse Diagnosis
Borderline personality disorders
Anxiety-tension states
Agitated depressions
Hypomanic states
Schizoaffective disorders

Causes

Established Causes
The primary definitive cause of AD/HD is unknown.

Theoretical Causes
Evidence suggests that there is a genetic predisposition for developing this disorder. There is a familial pattern. One-third of children with AD/HD have a parent or sibling with the same problem.

Positron emission tomography (PET scanning) of the brains of adults with AD/HD reveal reduced utilization of glucose (sugar), the brain's main energy source, in areas of the brain that regulate attention and movement. This implies an abnormality in brain function.

Known Risk Factors for Developing This Disorder

A strong family history of AD/HD or other personality disorders.

Despite many years of controversy, there is no proof that food allergies, food additives, sugar, head injuries, or fluorescent lights cause AD/HD.

Goals of Treatment

Can This Disorder Be Cured?

The primary definitive cause is unknown. No curative therapy is available.

Can This Disorder Be Treated Effectively?

Available drugs can significantly improve attention span and reduce hyperactivity.

Specific Goals

To allay disruptive behavior, improve ability to adjust and cope, and pursue academic achievement.

Health Professionals Who Participate in Managing This Disorder

Family physicians
Pediatricians
General internists
Psychiatrists
Neuropsychiatrists
Clinical psychologists
Pharmacists
Occupational therapists
Special education teachers

Currently Available Therapies for This Disorder

Nondrug Treatment Methods

- Family counseling
- Behavioral modification psychotherapy
- Appropriate academic or vocational education

Drug Therapy

- dextroamphetamine (Dexedrine)
- imipramine (Tofranil)

- methylphenidate (Ritalin)
- pemoline (Cylert)

Management of Therapy

AD/HD is now considered to be a neurological rather than a psychiatric disorder. It is amenable to appropriate drug therapy but does not respond to conventional psychotherapy alone. Since there is no specific test or "marker" that can identify AD/HD, the first major problem is correct diagnosis. It is now generally recognized that an acceptable defining syndrome is identifiable that permits the diagnosis of AD/HD with reasonable certainty. However, the practical utilization of this requires (1) the availability of reliable observations of behavior patterns, and (2) the consultation and interpretation of a qualified neuropsychiatrist who is experienced in this field. An anxious parent may suspect the diagnosis, and an exasperated teacher can bestow the diagnosis, but these are hardly adequate to consider committing a child to long-term therapy with stimulant drugs. When the behavior of a child with *suspected AD/HD* significantly interferes with social and academic performance, expert consultation should be sought. If the diagnosis is confirmed, a trial of stimulant drug therapy is appropriate and justified. Much publicity has been given to what is judged to be the hasty and often inappropriate use of Ritalin (methylphenidate) to medicate "unruly children" in the classroom. It is just as wrong and inexcusable to give Ritalin to a child who does not have AD/HD as it is to not provide a trial of Ritalin to the child who is shown to have AD/HD. These are critical decisions that can have profound influence of the life of the child *and* the adult he will become.

Adults do not spontaneously acquire AD/HD in adulthood. Adults found to have AD/HD have had it since early childhood. Recent studies disclose that mothers of children with this disorder were aware of the hyperactivity in the later stages of fetal development within the womb, and later still as newborns and toddlers. Approximately 25% of children with AD/HD retain the characteristic features of this disorder through adolescence and into adult life. Here again, the correct diagnosis may be very elusive. If good fortune brings the AD/HD adult to a perceptive and empathetic physician, the response to therapy is just as rewarding as it is with the affected child. Therapy for the adult consists of appropriate medication, behavioral psychotherapy, and academic education or vocational training. This program of combination interactive treatment requires close supervision by the therapist and total compliance and commitment by the patient. But the results can be dramatic.

A few caveats are in order:

- Some authorities consider AD/HD to be part of the constellation of neurological dysfunctions collectively referred to as Tourette syndrome (see the Profile of Tourette syndrome in this section). If the patient being treated for AD/HD develops "tics" consistent with TS, it may be necessary to add a tic-suppressant medication, such as clonidine. If clonidine is not effective, a tricyclic antidepressant may be tried. However, these drugs carry a risk of possible induction of serious heart rhythm disturbances. Their use must be monitored very closely.

- Although methylphenidate (Ritalin) and other psychostimulant drugs are generally considered to be the drugs of choice for treating AD/HD and are usually the first to be tried, it is acknowledged that approximately 30% of patients do not respond satisfactorily and that unpleasant side effects, such as broken sleep and weight loss, often lead to noncompliance. The search for alternatives to Ritalin has identified four drugs of different classes that are worthy of consideration and further clinical trials. These are clonidine (Catapres), guanfacine (Tenex), bupropion (Wellbutrin), and venlafaxine (Effexor). If your experience with Ritalin has not been satisfactory, ask your physician to consider the feasibility of trying one of these.

- Experience has confirmed that when the diagnosis of AD/HD is correct, the majority of children respond favorably to a trial of psychostimulant drugs, such as Ritalin. The normal child without AD/HD is overly stimulated and excited when given Ritalin—an expected pharmacological response to a psychostimulant drug. On the other hand, the AD/HD child is calmed and controlled by Ritalin—a paradoxical response. This trial-and-error aspect of therapy for AD/HD is inescapable. And so is the question of how long Ritalin therapy should be continued. There is evidence to suggest that in a substantial number of cases, Ritalin may be gradually withdrawn after two years of continual use. When necessary, Ritalin therapy can be resumed. However, it is altogether reasonable and practical to periodically introduce drug-free intervals to determine when the permanent discontinuation of Ritalin therapy is appropriate.

Possible Drug Interactions of Significance

Because of the nature of drugs that may be used to manage this disorder, adequate consideration of the volume and complexity of potential drug interactions is beyond the scope of this book. Consult *The Essential Guide to Prescription Drugs*, or similar drug reference book for possible interactions of significance (see Appendix 17, Drug Information Sources).

Special Considerations for Women

Women with AD/HD share many of the same features of this syndrome: impaired ability to focus, chronic disorganization, subtle problems with memory and information processing, and impulsiveness. They may also experience intensification of symptoms associated with PMS. However, women show less tendency to hyperactivity. Their response to appropriate therapy is equally rewarding. Some women report a most gratifying improvement in sexuality. Instead of mentally compiling the next day's shopping list while making love, they are able to focus on the pleasure of the moment and experience complete fulfillment. They are more productive in their professional roles, less moody and depressed, and feel more in control of their personal destiny.

Pregnancy

Methylphenidate is designated Pregnancy Category B, considered safe to use during pregnancy. There are anecdotal reports of this drug's calming effect on both mother and her hyperactive fetus. Ask your physician for guidance.

Breast-Feeding

The presence of this drug in breast milk is unknown. Consult your physician regarding the compatibility of nursing and all drugs you are taking.

Quality of Life Considerations

Adults who developed AD/HD in early childhood but were erroneously diagnosed and inadequately treated have great difficulty in just about every aspect of life. Their destructive patterns of behavior alienate family and associates. They seldom complete educational pursuits, they cannot maintain employment, and their marriages often fail. They are more prone to abuse alcohol or drugs, encounter accidents and trouble with the law, and commit suicide. Their salvation depends totally on the ultimate recognition of the true nature of their disorder. With appropriate treatment supervised by an empathetic and skillful therapist, most adults with AD/HD experience dramatic improvement in mood, concentration, and ability to cope successfully in a complex world.

Resources

Recommended Reading

Caring for the Mind: The Comprehensive Guide to Mental Health, Dianne Hales and Robert E. Hales, M.D. New York: Bantam Books, 1995. Highly recommended.

Driven to Distraction: Recognizing and Coping with Attention Deficit Disorder for Childhood Through Adulthood, E.M. Hallowell, M.D., and J.J. Ratey, M.D. New York: Pantheon Books, 1994. This is must reading.

Answers to Distraction, E.M. Hallowell, M.D., and J.J. Ratey, M.D. New York: Pantheon Books, 1994.

*Beyond Ritalin: Facts About Medication and Other Strategies for Help-
ing Children, Adolescents, and Adults with Attention Deficit Disorders,*
S.W. Garder, M.D. Garber, and R.F. Spizman. New York: Villard Books,
1996.

Additional Information and Services
National Mental Health Association
1021 Prince Street
Alexandria, VA 22314-2971
Phone: 1-800-969-NMHA, (703) 684-7722; Fax: 703-684-5968
    State groups: 650.

BREAST CANCER

Other Names Carcinoma of breast, ductal carcinoma, intraductal carcinoma, lobular carcinoma, carcinoma-in-situ

Prevalence/Incidence in U.S.
    Prevalence: 7 per 1,000 women; incidence: 3 per 1,000 per year
    Estimated new cases annually: 182,000
    Estimated deaths annually: 46,000
    One in every nine women who live to age 85 will develop some form
of breast cancer.

Age Group 20% of cases are under 50 years of age; 80% are over 50.

Male-to-Female Ratio 1 to 99

Principal Features and Natural History
Early breast cancer causes no symptoms to indicate its presence; in its
earliest stages it cannot be detected by self-examination. After a period
of slow growth, the aggregate of cancer cells causes local changes that
can be detected only by mammography. Most breast cancers begin in
the lining of small tubes (ducts) within one breast (ductal carcinoma).
Less frequently, cancer will develop within the lobes of breast tissue
(lobular carcinoma); this type may occur in both breasts simultaneously.
Early cancerous tumors that are locally confined to one site (in situ) can
be detected by mammography and totally removed surgically. The prognosis for "cure" is excellent. Undetected cancers continue to grow and
extend into adjacent tissues. Eventually, tumor cells may invade lymphatic
vessels and thus spread to regional lymph nodes in the armpits (axilla)
and neck. Invasion of blood vessels by cancer cells will result in spread to
other organs and tissues (metastasis). Untreated breast cancer characteristi-

cally spreads to the brain, lungs, liver, or bones. Very infrequently (1–4%), cancer will arise in the nipple tissues and adjacent skin of the breast (Paget's disease of the breast; not related to Paget's disease of bone).

The long-term course of every case of breast cancer is determined by many factors: the size and nature of the tumor at the time of discovery, the stage of the disease (see discussion of "staging" below), the patient's age and overall state of health, the choice of therapies, individual response to treatment. At this time, the overall 5-year-survival rates are as follows:

Stage 0 (in situ)	95%
Stage I	85%
Stage II	66%
Stage III	41%
Stage IV	10%

Diagnostic Symptoms and Signs

The presence of a discrete lump or thickening within the breast
The development of a lump in the armpit (axillary lymph node)
Change in size or shape of the breast, not due to weight gain or loss
Nipple retraction or discharge from the nipple
Change in color or texture of the skin of the breast
Pain in the breast not related to the menstrual cycle

Diagnostic Tests and Procedures

For early detection:
Breast self-examination monthly to detect changes over time
Periodic breast examination by physician or nurse
Screening mammography to detect tissue changes in the absence of symptoms
Ultrasonography to image abnormal tissue textures; to differentiate between cysts (hollow, fluid-filled) and tumors (solid)
For specific diagnosis:
Diagnostic mammography to evaluate breast symptoms
Fine-needle aspiration of fluid and/or tissue for pathological evaluation. This test has high specificity; rare false-positive results (see specificity in Glossary).
Core-needle biopsy. This nonsurgical test provides a larger tissue sample for examination.
Needle-localization biopsy and specimen radiography to confirm that suspicious lesions found on mammography are excised for examination.
Incisional biopsy (obtained surgically) provides a portion of the tumor for pathological evaluation and confirmation of diagnosis.
Estrogen receptor (ER) and progestin receptor (PR) tests of biopsy tissue cells (a guide to selection of therapy)

Genetic testing for markers thought to have prognostic value: c-erB-2
   (HER-2/neu), c-myc, and p53
Tests to determine the rate of tumor growth: rate of cell multiplication (a
   guide to selection of therapy and to prognosis)
Appropriate blood counts, blood chemistry tests, selective organ and
   bone scans

ALERT!

No imaging study can prove that a breast mass is or is not malignant
(cancer). If you can feel a mass (lump or thickening) in your breast that
is a new development, do not ignore it if a mammogram is reported to
be normal (negative). Insist that a biopsy be performed promptly. Do
not wait for a follow-up mammogram to be done sometime in the
future.

Diagnostic "Markers" for This Disorder

Specific cell changes in the biopsy specimen that indicate malignancy
(cancer), confirmed by pathological evaluation.

Similar Conditions That May Confuse Diagnosis

Benign conditions that may cause lumps in breast tissue and/or suspicious findings on mammograms:
fat necrosis (dead tissue) following breast trauma
fibroadenomas
fibrocystic breast disease
lipomas (aggregates of fatty tissue)
sclerosing adenosis
spontaneous bruising within breast tissue (capillary fragility)

Causes

Established Causes

The definitive cause that initiates breast cancer in unknown.

Theoretical Causes

Genetic predisposition: the presence of oncogenes (see Glossary)
thought to be conducive to some types of breast cancer.

Known Risk Factors for Developing This Disorder

Major risk factors:
History of previous breast cancer
Family history of breast cancer: If two first-degree relatives (mother, sis-
   ter, or daughter) have had breast cancer, risk is five times the average.
   If one grandmother, aunt, or cousin has had breast cancer, the risk is
   1.5 times the average.

Carrier of BRCA1 or BRCA2 genetic mutations (see Appendix 11, Genetic
    Disorders and Gene Therapy)
Over 50 years of age
Minor risk factors:
Onset of menstruation at age 12 or younger
No children, or first child after age 30
Onset of menopause after age 55
Breast cysts or precancerous breast disease
Potential (but unproven) risk factors:
High-fat diet (35% or more of daily calories)
Obesity (40% over ideal body weight)
Moderate to heavy alcohol consumption
Sedentary lifestyle
Radiation exposure
Estrogen replacement therapy in postmenopausal women who have a
    strong family history of breast cancer
Exposure to pesticides and other environmental pollutants

Drugs That Can Cause This Disorder

Some observations have raised the question of a possible association
between the use of oral contraceptives or estrogens and an increased
incidence of breast cancer. Published results of studies have been conflicting and inconclusive. One statistical association implied an
increased risk of premenopausal breast cancer if oral contraceptives
were used for at least 4 years prior to the first pregnancy. Another
implied an increased risk of postmenopausal breast cancer if estrogen
replacement therapy was used continuously for 6 years. Statistical association does not prove a causal relationship. To date, no definitive
cause-and-effect relationship has been established (see cause-and-effect
relationship in the Glossary).

Goals of Treatment

Can This Disorder Be Cured?

With early detection and prompt initiation of appropriate treatment,
85–95% of cases of breast cancer can achieve 5-year survival periods.
Some of these will experience no recurrence—a "cure."

Can This Disorder Be Treated Effectively?

Treatments that are known to be effective include surgery, irradiation
(X-ray therapy), chemotherapy, and hormonal therapy. The outcome of
treatment depends upon several factors:
• the cell type and grade of malignancy of the tumor at the time of discovery

- the presence of oncogenes (see Glossary) that imply a negative prognosis
- the stage of the cancer at the time of discovery: totally confined to the point of origin (in situ); local expansion only; spread to regional lymph nodes; spread to other parts of the body (metastasis) (see discussion of "staging" below)
- the type of surgical procedure used to remove the tumor
- the use of radiation therapy in conjunction with surgery
- the sensitivity of the tumor cells to radiation therapy, to antineoplastic (chemotherapeutic) drugs, and to appropriate hormonal therapy
- the state of the patient's general health, especially the immune system

Specific Goals
- Early detection and accurate staging of disease
- Comprehensive determination of an optimal plan of therapy
- Total elimination of all cancer cells (to the extent possible)
- Effective management of adverse effects of treatment
- Realistic consideration of the patient's quality of life—in the total context of the stage of the disease, life expectancy, current state of mental and physical health, and the anticipated burden of therapy-induced suffering

Health Professionals Who Participate in Managing This Disorder
Family physicians
General internists
Radiologists
Radiological technicians
Pulmonologists
General surgeons
Plastic surgeons
Thoracic surgeons
Gynecologists
Pathologists
Medical oncologists (chemotherapists)
Surgical oncologists
Radiation oncologists (radiotherapists)
Nurse oncologists
Medical geneticists
Genetic counselors
Psychiatrists
Clinical psychologists
Dietitians

Medical social workers
Pastoral counselors

Currently Available Therapies for This Disorder

Surgical Procedures
Primarily for removal of the tumor:
- lumpectomy: removal of small, well-localized tumors and removal of some axillary lymph nodes
- segmental resection: wedge-shaped removal of larger tumors—a partial mastectomy; removal of some axillary lymph nodes
- breast conservation surgery: local excision of the primary tumor; removal of some axillary lymph nodes; postoperative breast irradiation (X-ray therapy). This is the currently recommended procedure for stages I and II breast cancer.

For removal of the breast:
- simple or total mastectomy: removal of the breast only, all adjacent tissues left intact; removal of some axillary lymph nodes
- modified radical mastectomy: removal of the entire breast, the adjacent covering of the chest muscles, and (if necessary) any muscle involved by tumor spread; removal of some or all axillary lymph nodes
- radical mastectomy: removal of the entire breast, adjacent muscles that support the breast, the fatty tissues of the chest wall and armpit, and all axillary lymph nodes. This procedure results in significant pain and swelling, major disfigurement of the chest, and weakness of the arm.

For removal of the ovaries:
- In premenopausal women, surgical removal of the ovaries may be done to remove the principal source of estrogen that stimulates the proliferation of breast cancer cells.

Radiation Therapy
This is generally used postoperatively in conjunction with all of the surgical procedures described above. In selected cases, it may be used before and after surgery. Localized irradiation is either by external source (high-dose X-ray) or internally (radioactive implants).

Drug Therapy
The use of drugs following surgery and radiation therapy is referred to as "adjuvant" therapy. The following classes of drugs are currently used:
1. Hormonal agents to block the availability of hormones that sustain the growth of cancer cells—"cytostatic" effect
   - aminoglutethimide (suppresses adrenal gland production of estrogen)
   - diethylstilbestrol (DES)
   - tamoxifen (Nolvadex)

2. Chemotherapeutic agents: the use of potent anticancer drugs that destroy cancer cells—"cytotoxic" effect
   - cisplatin (Platinum, Platinol)
   - cyclophosphamide (Cytoxin, Endoxan)
   - doxorubicin (Adriamycin)
   - 5-fluorouracil (5-FU, Adrucil)
   - melphalan (Alkeran, phenylalanine mustard)
   - methotrexate (Amethopterin, Mexate, Folex)
   - mitomycin (Mutamycin)
   - paclitaxel (Taxol)
   - triethylene thiophosphoramide (Thiotepa)
   - vinblastine (Velban)
   - vincristine (Oncovin)

   Note: These drugs are used in carefully selected combinations and given in cycles judged to be most effective for each patient individually.
3. Biological agents: natural constituents of the blood that are used to stimulate the bone marrow that is severely depressed by chemotherapeutic drugs (see bone marrow depression in the Glossary)
   - filgrastim (Neupogen): granulocyte colony stimulating factor—increases production and activities of certain white blood cells
   - sargramostim (Leukine, Prokine): granulocyte-macrophage colony stimulating factor—increases production and activities of certain white blood cells
   - epoetin-alfa (Epogen, Procrit): erythrocyte stimulating factor—increases production of red blood cells; reduces the need for blood transfusions

New Drugs in Development for Treating This Disorder

- Gonadotropin-releasing hormone agonists (GNRHAs) given to premenopausal women to reduce the amount of estrogen produced by the ovary to levels found in postmenopausal women. These drugs are designed to provide an effective contraceptive in premenopausal women that will also reduce ovarian and uterine cancer risk and prevent breast cancer.
- Monoclonal antibodies that are designed to block the action of certain growth factors that stimulate the proliferation of breast cancer cells.

Management of Therapy

The first essential requirement for planning the treatment of any cancer is a precise pathological diagnosis: the tissue of origin (histology and cytology), and the estimated degree (grade) of malignancy. The pathologist makes these determinations by examining cell and tissue samples (biopsies) of the tumor. The second essential requirement for planning treatment is determining the basic characteristics of the primary tumor and the extent of spread (metastasis) from its point of origin. This process is called "staging."

Tests performed to establish the diagnosis and overall status of the cancer provide the information used to characterize the stage of the disease to be treated. At the time of diagnosis, breast cancer can be found to exist in any one of the following stages:

Stage 0

Breast cancer in situ: Very early cancer, confined within a duct (a small tube that carries milk from a milk gland to the nipple). Also called intraductal cancer.

Stage I

Cancer is confined within the breast:
T1—the tumor is less than 2 cm in diameter
T2—the tumor is 2–5 cm in diameter
T3—the tumor is more than 5 cm in diameter, but not invading the skin or chest wall

Stage II

Primary tumor of any size, with spread (metastasis) to axillary lymph nodes (in the armpit). This is referred to as node-positive cancer.

Stage III

Advanced regional metastatic disease, involving lymph nodes under the arm and in the neck, and muscles of the chest wall

Stage IV

Distant spread to other organs (brain, lungs, liver, bones)

Once the exact type of cancer and its stage are established, an appropriate treatment plan can be initiated. In addition, an attempt at prognosis is possible, should the patient and/or family wish to consider this.

Treatment of Stage 0: Breast Cancer in situ

Local excision of the tumor, with ample margin of normal tissue; radiation therapy to the breast.

Treatment of Stage I Breast Cancer

Breast conservation surgery: local excision of the primary tumor with clear margins (all cancerous tissue removed); selective removal of axillary lymph nodes; radiation therapy to the breast.

A second option is total mastectomy, with selective axillary node removal and radiation therapy to the breast.

Adjuvant therapy: selective use of postoperative tamoxifen and/or chemotherapy; selective removal of the ovaries. This procedure is currently under clinical evaluation.

Treatment of Stage II Breast Cancer

When feasible, breast conservation surgery and postoperative radiation therapy to the breast as in Stage I. When not feasible, total mastectomy or modified radical mastectomy with axillary lymph node removal. Postoperative radiation therapy to the chest wall and regional lymph nodes as warranted; adjuvant combination chemotherapy in pre- and postmenopausal patients; adjuvant tamoxifen therapy in postmenopausal patients with positive estrogen receptors. Tamoxifen may be given alone or with combination chemotherapy.

The use of combination chemotherapy given before surgery is currently under clinical evaluation.

The use of high-dose chemotherapy with bone marrow transplantation is currently under clinical evaluation.

Treatment of Stage III Breast Cancer

Stage III is divided into stage IIIA (operable) and stage IIIB (inoperable) breast cancer.

For treatment of stage IIIA:

If the tumor is very large or axillary lymph nodes are grown together (fixed), combination chemotherapy is given before surgery to shrink the tumor. Surgery is either a modified radical mastectomy or a radical mastectomy with postoperative radiation therapy to the chest wall.

Treatment of stage IIIB:

Surgery is initially limited to obtaining biopsy tissue for diagnosis and tumor analysis; radiation therapy for local-regional disease; combination chemotherapy for systemic treatment of distant metastases.

If response to treatment is adequate after radiation therapy and chemotherapy, surgical removal of residual tumor is considered.

Treatment of Stage IV Breast Cancer

Surgical biopsy to obtain tissue for diagnosis and tumor analysis; hygienic (clean-up) mastectomy or radiation therapy to control local disease.

If no evidence of metastases to brain, lung, liver, or bone, and estrogen receptor and progestin receptor tests are positive, hormonal therapy may be tried. If there is evidence of distant organ metastases or estrogen and progestin tests are negative, combination chemotherapy may be tried.

Ancillary Drug Treatment (as required)

For hot flashes due to tamoxifen:
• clonidine (Catapres)
For relief of pain:
　see Appendix 3

For control of nausea and vomiting due to chemotherapy:

see Appendix 4

Note: Drug selection, dosage, and administration schedule must be determined by the physician for each patient individually.

Current Controversies in Management

The conventional wisdom of withholding estrogen replacement therapy for menopausal women following chemotherapy for breast cancer is being challenged. The established belief has been that estrogen medication could contribute to the recurrence of breast cancer in remission. A recent review of pertinent studies by oncologists found no evidence to support the theory that estrogen replacement therapy reactivates dormant cancer cells, enhances the development of tumors in high-risk women, or alters the ability of mammograms to detect early breast cancer. The study group recommends that estrogen replacement should be made available to breast cancer patients who have no evidence of cancer activity following treatment and are experiencing significant symptoms of menopausal estrogen deficiency.

Important Points to Consider

1. Women with early stage breast cancer who consider breast-conservation surgery should also consult their surgeon regarding the feasibility of breast reconstruction as part of the initial surgical procedure. Plastic surgery for cosmetic purposes can also be done later as circumstances warrant. However, concerns regarding the cosmetic consequences of surgery and radiation therapy should be discussed at the beginning of treatment. For current information on breast implants, call the Food and Drug Administration (FDA): 1-800-532-4440, Monday through Friday, 9 A.M. to 7 P.M., EST.

2. In spite of aggressive therapy that is designed to be "curative," breast cancer can recur. Routine periodic follow-up examinations are mandatory for the preservation of health. Ask your physician for guidance regarding the nature and frequency of follow-up tests.

Special Considerations for the Elderly

For early stage breast cancer, lumpectomy and radiation therapy in women 65 years of age and older produces freedom-from-recurrence rates and survival similar to those of women younger than 65 years of age.

Quality of Life Considerations

• You, the patient, should insist on being fully informed about the nature of your cancer, and plan to participate in all decisions regarding treatment. Seek a knowledgeable physician who will understand your concern and honor your requests.

- Insist that the guidelines for breast-conservation treatment be followed as closely as possible.
- Insist that surgical incisions for tumor biopsy or excision conform with currently recommended standards.
- Insist that a separate incision be used to obtain axillary lymph nodes for examination; this will prevent avoidable disfigurement and yield an acceptable cosmetic result.
- Discuss thoroughly the anticipated benefits and risks of any chemotherapy that is offered. What is the probability that the benefits will justify the burden of suffering that chemotherapy imposes?
- Discuss thoroughly the alternative use of tamoxifen. Is it appropriate for you? What are its advantages and disadvantages?

Controversies! Dilemmas! Resolutions?

Breast cancer is the most common type of cancer in women and the second most common cause of death due to cancer. Of all disorders that afflict women, it is one of the most difficult to detect, diagnose, and manage satisfactorily. In spite of substantial progress made within the past 50 years, many aspects of breast cancer diagnosis and treatment remain controversial. Physicians and their women patients alike are keenly aware of the many uncertainties that must be acknowledged and dealt with as they cope with this elusive and haunting disease. The following issues are outlined for your consideration. They are presented here to help focus your attention and affirm your resolve to make decisions that best serve your physical and emotional well-being.

Breast cancer is a disease of uncertainties. The only element of reasonable certainty within the scope of its management is the pathological determination of its diagnosis. Everything that precedes and follows is tainted with uncertainty. The most knowledgeable and skilled clinicians that confront this disease must make decisions and pursue attempts at therapy with incomplete understanding of the actual status of the disease process and the eventual outcome of treatments proposed.

The woman with breast cancer (and her family) must recognize and understand and share the collective dilemma that all involved are obliged to cope with. Health care professionals should do all in their power to inform the patient regarding the current state of knowledge and the particulars of the patient's status, but they do not wish to and cannot be expected to make critical decisions without the patient's active participation. It is the patient's responsibility to ask questions and to learn all that she can about her disease and herself in order to provide "informed consent" or elect "informed refusal" as recommendations are made. She will need five kinds of information:

1. General information about breast cancer
2. Available options for diagnosis and treatment

3. Potential risks of diagnostic procedures
4. Potential risks of each type of therapy
5. Realistic prediction of treatment outcomes

As each new issue arises for resolution, the patient must evaluate her response to the situation at hand and find the level of uncertainty that is acceptable to her. Open discussions with family members, close friends, and her personal physician will facilitate this.

For women who experience concern regarding the possible development of breast cancer and for those who are presently coping with its presence, the following issues deserve consideration.

Personal Risk Assessment

This is the logical starting point. You have a 5-in-1,000 chance of developing breast cancer. Is it likely or unlikely that you will develop it? Should you worry about it or forget it?

Uncertainty factor: Approximately 80% of women who develop breast cancer have no known risk factors.

Pragmatic approach: Study all of the risk factors cited above and make a personal judgment as to whether you are at high, average, or low risk. This may help you to relate individually to subsequent issues and find comfortable resolutions.

Breast Self-Examination (BSE)

Only 25% of American women practice breast self-examination on a regular basis. Preventive medicine specialists urge all women to perform BSE monthly beginning at age 20. Approximately 85% of breast masses (benign and malignant) are discovered by the patient before physician examination or mammography. One of every two women will consult a physician in her lifetime to evaluate a breast problem; one in three women will have a biopsy; one in nine women will be found to have breast cancer.

Uncertainty factors: Normal breast tissue has a somewhat lumpy texture. Detectable changes in breast tissue occur naturally during each menstrual cycle. How does a woman recognize a "suspicious" mass that warrants physician examination? How soon should she obtain physician examination?

Pragmatic approach: If your "uncertainty tolerance" causes you to be concerned, a few simple procedures may ease your anxiety and make the situation tolerable.

- Ask your personal physician or his trained nurse to teach you how and when to perform BSE. Ask for an illustrated brochure of instructions to use at home.
- Practice this regularly so that you will become familiar with the "normal" texture of your breast tissues.
- While performing BSE on a regular monthly schedule, if you find a definite and persistent change from your familiar pattern, consult your

physician promptly for evaluation and guidance. Do not wait to see if "it will go away" over the next few weeks or months.

Periodic Breast Examination by Physician

Preventive medicine specialists urge women to have clinical breast examinations by their personal physician every three years from age 20 to 39 years, then annually for the rest of their lives. Approximately 15% of all breast masses are first detected by the physician or by screening mammography. Breast surgeons are credited with being more astute in detecting early, borderline changes that warrant investigation.

Uncertainty factors: The density of breast tissue in women under 30 years of age limits the ability of mammography to detect early breast cancer. Significant breast changes in this age group are best detected by a physician skilled in physical diagnosis. However, in this or any age group, it is impossible to be certain that a mass is benign on physical examination. A biopsy is required to determine whether the mass is benign or malignant.

Pragmatic approach: If you consider yourself to be at high risk for breast cancer, or the nature of your breast tissue makes it difficult for you to be certain that you have no suspicious changes, allow your "uncertainty tolerance" to determine how often you have physician breast examination. On the other hand, if you consider yourself to be at low risk and you perform BSE on a regular basis with ease and assurance, seek an agreement with your physician regarding an appropriate schedule for clinical examination.

Periodic Screening Mammograms

Recognizing that early diagnosis is the key to reducing the high morbidity and mortality due to breast cancer, the majority of national medical organizations recommend that 40- to 49-year-old women have screening mammography every one to two years, then annually for the rest of life beginning at age 50. Recently some biostatisticians determined that screening mammography in the 40- to 49-year age group produced no significant reduction in long-term mortality due to breast cancer. As a result of this, some organizations dropped the recommendation for routine mammographic screening of 40- to 49-year-old women. Other organizations observed that the number of cases of newly discovered breast cancer in 40- to 49-year-old women was not significantly less than those discovered in the 50- to 59-year age group. The delayed diagnosis resulting from delayed mammography may impact quite negatively on those women who are found to have breast cancer some years after its inception. Some figures to put this in perspective: Of 1,000 women having screening mammograms, 90% will have negative (normal) films; 10% will have positive (abnormal) findings that require further evaluation. Of this 10%, 8% will be shown to have a benign tumor without surgical biopsy; only 2% will require surgical biopsy to detect five expected cancers.

Uncertainty factors: Mammography can correctly identify 85–90% of potential breast cancers; it can yield false-negative results in 10–15% of cases. Mammography is capable of detecting very early changes (possibly cancerous) that will not be detectable by BSE or physician examination for two years. However, it can also fail to demonstrate diagnostic features of cancer in malignant tumors that are easily felt by the patient and the physician. Just as no physical examination can prove that a breast mass is benign, no imaging study can prove that a breast mass is malignant.

Pragmatic approach:

- For women with low "uncertainty tolerance" it is advisable to obtain a good quality baseline mammogram between 35 and 40 years of age. This can be used to compare with findings in later mammograms that pose problems in interpretation. All mammograms should be performed in facilities that are fully certified by the American College of Radiology.
- If a persistent breast mass is found by BSE, physician examination, or mammography, insist that a definitive biopsy procedure be done promptly. A delay of more than two months between detection of the tumor and a diagnosis of cancer increases the risk of advanced stage disease and shortened survival. Regardless of your "uncertainty tolerance," the earliest diagnosis is definitely in your best interest.

Biopsy Procedures

Several methods of obtaining tissue samples (biopsies) are available. Diagnostic mammograms are used to locate the target tissue within the breast and to facilitate the placement of tissue markers and biopsy needles with precision. Fine-needle aspiration and large-bore needle sampling are minimally invasive and may provide adequate material for diagnostic evaluation. If a larger tissue sample is required, surgical biopsy is performed. Incisional biopsy removes a portion of the tumor that is adequate for complete pathological evaluation and initial therapeutic planning. Excisional biopsy involves removal of the entire tumor (lumpectomy) and axillary (armpit) lymph nodes for detailed pathological study and staging.

Uncertainty factors: At this point, circumspect consideration should be given to several issues simultaneously:

- obtaining adequate biopsy samples with minimal invasive procedures. What is the optimal biopsy procedure in each case individually?
- using surgical techniques that minimize cosmetic disfigurement. Can this be accommodated with later curative surgery and breast reconstruction?
- providing adequate time for careful and thorough pathological studies of biopsy specimens. Is the delay reasonable and acceptable?

- planning a comprehensive, individualized treatment program that optimizes the nature and timing of therapeutic procedures. Can this be conveyed to the patient in such a way that she can make informed and rational decisions?

Pragmatic approach: Ask your surgeon to select the best single biopsy procedure that will provide an optimal tissue sample for thorough pathological study. Request that incisions conform with current state-of-the-art recommendations that minimize pain and disfigurement. State clearly that you prefer a two-stage procedure: stage 1—biopsy only; stage 2—definitive therapy. Ask your surgeon to explain any problems you may be creating with your requests.

Selection of Optimal Treatment

The currently available therapies for breast cancer and the goals of treatment are outlined in the breast cancer Profile. Information derived from (1) detailed pathological studies of biopsy specimens and (2) staging procedures will be used to formulate a comprehensive treatment program that is designed to provide the best possible outcome. The major determinants of treatment selection include the following:

the cancer cell type and grade of malignancy

the rate of cell multiplication (tumor growth)

the presence of estrogen receptors (ER) and progestin receptors (PR) on tumor cells

the presence of cancer cells in axillary lymph nodes: node positive or node negative

the extent of cancer within the breast and adjacent structures

the presence of metastases in brain, lung, liver, or bone

Uncertainty factors: The various tests conducted by tumor pathologists can determine the critical characteristics of cancer cells with reproducible accuracy and precision. However, the analysis of lymph nodes for the presence of cancer cells does not attain total accuracy. Axillary lymph nodes judged to be disease-free (node negative) after routine examination have been found to contain micrometastases (tiny clusters of cancer cells) in 9% of cancer patients. It is also recognized that many patients undoubtedly have micrometastases in other body tissues that cannot be identified. In view of this possibility, should all patients with stage I and higher cancer be given systemic chemotherapy? How accurately can current staging procedures identify those patients who should receive systemic therapy?

Pragmatic approach: After your diagnostic assessment is completed and recommendations for therapy are made, ask your physician to explain their rationale. Recognize that all current therapies—surgery, radiation, adjuvant chemotherapy, and hormonal therapy—are based on results obtained from earlier therapeutic trials, results obtained by trial and error. In order to make informed judgments and rational decisions *that are right for you,* ask the following questions:

- What is my prognosis if I receive no treatment?
- What is the minimal therapy I can receive and reasonably expect to have an acceptable quality of life? And for how long?
- What are the predictable benefits I may receive from the therapies recommended?
- What are the predictable adverse effects I may experience from the therapies recommended?
- Can you give me an objective assessment of whether the anticipated benefits of treatment will justify the burden of its adverse effects?
- If I begin the recommended treatment program and decide later that I want to withdraw, will you honor my decision without prejudice or penalty?

As you review these considerations with your physicians, you will undoubtedly recognize the unavoidable uncertainties in their answers. An important part of your therapy will be the recognition and acceptance of the reality of your situation. Do what you can to muster your own inner strengths. Accept the support of your family and friends. Develop a philosophy that is a blend of the realistic and the positive. You should become your own best therapist.

The Role of Prevention in This Disorder

Primary Prevention

At this time there is no known way to prevent the development of primary breast cancer. However, a study is in progress to determine if the use of tamoxifen by healthy women at high risk for breast cancer can prevent its development. It has been shown that tamoxifen, when taken by women who had breast cancer surgery, reduces the occurrence of cancer in the remaining breast by 38%.

Secondary Prevention

Early detection of breast cancer by regular breast self-examination, periodic breast examination by a physician or nurse, and screening mammograms is the most effective method currently available to minimize the impact of this disease.

Early diagnosis and prompt initiation of appropriate therapy provide the best means for disease control and long-term cure.

Resources

Recommended Reading

What You Need To Know About Breast Cancer, National Cancer Institute, NIH Publication No. 94-1556, July 1993. For a copy call the Cancer Information Service: 1-800-4-CANCER.

Tamoxifen and Breast Cancer, M.W. DeGregorio, M.D., and V.J. Wiebe, M.D. New Haven: Yale University Press, 1994.

The Cancer Patient's Handbook, Mary-Ellen Siegel, M.S.W. New York: Walker and Co., 1986.

Cancer Free: The Comprehensive Cancer Prevention Program, S.J. Winawer, M.D., and Moshe Shike, M.D., New York: Simon & Schuster, 1995.

Additional Information and Services
Office of Cancer Communications
National Cancer Institute
National Institutes of Health
9000 Rockville Pike
Building 31, Room 10 A 31
Bethesda, MD 20892
Phone: (301) 496-6631

Provides a list of available written materials on cancer in general and on specific types of cancer.

Cancer Information Service (CIS)
National Cancer Institute
Phone: 1-800-4-CANCER

The caller is connected with the regional office serving the caller's area. Trained information specialists provide accurate, personalized answers to cancer-related questions; referrals to community agencies and services; referrals to Comprehensive Cancer Centers and current clinical trials.

American Cancer Society
1599 Clifton Road, NE
Atlanta, GA 30329-4251
Phone: 1-800-ACS-2345, (404) 320-3333

Disease Management Expertise
See Appendix 2, Part One: The National Cancer Institute (NCI) Designated Cancer Centers; Part Two: Clinical Trials.

CHOLESTEROL DISORDERS

Other Names
Dyslipidemia, hypercholesterolemia, hyperlipidemia, hyperlipoproteinemia, hypertriglyceridemia, lipid transport disorder, lipoprotein disorder

Prevalence/Incidence in U.S.
An estimated 60 million adults are thought to have a total cholesterol level in the "too high" range: over 200 to 240 mg (current standard).

0.1% of the population has congenital (familial) hypercholesterolemia.
1.0% of the population has congenital (familial) hypertriglyceridemia.

Age Group
In the U.S., the low-density lipoprotein (LDL) cholesterol begins to rise after adolescence and continues to rise for 30 years. Significant elevations of LDL-cholesterol levels are found in the 20- to 50-year age group.

Male-to-Female Ratio
25 to 54 years of age: men show moderately higher levels of total cholesterol and LDL cholesterol; 55 years and older: women show moderately higher levels of total cholesterol and LDL cholesterol.

Principal Features and Natural History
The principal blood fats (lipids)—notably cholesterol and triglycerides—are combined in the liver with proteins (to form lipoproteins) that facilitate their transport to body tissues. There are normally three major classes of lipoproteins: very low-density lipoproteins (VLDL), low-density lipoproteins (LDL), and high-density lipoproteins (HDL). Each class contains differing proportions of fat and protein. VLDL consists of five-sixths triglycerides and one-sixth cholesterol. While circulating in the blood, VLDL is transformed first to intermediate-density lipoprotein (IDL), which is 30% cholesterol and 40% triglyceride, and then to low-density lipoprotein (LDL), which carries from 60–75% of the total blood cholesterol. High levels of LDL cholesterol are associated *statistically* with an increased risk of coronary heart disease—the higher the level, the higher the risk. HDL carries less than 25% of the total blood cholesterol. It is thought to assist with the removal of LDL cholesterol from the blood and body tissues. High levels of HDL cholesterol appear to be protective against coronary heart disease—the higher the HDL level, the lower the risk.

The principal cholesterol disorders are classified into five major types according to the nature of the lipoprotein abnormality and associated clinical features. Types I and V do not predispose to the development of atherosclerosis. Types II, III, and IV are high-risk factors for accelerating the atherosclerotic process that causes coronary heart disease and peripheral vascular disorders. The lipoprotein features of these classes are as follows:

Type IIa: increased total cholesterol and LDL cholesterol; normal triglycerides

Type IIb: increased total cholesterol, LDL cholesterol, and VLDL; moderately increased triglycerides

Type III: increased total cholesterol and IDL cholesterol (abnormal form); increased triglycerides

Type IV: normal or moderately increased total cholesterol, increased VLDL, decreased HDL cholesterol; increased triglycerides

Diagnostic Symptoms and Signs

In the majority of cases, there are no symptoms or signs directly attributable to the elevated blood levels of cholesterol or triglycerides. In the rare congenital forms of hypertriglyceridemia (Types I and V hyperlipoproteinemia), affected individuals may develop nodules of fat-containing cells (xanthomas) on the extremities and also be prone to pancreatitis. Those with Type II and III hyperlipoproteinemia may develop xanthomas on the extremities; xanthomas on the palms are diagnostic of Type III.

Diagnostic Tests and Procedures

Measurements of blood levels of the blood lipids: total cholesterol, LDL cholesterol, HDL cholesterol, and triglycerides

Analysis of blood lipids to determine the type of hyperlipoproteinemia

Appropriate physical examinations to determine the presence of atherosclerotic disease

Diagnostic "Markers" for This Disorder

Blood Levels:	Low	Borderline	High
Total cholesterol	under 200	200–240	240+
LDL cholesterol	under 130	130–160	160+
HDL cholesterol	under 35	35–45	45+
Triglycerides	under 200	200–400	400+

Formula for computing LDL cholesterol (with triglyceride level under 400): LDL = total cholesterol – HDL – (triglyceride/5)

Causes

The major cholesterol disorders are primarily hereditary (familial) and therefore genetically determined. Secondary causes can contribute to congenital lipid disorders or can independently account for abnormalities of blood lipid metabolism. Among the secondary causes are the following conditions: hypothyroidism, biliary cirrhosis, nephrosis, anorexia nervosa, and acute intermittent porphyria can cause significant increases in blood cholesterol levels. Diabetes, chronic alcoholism, chronic kidney failure, and acute hepatitis can cause significant increases in blood triglyceride levels. However, the most apparent secondary cause of lipid disorders is the high dietary cholesterol and fat content consumed by the American public.

Drugs That Can Cause This Disorder

The following drugs have been reported to cause abnormal increases in LDL-cholesterol blood levels: amiodarone, anabolic (male hormonelike) steroids, some beta-blockers, corticosteroids, cyclosporine, isotretinoin, mitotane, progestin, retinoids, thiazide diuretics (see Appendix 16, Drug Classes).

The following drugs have been reported to cause abnormal increases in triglyceride blood levels: cimetidine, corticosteroids, estrogens, furosemide, isotretinoin, oral contraceptives, phenothiazines, timolol, thiazide diuretics (see Appendix 16, Drug Classes).

The following drugs have been reported to cause reductions of HDL-cholesterol blood levels: anabolic steroids, androgens, some beta-blockers, phenothiazines, probucol, progestins, retinoids.

Goals of Treatment

Can This Disorder Be Cured?

The pattern of individual cholesterol metabolism is genetically determined. There is no current therapy to alter this.

Can This Disorder Be Treated Effectively?

Blood levels of total cholesterol, cholesterol fractions, and triglycerides can be favorably modified by dietary changes, regular exercise, and selected medications.

Specific Goals

- Normalization of blood lipid levels to currently accepted standards: total cholesterol of less than 200 mg; LDL cholesterol of less than 130 mg; HDL cholesterol of more than 35 mg; triglycerides of less than 200 mg (in the absence of other significant lipid abnormalities)
- Avoidance or reduction of adverse drug effects
- Prevention, retardation, or reversal of atherosclerotic arterial changes throughout the body to reduce the risk of coronary heart disease, peripheral vascular disease, and stroke
- Laboratory values in current use to assess "risk" for coronary heart disease:

HDL Cholesterol

Low risk	over 60 mg
Moderate risk	35–60 mg
High risk	under 35 mg

Cholesterol/HDL Ratio

Low risk	3.3–4.4
Average risk	4.4–7.1
Moderate risk	7.1–11.0
High risk	over 11.0

LDL/HDL Ratio

Low risk	0.5–3.0
Moderate risk	3.0–6.0
High risk	over 6.0

Health Professionals Who Participate in Managing This Disorder

Family physicians
General internists
Pediatricians
Cardiologists
Vascular disease physicians
Endocrinologists
Pharmacists
Nutritionists
Registered dietitians
Physical therapists

Currently Available Therapies for This Disorder

Nondrug Treatment Methods

1. Diet modification: Ask your physician or dietitian to provide you with printed diet plans that include the following features:
   - total dietary fat—30% or less
   - saturated fats—8–10%
   - polyunsaturated fats—up to 10%
   - monounsaturated fats—up to 15%
   - dietary cholesterol—less than 300 mg daily
2. Weight reduction: Total daily calories should be adjusted to achieve and maintain normal weight for sex, height, and body build.
3. Exercise program: Consult your physician and physical therapist regarding the nature and amount of aerobic exercise that will be safe and effective for you.

Drug Therapy

- Drugs that inhibit synthesis of cholesterol and lipoprotein: fluvastatin (Lescol), lovastatin (Mevacor), pravastatin (Pravachol), simvastatin (Zocor), niacin (nicotinic acid, Nicobid, Nicolar, Nicotinex, etc.)
- Drugs that hasten the clearance of lipoproteins in the bloodstream: clofibrate (Atromid-S), fenofibrate (Lipidil), gemfibrozil (Lopid)
- Drugs that accelerate breakdown and elimination of lipoproteins: cholestyramine (Questran), colestipol (Colestid), probucol (Lorelco)
- Estrogen replacement therapy for selected women
- Other drugs used less often: dextrothyroxine (Choloxin), neomycin

New Drugs in Development for Treating This Disorder

- A drug of the statin class: mevastatin (Compactin). Drugs of this class, for the most part, significantly reduce total and LDL cholesterol and raise HDL cholesterol. They may prove to be effective in lower dosage and therefore less likely to cause adverse effects.
- Drugs of the fibric acid class: bezafibrate. This drug effectively reduces LDL cholesterol and triglycerides, raises HDL cholesterol and is well tolerated. Benefits were maintained in trials lasting up to 4.5 years.

Management of Therapy

Our present understanding of how cholesterol disorders are causally related to the development of atherosclerosis (coronary and peripheral vascular disease) is incomplete and controversial. Although large population studies have demonstrated that high cholesterol blood levels are associated statistically with an increased incidence of atherosclerosis, total cholesterol (TC) values alone have low predictability for the actual development of coronary heart disease on an individual basis. The somewhat exaggerated emphasis on "statistical significance" has resulted in the creation of unrealistic risk ratios based on minor changes in blood lipid levels that are meaningless in the light of wide individual variability and the irreproducibility of laboratory test results as currently obtained. Determination of isolated blood lipid levels provides at best an incomplete appraisal of an individual's status regarding an inclination to develop atherosclerosis. They represent only one aspect of a disease process in which many other causative factors are involved. An understanding of the complex interactions of the numerous cholesterol-triglyceride-apoprotein linkages (lipoprotein fractions) is the key to learning which components and what concentrations can be relied upon to predicate an increased risk for the consequent development of atherosclerosis. For example, high levels of apolipoprotein (a) are thought to be a much stronger predictor than total cholesterol values for identifying those at high risk for atherosclerotic heart disease. Anyone who has reason to be concerned about a possible cholesterol disorder is well advised to reduce dietary fat and cholesterol intake. The majority of individuals with elevated blood lipid values do not require drug therapy to manage their disorder. Before starting a long-term, expensive, and somewhat risky program of drug treatment, the concerned individual should first seek a detailed evaluation at a reputable lipid research center, either in person or by submission of appropriate blood samples and medical information.

Determining the Need for Treatment

Observe the following procedures for the measurement of blood lipid values:

1. Do not alter your regular diet during the week prior to testing. You should not be on a reducing diet.
2. You should be free of any kind of infection.
3. Avoid all alcoholic beverages for 24 hours prior to testing.
4. Fast for 12 to 14 hours prior to testing.
5. Your blood samples should be examined by a reliable laboratory that has established a record for providing accurate, precise and reproducible test results.
6. For proper evaluation, a blood lipid profile should include values for total cholesterol, LDL- and HDL-cholesterol fractions and triglycerides.
7. Obtain blood lipid measurements on at least two separate occasions (three if in doubt) and use the average of the test results.

When to Treat

Current recommendations regarding initiation of treatment are based on the following guidelines. Either diet therapy alone or diet plus drug therapy is recommended when the blood lipid values exceed those stated in the table below:

	Diet Alone		Diet and Drugs	
Age Group	*Cholesterol*	*LDL*	*Cholesterol*	*LDL*
20–29	200	140	220	160
30–39	220	155	240	175
Over 40	240	160	260	185

Based upon sophisticated analyses of numerous studies, some experts conclude that cholesterol-lowering drugs should be used only in patients with established coronary heart disease or in those who demonstrate significantly high-risk factors for coronary heart disease death.

How to Treat

Note: In a field as complex and changeable as this one, it is not surprising that experts differ in their opinions regarding the "best" treatment approach and the "drugs of choice" recommended for each type of cholesterol disorder. Based upon the current literature covering this subject, the following guidelines appear to represent the most knowledgeable and prudent approach to the management of common cholesterol disorders.

Diet modification is the initial primary treatment for all individuals with elevated blood lipid levels. The total caloric intake should be designed to achieve ideal body weight. The initial diet should restrict saturated fats to 10% of the total calories and restrict cholesterol to less than 300 mg daily. This low-fat, low-cholesterol diet should be adhered to for six months to fully evaluate its effectiveness. Individuals with severe blood lipid disorders may require the guidance of a registered dietitian.

If an adequate trial of dietary therapy fails to lower blood lipid values to acceptable levels, consideration may be given to adding a trial of drug therapy while dietary modification continues. No single drug is appropriate for treating all blood lipid disorders. The choice of the initial drug depends upon the specific nature of the lipoprotein abnormality. Begin with an adequate trial of a single drug. If the response is insufficient, substitute another drug or add a second drug as appropriate. Measure blood lipid levels four to six weeks after starting drug treatment and at 3-month intervals until a stable response is obtained.

To reduce elevated LDL cholesterol (the most common form of cholesterol disorder in the U.S.):
- weight reduction if necessary
- diet low in saturated fats and cholesterol
- effective drugs:
  cholestyramine (Questran)
  colestipol (Colestid)
  fluvastatin (Lescol)
  lovastatin (Mevicor)
  simvastatin (Zocor)
  niacin (nicotinic acid)

To reduce elevated VLDL cholesterol:
- weight reduction
- diet low in saturated fats and cholesterol
- alcohol restriction
- strict control of diabetes (if present)
- effective drugs:
  niacin (nicotinic acid)
  gemfibrozil (Lopid)

To reduce elevated LDL and VLDL cholesterol:
- weight reduction
- diet low in saturated fats and cholesterol
- effective drugs:
  niacin (nicotinic acid)
  gemfibrozil (Lopid)
  clofibrate (Atromid-S), not recommended due to serious adverse drug
     effects

To raise HDL cholesterol:
- weight reduction
- smoking cessation
- regular exercise
- modest use of alcohol (no more than one to two drinks daily)
- avoidance of progestin-containing contraceptives
- the currently recommended drug is niacin

Ancillary Drug Treatment (as required)

For constipation (due to cholestyramine or colestipol):
• docusate (Colace, Dialose, Doxidan, Surfak, etc.)
• Citrucel
• Metamucil

For diarrhea (due to probucol):
• diphenoxylate (Lomotil)
• loperamide (Imodium)

For associated diabetes mellitus:
    see Profile of diabetes in this section

For associated hypertension:
    see Profile of hypertension in this section

For associated hypothyroidism:
    see Profile of hypothyroidism in this section

Note: Drug selection, dosage, and administration schedule must be determined by the physician for each patient individually.

Important Points to Consider

1. A do-it-yourself home test kit is now available for measuring your total cholesterol blood level: CholesTrak Home Cholesterol Test, ChemTrak, Sunnyvale, CA, 1-800-927-7776. The test range is from 125 mg to 400 mg. The kit provides complete instructions for performing and interpreting the test. It is important to note that blood levels of *total cholesterol* are adequate for screening purposes but are not adequate for making decisions about treating levels above the normal range.

2. All patients being evaluated for potential atherosclerotic cardiovascular disease should have measurements of total cholesterol, LDL cholesterol, HDL cholesterol, and triglycerides.

3. Multiple studies have demonstrated that appropriate treatment of some cholesterol disorders can arrest progression and promote regression of existing atherosclerosis in arterial blood vessels.

4. Every individual who is shown to have a significant cholesterol disorder should also have an assessment of risk factors for coronary heart disease. Aggressive treatment to lower cholesterol is likely to benefit only those who have substantial risk for developing coronary artery disease—a relatively small portion of the population. Other coronary heart disease risk factors include:
   • family history of coronary heart disease (CHD) before age 55
   • atherosclerotic disease of other arteries: cerebral, carotid, peripheral
   • diabetes
   • hypertension
   • cigarette smoking

- severe obesity
- HDL-cholesterol level below 35 mg/dl

5. Some experts now recommend that aggressive drug therapy be reserved for those at high risk for developing CHD. It is prudent to delay drug treatment in most men under 35 and in premenopausal women with LDL-cholesterol levels of 160 to 220 mg and at low risk for CHD.
6. Individuals with isolated low HDL-cholesterol levels should receive drug treatment only if they are known to have CHD or have additional risk factors for CHD.
7. Every individual has a different level of responsiveness to every medication. Drug treatment must be carefully monitored and individualized.
8. Multiple drug treatment is often preferable and more effective than using maximal doses of a single drug. The adverse effects of lipid-lowering drugs usually increase at high doses faster than the therapeutic effects.

Possible Drug Interactions of Significance

Niacin *taken concurrently* with lovastatin (Mevacor) and other cholesterol-lowering drugs may cause muscle damage.

Special Considerations for Women

Postmenopausal women with significant risk factors for atherosclerotic disorders should consult their physicians regarding the benefits of estrogen replacement therapy. The results of clinical trials indicate that estrogen therapy significantly reduces the development of coronary heart disease. It lowers total cholesterol and LDL-cholesterol levels and raises HDL-cholesterol levels. Oral estrogen preparations are more effective than estrogen patches in treating cholesterol disorders.

Pregnancy

Lovastatin is designated Pregnancy Category X (see Appendix 15, FDA Pregnancy Categories).

Breast-Feeding

Lovastatin is probably present in breast milk. Avoid drug or refrain from nursing.

Special Considerations for the Elderly

Some studies suggest that elevated total cholesterol levels have less clinical significance after the age of 70 years. If you have no significant risk factors (other than age) for coronary or cerebral vascular disease, consult your physician regarding the advisability of taking cholesterol-lowering drugs. Some authorities believe that the risks of such medications exceed their benefits in older persons.

The Role of Prevention in This Disorder

Primary Prevention

Genetically determined cholesterol disorders are not preventable. However, many cases of acquired cholesterol disorder are amenable to varying degrees of prevention. Although sometimes difficult to maintain, preventive measures are simple and straightforward. A preventive lifestyle should be established as early in life as possible: moderate exercise on a regular basis; a low-fat, low-cholesterol diet; maintenance of normal weight; moderate consumption of alcohol (no more than one or two drinks daily); avoidance of harmful stress. There is ample evidence to confirm that such a lifelong program can deter harmful levels of blood lipids that lead to atherosclerotic disease.

Secondary Prevention

In the presence of established atherosclerosis, appropriate measures to stabilize the process are in order. Recent studies confirm that treatments currently available can slow the progression of vascular disease and, in some cases, reverse it. Refer to the above category "How to Treat."

Resources

Recommended Reading

Beyond Cholesterol: The Johns Hopkins Complete Guide for Avoiding Heart Disease, Peter O. Kwiterovich, Jr., M.D. Baltimore: Johns Hopkins University Press, 1989.

Good Cholesterol, Bad Cholesterol, Eli M. Roth, M.D., and Sandra L. Streicher, R.N. Rocklin, CA: Prima Publishing & Communications, 1989.

Additional Information and Services

Council on Arteriosclerosis of the American Heart Association
c/o The American Heart Association
7320 Greenville Avenue
Dallas, TX 75231
Phone: (214) 706-1293; Fax: (214) 706-1341
Publications available.

Citizens for Public Action on Blood Pressure and Cholesterol
7200 Wisconsin Avenue, Suite 1002
Bethesda, MD 20814
Phone: (301) 907-7790
Telecommunications services: Fax: (301) 907-7792
Publications available: *Cholesterol Update* bimonthly, newsletters, educational literature.

Disease Management Expertise

National Institutes of Health

National Heart, Lung, and Blood Institute
Division of Heart and Vascular Diseases
Lipid Metabolism Atherogenesis Branch
Basil M. Rifkind, M.D., Chief
National Cholesterol Education Program
9000 Rockville Pike
Bethesda, MD 20824
Phone: (301) 435-0545, (301) 435-4555; Fax: (301) 480-2849

CHRONIC BRONCHITIS

Other Names COPD, chronic obstructive pulmonary disease

Prevalence/Incidence in U.S.
Current estimate: Approximately 13 million
Estimated deaths annually: 4,000

Age Group Over 40 years of age

Male-to-Female Ratio More common in men

Principal Features and Natural History
Chronic bronchitis refers to a condition that is characterized by perpetual
inflammation in the lining tissues of bronchial tubes, the air passages that
connect the windpipe (trachea) with the lungs. It is usually the result of several factors that serve as continual irritants to the respiratory tract. Episodes
of acute bronchitis (chest colds) in early life may sensitize the tissues to
other irritants that prevent complete healing and foster chronic inflammation. The most common irritant by far is tobacco smoke—inhaled actively
by cigarette smokers and passively by those close by. Other irritants include
ambient air pollutants and certain industrial dusts and fumes. Continuous
irritation perpetuates the inflammatory response, causing thickening of the
bronchial tissues and excessive production of mucus. This, in turn, is conducive to low-grade bacterial infections that compound the underlying
inflammation and create a progressive pattern of tissue destruction.

The cardinal features of chronic bronchitis are chronic coughing
("smoker's cough"), production of thick phlegm (mucus), and recurring
episodes of superimposed acute bronchitis. Eventually the diseased
bronchial passages become narrowed, producing obstruction to the flow
of air, hence the designation chronic obstructive pulmonary disease
(COPD). Because of its insidious onset and slow progression, chronic
bronchitis is often ignored until it reaches an advanced and irreversible
state. Eventually cough and mucus production become chronic through-

out the year, usually worse in the morning and in cold, damp weather. As a consequence of years of progressive lung deterioration, the heart enlarges and begins to fail (cor pulmonale), resulting in shortness of breath and fluid retention in the legs.

Diagnostic Symptoms and Signs
Criteria: A mucus-producing cough most days of the month, three months of the year, for two successive years; no other underlying disease to explain the cough.

Diagnostic Tests and Procedures
X-ray examinations of the lungs
Lung function tests
Arterial blood gas analysis

Similar Conditions That May Confuse Diagnosis
Asthmatic bronchitis
Bronchiectasis

Causes

Established Causes
Repeated episodes of acute bronchitis
Cigarette smoking
Occupational exposures: coal miners, grain handlers, metal molders
Air pollutants: sulfur dioxide, etc.

Goals of Treatment

Can This Disorder Be Cured?
Irreversible damage to lungs and heart cannot be cured.

Can This Disorder Be Treated Effectively?
Available drugs can provide some measure of symptomatic relief.

Specific Goals
- Prudent control of coughing
- Liquefaction of mucus
- Suppression of acute, recurrent bronchial infections
- Bronchodilator therapy to ease breathing
- Treatment of congestive heart failure

Health Professionals Who Participate in Managing This Disorder
Family physicians
General internists

Geriatricians
Pulmonologists
Behavioral psychologists
Pharmacists
Physician assistants
Nurse practitioners
Medical social workers

Currently Available Therapies for This Disorder

Drug Therapy
- albuterol (Proventil, Ventolin)
- metaproterenol (Alupent, Metaprel)
- theophylline
- ipratropium (Atrovent)
- cortisonelike drugs (corticosteroids)
- anti-infectives (for acute exacerbations)
- oxygen
- diuretics

Nondrug Treatment Methods
- Pneumococcal and influenzal vaccinations
- Exercise training programs
- Pulmonary rehabilitation programs

Management of Therapy

For Acute Exacerbations of Chronic Bronchitis
Oral anti-infectives with broad antibacterial activity:
- amoxicillin/clavulanic acid (Augmentic)
- azithromycin (Zithromax)
- cefixime (Sprax)
- cefpodoxime (Vantin)
- cefprozil (Cefzil)
- cefuroxime axetil (Ceftin)
- loracarbef (Lorabid)

Oral anti-infectives with limited antibacterial activity:
- amoxicillin
- ampicillin
- cefaclor (Ceclor)
- ciprofloxacin (Cipro)
- clarithromycin (Biaxin)
- doxycycline
- erythromycin
- trimethoprim-sulfamethoxazole (Bactrim, Septra)

Therapeutic Drug Monitoring (Blood Levels)
Recommended blood level range for theophylline: 10–15 mcg/ml

Ancillary Drug Treatment (as required)
For congestive heart failure:
- diuretics
- digoxin (controversial)
(See Profile of congestive heart failure in this section.)
Note: Drug selection, dosage, and administration schedule must be determined by the physician for each patient individually.

Possible Drug Interactions of Significance

Because of the number of drugs that may be used to manage this disorder, adequate consideration of the volume and complexity of potential drug interactions is beyond the scope of this book. Consult *The Essential Guide to Prescription Drugs*, or similar drug reference book for possible interactions of significance (see Appendix 17, Drug Information Sources).

Special Considerations for the Elderly

In older persons with breathing difficulties it is often difficult to distinguish between the possible causes—asthma, chronic bronchitis, or emphysema. Asthma, which is reversible with medication, occurs much more frequently in the elderly than was originally thought. Recent studies have documented that between 15% and 50% of older people may have airway obstruction (COPD) that is reversible and therefore treatable. Simple tests of pulmonary function can readily determine this.

The Role of Prevention in This Disorder

Primary Prevention
- Total and permanent cessation of smoking
- Avoidance of harmful industrial dusts and fumes

Secondary Prevention
Prompt treatment of intercurrent acute exacerbations of bronchial infections.

Resources

Recommended Reading
Around the Clock with C.O.P.D.: Helpful Hints for Respiratory Patients, American Lung Association, 1994. For a copy call 1-800-LUNG-USA (1-800-586-4872).

Additional Information and Services
American Lung Association

1740 Broadway
New York, NY 10019-4374
Phone: 1-800-LUNG-USA, (212) 315-8700; Fax: (212) 265-5642
  State groups: 59. Local groups: 72. Publications and videotapes available.

COLON CANCER

Other Names Carcinoma of colon, adenocarcinoma of colon

Prevalence/Incidence in U.S.
Estimated new cases annually: 160,000
Estimated deaths annually: 51,000

Age Group
For colon cancer associated with familial polyposis or ulcerative colitis—
  under 50 years old
For colon cancer not associated with other disorders—over 50 years old

Male-to-Female Ratio Incidence is equal.

Principal Features and Natural History
The colon (large bowel or large intestine) is the 5-foot-long lower segment of the intestinal tract. It begins in the right lower corner of the
abdomen at its junction with the small intestine. From there it extends
upward (ascending colon) to the right upper corner of the abdomen,
turns sharply to the left, and extends across the upper abdomen (transverse colon) to the left upper corner. There it turns sharply downward
and extends to the left lower abdomen (descending colon) where it
makes an S-shaped curve (sigmoid colon) to join the rectum. Cancer
can develop in any portion of the colon; the usual distribution is:
ascending, 24%; transverse, 16%; descending, 7%; sigmoid, 38%; rectum, 15%. Sites of origin are important diagnostically: More than half
(53%) of colon-rectal cancers can be found by sigmoidoscopic examination.
  The primary site for the initiation of cancer is usually well localized
within the surface tissues that cover the inner wall of the colon (the
mucosa). Some cancers originate in small benign polyps (tissue mounds)
that develop on the mucosa. The characteristic growth pattern of colon
cancer is to first invade the layers of tissue that constitute the colon wall,
and then to extend concentrically around the wall and longitudinally
along the wall.
  Like most internal cancers, early colon cancer produces no symptoms
or signs. It is often painless until it is well advanced. The first detectable

sign of its presence may be the finding of traces of blood in a stool (fecal) sample due to occult (hidden) bleeding from the tumor. Over time this can cause significant anemia, weakness, and fatigue.

In time, the invasive nature and increasing size of the tumor begin to cause symptoms that indicate its presence. The more prominent symptoms and signs clearly reflect disturbances of colon function. Other symptoms may be related to spread (metastasis) of the cancer to the liver, brain, lungs, kidneys, ovaries, or bladder.

At the time of discovery, colon cancer can be found in any of the following stages:

Stage 0, carcinoma-in-situ: Localized within surface cells (polyps); no spread to lymph nodes; no distant metastases

Stage I (8%): Tumor invades into the muscle layer of the colon wall and extends around and along one segment of the colon; no spread to lymph nodes; no distant metastases

Stage II (39%): Tumor penetrates through all layers of the colon wall and extends a greater distance around and along one segment of the colon; no spread to lymph nodes; no distant metastases

Stage III (28%): Tumor of any size; spread to regional lymph nodes; no distant metastases

Stage IV (25%): Tumor of any size; spread to regional lymph nodes; distant metastases to liver, lung, etc.

Diagnostic Symptoms and Signs

A change in the pattern of bowel movements: diarrhea or constipation

Blood on the surface or mixed in the stool: either bright red or dark reddish-brown

Stools of a smaller caliber than usual: may be rodlike or ribbon-shaped

General abdominal discomfort: bloating, gas pains, cramping, persistent localized pain

A feeling that the bowel does not empty completely on defecation

Unexplained weight loss

Progressive fatigue and weakness

A mass that can be felt in any segment of the colon

Diagnostic Tests and Procedures

Battery of laboratory tests: complete blood cell counts, urine analysis, liver function tests, appropriate blood chemistries, CEA assay (carcinoembryonic antigen)

Fecal occult (hidden) blood tests

Digital rectal examination

Proctoscopic and sigmoidoscopic examinations

Colonoscopic examinations

X-ray studies of the colon: barium enemas with air contrast to outline
   polyps and tumors
X-ray studies of the lungs for metastases
CT scans of the colon for tumor extension and of the liver for metastases

ALERT!

The carcinoembryonic antigen (CEA), although present in the blood of
some patients with colon cancer, is not a specific test for this disease.
Many conditions can cause increased levels of CEA: cancer in other sites,
stomach inflammation (gastritis), kidney disease, smoking. Also, not all
colon cancers secrete CEA. If an elevated CEA level is found before surgical removal of the tumor, it usually declines following surgery. Monitoring CEA levels postoperatively may be a useful guide to evaluate therapy.
Rising CEA levels may indicate recurrence of cancer.

Diagnostic "Markers" for This Disorder

The identification of cancer cells in biopsy specimens obtained during
sigmoidoscopic or colonoscopic examination.

Similar Conditions That May Confuse Diagnosis

Benign (noncancerous) polyps
Diverticulitis
Active ulcerative colitis
Active Crohn's disease of the colon

Causes

Established Causes

The definitive cause of colon cancer is not known at this time.

Theoretical Causes

Genetic predisposition
High-animal fat, low-fiber diet: causes increased concentration of bile
   acids in the colon, slows passage of food residues, enhances the
   action of carcinogenic (cancer-causing) agents

Known Risk Factors for Developing This Disorder

Family history of colon or rectal cancer in a parent or sibling (25% of
   patients)
Family history of familial polyposis (very strong risk factor)
Personal history of ulcerative colitis or Crohn's disease of the colon
   (strong risk factor)
Personal history of colon or rectal polyps
For women: personal history of breast, ovarian, or uterine cancer

High intake of salt-cured, salt-pickled, and smoked foods
Excessive alcohol consumption

Goals of Treatment

Can This Disorder Be Cured?
Disease-free periods of 5 to 10 years ("cures") can be achieved when:
- the cancer has been detected early
- the cancer is confined to a single segment of the colon
- the affected segment is carefully removed with wide clear margins at both ends
- there has been no spread to regional lymph nodes
- there has been no distant spread to other organs
- postoperative radiation therapy or chemotherapy was used when warranted

Can This Disorder Be Treated Effectively?
Appropriate use of surgery, radiation therapy, and adjuvant chemotherapy can significantly reduce morbidity and improve survival in selected patients.

Specific Goals
- Early diagnosis of operable cases
- Accurate staging to determine optimal therapy
- Successful removal of all malignant tissues
- Optimal use of radiation therapy and adjuvant chemotherapy
- Maximal periods of disease-free postoperative life
- Maintenance of an acceptable quality of life

Health Professionals Who Participate in Managing This Disorder
Family physicians
General internists
Gastroenterologists
Radiologists
General surgeons
Proctologists
Colon-rectal surgeons
Pathologists
Medical oncologists
Surgical oncologists
Radiation oncologists
Nurse oncologists
Enterostomal therapists
Psychiatrists

Dietitians
Medical social workers
Pastoral counselors

Currently Available Therapies for This Disorder

Surgery
- Polypectomies: removal of polyps from the colon or rectum
- Partial colectomy: segmental resections of the colon
- Total colectomy: removal of the entire colon
- Colostomy: surgical creation of an opening (stoma) between the colon and the surface of the abdomen to facilitate defecation
- Resection of selected metastases in liver, lung, or ovary

Radiation Therapy
- Preoperative X-ray treatment to reduce the size of tumors in preparation for removal
- Postoperative X-ray treatment to destroy cancer cells remaining in the operative area
- Palliative X-ray treatment to relieve pain in patients whose tumors cannot be removed

Chemotherapy
The following drugs are used in various combinations to kill cancer cells:
- 5-fluorouracil
- folinic acid
- leucovorin
- levamisole

Management of Therapy
The optimal treatment of colon cancer is determined by the stage of disease at the time of discovery. The following treatment options are those in current use.

For Stage 0: Carcinoma-in-situ
Local excision (tissue removal) or simple polypectomy (polyp removal) with clear margins.

Partial colectomy: segmental resection (removal of colon segment) for larger tumors not amenable to local excision.

For Stage I
Partial colectomy: wide segmental resection and anastomosis (reconnection of healthy sections of colon following removal of cancerous segment). This stage has a high cure rate. No adjuvant (auxiliary) radiation therapy or chemotherapy is used.

For Stage II

Partial colectomy: wide segmental resection and anastomosis. Following surgery, patients should be considered for entry into carefully controlled clinical trials evaluating the use of regional or systemic chemotherapy, radiation therapy, or biological therapy.

For Stage III

This stage denotes cancer spread to regional lymph nodes. The number of lymph nodes involved affects prognosis: Patients with one to three involved nodes have a significantly better survival than those with four or more nodes involved.

Partial colectomy: wide segmental resection and anastomosis. Removal of regional lymph nodes. Postoperative chemotherapy with 5-fluorouracil and levamisole.

Eligible patients should be considered for entry into carefully controlled clinical trials comparing postoperative chemotherapy, radiation therapy, or biological therapy.

For Stage IV

This stage denotes significant local disease and spread (metastasis) to distant organs.

Surgical resection of involved colon with anastomosis; or creation of a bypass in selected cases with obstructing primary tumors. Surgical resection of isolated metastases in the liver, lungs, or ovaries.

Palliative radiation therapy to control pain. Palliative chemotherapy to control tumor growth.

Referral to clinical trials investigating new drugs and biological therapies.

Ancillary Drug Treatment (as required)

For pain management:
   see Appendix 3
For control of nausea and vomiting:
   see Appendix 4
Note: Drug selection, dosage, and administration schedule must be determined by the physician for each patient individually.

Treatment Outcomes

For localized disease—5 year survival is over 80%
For disseminated disease—5-year survival is less than 35%

Special Considerations for Women

A personal history of breast, ovarian, or uterine cancer may increase your risk for developing colon cancer. Observe all preventive measures. Utilize early detection procedures.

Pregnancy

Drugs used for cancer chemotherapy are contraindicated during pregnancy (see Appendix 15, FDA Pregnancy Categories).

Breast-Feeding

Avoid chemotherapeutic drugs or refrain from nursing.

Special Considerations for the Elderly

Age greater than 70 years is not a contraindication for standard treatments for colon cancer. Long-term survival is clearly achievable in the elderly.

Quality of Life Considerations

For those patients who undergo colon resections that are not amenable to anastomosis, a permanent colostomy may be unavoidable. Enterostomal therapists are available to teach patients how to manage colostomies properly and how to resume a fully active and acceptable way of life. The United Ostomy Association is a national support group that provides information and services for ostomy patients. See Resources below.

The Role of Prevention in This Disorder

Primary Prevention
- Eat a low-fat, high-fiber diet: fruits, vegetables, and whole grain cereals.
- Avoid salt-cured, salt-pickled, and smoked foods.
- Avoid excessive alcohol consumption.
- Maintain bowel regularity with diet and fiber; avoid constipation.
- Obtain prompt removal of all polyps when found.

Secondary Prevention
- Fecal test for occult (hidden) blood annually beginning at age 40 years (of limited value because of frequent false-positive and false-negative test results)
- Digital rectal examination annually beginning at age 40 years
- Sigmoidoscopy every three to five years beginning at age 50 years
- Colonoscopy every three to five years beginning at age 18 years if there is a history of familial polyposis, or a personal history of adenomatous polyps or ulcerative colitis; beginning at 40 years of age if there is a history of two or more first-degree relatives with colon cancer

Resources

Recommended Reading

What You Need To Know About Cancer of the Colon and Rectum, National Cancer Institute, NIH Publication No. 94-1552, April 1994. For a copy call the Cancer Information Service, 1-800-4-CANCER.

The Cancer Patient's Handbook: Everything You Need to Know About Today's Care and Treatment, Mary-Ellen Siegel, M.S.W. New York: Walker and Company, 1986.

Additional Information and Services
The Cancer Information Service
Phone: 1-800-422-6237, 1-800-4-CANCER
Questions answered in English or Spanish.

American Cancer Society (ACS)
1599 Clifton Road, NE
Atlanta, GA 30329
Phone: 1-800-ACS-2345

United Ostomy Association
36 Executive Park, Suite 120
Irvine, CA 92714
Phone: (714) 660-8624

Disease Management Expertise
See Appendix 2, Part One: The National Cancer Institute (NCI) Designated Cancer Centers; Part Two: Clinical Trials

CONGESTIVE HEART FAILURE

Other Names
Chronic heart failure, heart failure, cardiac decompensation, myocardial decompensation, left ventricular diastolic dysfunction, left ventricular systolic dysfunction

Prevalence/Incidence in U.S.
Current estimate: 2.3 million
Estimated new cases annually: 400,000
Estimated deaths annually: 200,000

Age Group 45 to 54 years—2.6/1000 population; 55 to 64 years—7/1000 population; 65 to 74 years—15/1000 population

Male-to-Female Ratio 1.5 to 1

Principal Features and Natural History
The designation "congestive heart failure" refers to a condition in which the heart is unable to pump enough blood to satisfy the needs of the body. Diseased heart muscle loses its contracting power, allowing increased filling pressures inside the heart chambers (ventricles); further

stretching and weakening of muscle tissue leads to muscle exhaustion and reduced pumping capacity; the forward flow of blood is impaired and excessive volumes of blood accumulate in vital areas throughout the body, producing congestion. Resulting symptoms include shortness of breath (dyspnea), first with exertion and later at rest; inability to breathe comfortably while lying down (orthopnea); fatigue and weakness, especially in the legs; a dry cough; night urination; swelling of the feet and ankles at the end of the day; and vague discomfort in the chest and abdomen.

It is important to understand that while the term "heart failure" primarily indicates impaired function of the left ventricle (lower left heart chamber), failure can result from dysfunction during either the systolic (contracting or pumping) phase, or the diastolic (relaxing or filling) phase of heart activity. This distinction is significant because the optimal drug therapies are specific for each type of failure. Drugs used to treat systolic dysfunction can be deleterious to patients with diastolic dysfunction, and vice versa.

Diagnostic Symptoms and Signs

Shortness of breath on exertion (dyspnea)
Arousal from sleep by shortness of breath (paroxysmal nocturnal dyspnea)
Shortness of breath while lying flat (orthopnea)
Decreased ability to remain active (reduced exercise tolerance)
Swelling of the feet and ankles (pedal edema)
Abdominal discomfort due to fluid accumulation (liver congestion, ascites)

Diagnostic Tests and Procedures

Complete blood cell counts, appropriate blood chemistries, urine analysis
Chest X-rays
Electrocardiograms (ECGs, EKGs), resting and with exercise
Echocardiograms
Radionuclide ventriculograms
Thallium scans (myocardial perfusion scintigrams)
Radionuclide angiocardiograms
Positron emission tomograms (PET)
Coronary artery angiograms

Diagnostic "Markers" for This Disorder

Heart enlargement on chest X-ray
Left ventricular dysfunction confirmed by echocardiogram
Left ventricular ejection fraction of less than 35–40%

Similar Conditions That May Confuse Diagnosis

Chronic obstructive pulmonary disease (COPD): Emphysema can cause marked shortness of breath (dyspnea).

Certain diseases of the liver and kidneys can cause swelling of the feet and ankles.

Varicose veins in the legs can cause swelling of the feet and ankles.

Certain antihypertensive medications may cause shortness of breath and swelling of the feet and ankles: doxazosin (Cardura), prazosin (Minipress), terazosin (Hytrin).

Causes

Primary causes of heart disease that ultimately lead to congestive heart failure:

hypertension (55%)
coronary artery disease (50%)
alcoholism (34%)
diabetes (23%)
idiopathic cardiomyopathy (unknown cause) (17%)
valvular heart disease (2%)
emphysema

Precipitating causes in predisposed individuals: inadequate compliance with therapy (most common), heart rhythm disorders, severe infections, obesity, pregnancy, anemia, hyperthyroidism, excessive heat and humidity.

Drugs That Can Cause This Disorder

In individuals with borderline heart function, the following drugs can precipitate congestive heart failure:

amantadine (Symmetrel)
beta-adrenergic-blocking drugs (beta-blockers) (see Appendix 16, Drug Classes)
cortisonelike drugs (corticosteroids) (see Appendix 16, Drug Classes)
estrogens
disopyramide (Norpace)
nonsteroidal anti-inflammatory drugs (NSAIDs) (see Appendix 16, Drug Classes)

Goals of Treatment

- Improvement of the heart's pumping performance by the use of digoxin (in left ventricular systolic dysfunction)
- Reduction of the heart's workload by the use of arterial and venous vasodilators: ACE inhibitors, hydralazine, nitrates

- Removal of excess salt and water from the body by the use of diuretics
- Relief of symptoms—fatigue, shortness of breath, ankle swelling, etc.—by means of the above procedures

Health Professionals Who Participate in Managing This Disorder

Family physicians
General internists
Pediatricians
Geriatricians
Cardiologists
Pulmonologists
Radiologists
Psychiatrists
Clinical psychologists
Cardiac surgeons
Thoracic surgeons
Transplant surgeons
Clinical nurse specialists
Nurse practitioners
Nurse educators
Pharmacists
Dietitians
Medical social workers

Currently Available Therapies for This Disorder

Drug Therapy

- Digitalis preparations: digitoxin, digoxin
- Angiotensin-converting enzyme (ACE) inhibitor drugs (see Appendix 16, Drug Classes)
- Diuretics (see Appendix 16, Drug Classes)
- Vasodilators: arterial dilator—hydralazine; venous dilators—isosorbide dinitrate, nitroglycerin
- Beta-adrenergic-blocking drugs (see Appendix 16, Drug Classes)
- Calcium-channel-blocking drugs (see Appendix 16, Drug Classes)
- Alpha-adrenergic-blocking drugs (see Appendix 16, Drug Classes)
- Oxygen

Nondrug Treatment Methods

- Prescribed aerobic exercise programs as appropriate: walking, bicycling, swimming
- Dietary modifications: sodium restriction to 2 grams daily; avoidance of alcoholic beverages; calories adjusted to achieve and maintain normal body weight; low-fat, low-cholesterol food selections

- Total and permanent abstention from cigarette smoking
- Surgical procedures:
    pacemaker implantation
    percutaneous transluminal coronary angioplasty (PTCA)
    coronary artery bypass graft (CABG)
    cardiomyoplasty
    myocardial wall resection (investigational)
    heart transplantation

New Drugs in Development for Treating This Disorder

- Xamoterol (Carwin), a new heart muscle stimulant under study in Europe and in the U.S., has been shown to be significantly better than digoxin in treating chronic heart failure. This drug is not yet available for general use.
- Carvedilol (Kredex), a new alpha/beta-blocker drug, is effective in the treatment of severe congestive heart failure when used in conjunction with digoxin, ACE inhibitors, and diuretics.

Management of Therapy

For Early, Mild Congestive Heart Failure

Three variations of initial treatment are used currently:
1. Treatment is started with digitalis (digoxin or digitoxin). This may be the only drug used if response is satisfactory. If necessary, a thiazide diuretic (or equivalent) is added.
2. Treatment is started with a thiazide diuretic (or equivalent), given alone. This may give a very adequate response, especially in the elderly. If necessary, digoxin (or digitoxin) is added.
3. Treatment is started with an ACE inhibitor. If significant fluid retention is present, a thiazide diuretic is added. If symptoms are not relieved, digoxin may be added.

For Moderate to Severe Congestive Heart Failure

- ACE inhibitor drugs are used in maximal tolerated dosage.
- Digoxin and thiazide diuretics are used in maximal tolerated dosage.
- As necessary, a stronger diuretic, such as furosemide, is used to replace the thiazide diuretic.
- If the response is inadequate, other vasodilators are added: isosorbide dinitrate or nitroglycerin patches for venous dilation; hydralazine for arterial dilation.
- For congestive heart failure with angina and/or hypertension, the addition of a calcium-channel-blocking drug may be tried.

Use of Digitalis

- Should be started only when there is a firm diagnosis of heart failure due to left ventricular systolic dysfunction. Periodic reassessment is necessary to determine continued need. Maintenance digitalis may not be necessary for life. Following correction of congestive heart failure, stable heart function may be achieved by using only diuretics and ACE inhibitor drugs.

- Digoxin is the form of digitalis most frequently used. Because digoxin products vary in their absorbability, refill your prescriptions with the same brand to ensure uniform drug effects.
- Take the exact dose at the same time each day.
- Learn to count your pulse and check its regularity. Notify your physician if your pulse rate is below 60 beats/minute or your pulse rhythm changes significantly.
- The elderly and individuals with hypothyroidism often have a reduced tolerance for digitalis; smaller doses are advisable.
- Digitalis (digoxin) toxicity (overdosage) occurs in 20% of users; it is more common in the elderly. The earliest indications of toxicity are usually loss of appetite, nausea, and vomiting; other indications include headache, facial pains, blurred vision, seeing "snowflakes" or yellowish-green halos, fatigue, weakness, and disturbances of heart rhythm. The elderly may show confusion; rarely, seizures may occur.
- Periodic blood levels can help to determine optimal dosage, especially if kidney function is impaired. The blood sample should be taken no less than six hours after the last dose.
- For complete information, see the Drug Profile of digoxin in Section Two of *The Essential Guide to Prescription Drugs*, or a similar drug reference book. Monitor for significant drug interactions.

Use of Diuretics ("Water Pills")

- Thiazide (or equivalent) diuretics may suffice as the only drug treatment for mild heart failure in many elderly patients.
- When possible, diuretics should be taken in the morning to minimize nighttime urination.
- If your diuretic is one that increases the excretion of potassium in the urine, it is important that your blood level of potassium be checked periodically. An abnormally low potassium level can increase the risk of digitalis toxicity. Consult your physician regarding the advisability of omitting your diuretic every third day to minimize the loss of potassium.
- If your diuretic is one that does not increase the excretion of potassium (amiloride, spironolactone, triamterene), you should not take a potassium supplement or eat excessive amounts of high-potassium foods (see Appendix 10).
- If you use diuretics on a regular basis, consult your physician regarding the degree of salt restriction he recommends for you. Many salt

substitutes have a high potassium content. Ask your physician for guidance regarding the selection and use of commercially available salt substitutes.

- In advanced congestive heart failure, you may be advised to use a thiazide diuretic concurrently with a stronger "loop" diuretic (furosemide, ethacrynic acid, bumetanide, or torsemide) and a potassium-saving diuretic (spironolactone or triamterene); the combined actions of the three types of drugs give a maximal diuretic effect.

Use of Angiotensin-Converting Enzyme (ACE) Inhibitors

ACE inhibitors (captopril, enalapril, lisinopril, others) are now considered to be the best tolerated and most useful vasodilators for the management of congestive heart failure. They are "balanced" vasodilators—affecting both arterial and venous circulation. Recent studies have confirmed that the routine use of ACE inhibitors in all degrees of heart failure has increased survival significantly.

Experts emphasize that full therapeutic doses of these drugs are required to obtain optimal benefits—make sure you understand how and when to take these drugs and follow the prescribed regimen faithfully.

Use of Direct Vasodilators

- These are generally used when heart failure does not respond adequately to digitalis, ACE inhibitors, and diuretics. These may be used earlier for those who cannot tolerate digitalis, and for those who need a vasodilator to treat hypertension (hydralazine) or angina (nifedipine).
- Nitrate vasodilators (primarily venous dilators) contribute to the relief of shortness of breath.
- Hydralazine (primarily an arterial dilator) contributes to the relief of fatigue and weakness.
- Isosorbide dinitrate (venous) and hydralazine (arterial) vasodilators are best used concurrently; they are quite effective in the majority of cases of chronic congestive failure.
- Alpha-adrenergic-blocking drugs (doxazosin, prazosin, terazosin) are both arterial and venous dilators; they are alternate choices. However, they may cause fluid retention and require additional diuretics with continued use.

Use of Calcium-Channel-Blockers

- These drugs are excellent vasodilators, but their utility in congestive heart failure is still being evaluated.
- Amlodipine (Norvasc) has been found to increase capacity for exercise in mild to moderate CHF when added to conventional treatment.
- These drugs may be tried if angina persists after relief of congestive heart failure. Monitor effects closely; calcium-channel-blockers may decrease the effects of digoxin.

Use of Beta-Adrenergic-Blockers
- These drugs may be tried if hypertension persists after relief of congestive heart failure.
- Beta-blockers may decrease the effects of digoxin; monitor effects closely.

Use of Oxygen
Oxygen must be properly humidified to prevent drying of tissues of the respiratory tract. It's best to administer by nasal prongs; avoid a mask.

Therapeutic Drug Monitoring (Blood Levels)
After the optimal dose of digoxin is determined, blood levels should be checked if:
- heart function deteriorates; symptoms of heart failure worsen
- kidney function deteriorates
- new medications are added that could affect digoxin blood levels
- signs of digoxin toxicity develop: see above

Recommended digoxin blood level: 0.5–2.0 ng/ml.

Ancillary Drug Treatment (as required)
For anxiety:
- buspirone (BuSpar)

For insomnia:
- doxylamine (Unisom)
- zolpidem (Ambien)

For anemia:
- iron preparations

For angina:
see Profile of coronary artery disease in this section

For hypertension:
see Profile of hypertension in this section

Note: Drug selection, dosage, and administration schedule must be determined by the physician for each patient individually.

Current Controversies in Management
With the advent of new drugs and improved understanding of the altered physiology associated with congestive heart failure, controversy regarding drug selection for its treatment has increased. A consensus is now emerging that holds the traditional "stepped-care" approach—diuretic, digoxin, then vasodilator—is no longer valid.

New studies show that angiotensin-converting enzyme (ACE) inhibitors (see above) can enhance treatment and prolong survival. They are now the vasodilators of choice, and their use is recommended for initiating treatment of CHF, given concurrently with digoxin and diuretics as indicated by the patient's condition.

Further experience and detailed analysis of drug performance are required to resolve current controversies. Drug choices will remain a matter of individual physician preference for some time to come.

Special Considerations for Women

Pregnancy
ACE inhibitor drugs (see Appendix 16, Drug Classes, for specific drug names) are designated Pregnancy Category D (see Appendix 15, FDA Pregnancy Categories, for explanation).

Breast-Feeding
Some ACE inhibitor drugs are known to be present in breast milk. Avoid drug or refrain from nursing.

Special Considerations for the Elderly

Instead of shortness of breath with exertion, older persons with heart failure may first develop insomnia, lethargy, weakness, agitation, or confusion.

Older persons are more likely to experience the toxic effects of digoxin: headache, dizziness, fatigue, weakness, depression, confusion, delusions, difficulty in reading. Report these symptoms promptly; a digoxin blood level measurement may be indicated.

Older persons are more sensitive to any drug that lowers blood pressure. If you are advised to take a diuretic, angiotensin-converting enzyme (ACE) inhibitor, vasodilator, or calcium-channel-blocking drug, start with small doses until your full response is known. Avoid rapid and excessive drops in blood pressure (see Appendix 16, Drug Classes, for specific drug names).

Quality of Life Considerations

The customary emphasis on determining the cause and optimal treatment of heart failure often precludes consideration of other aspects of the patient's illness. Although appropriate treatment may well relieve shortness of breath and improve tolerance for exercise, attention must also be given to the individual's emotional and mental state. The proper management of anxiety and depression, the provision of a beneficent support system, and the maintenance of social roles and relationships can significantly improve the patient's well-being and survival.

The Role of Prevention in This Disorder

Primary Prevention
The most effective primary measures for the prevention of congestive heart failure are those that prevent or control the principal causes of heart failure:

- hypertension: early detection and effective long-term control
- coronary artery disease: early detection and reduction of risk factors; prevention of heart attack (myocardial infarction)
- alcoholism: effective counseling and total abstention from drinking
- diabetes: early detection and strict control of blood sugar levels for life
- life-long avoidance of the following:
  sedentary lifestyle
  high-fat, high-cholesterol diet
  excessive use of salt
  obesity
  cigarette smoking

Secondary Prevention

- If left ventricular dysfunction (incipient heart failure) is documented by appropriate testing, the early use of ACE inhibitor drugs may prevent or delay the onset of symptoms.
- If symptoms of heart failure develop, *comply fully* with all treatment recommendations, especially the proper use of medications.

Resources

Recommended Reading

Living with Heart Disease: Is It Heart Failure? Consumer Version, Clinical Practice Guideline Number 11, U.S. Department of Health and Human Services, Agency for Health Care Policy and Research, Executive Office Center, Suite 501, 2101 East Jefferson Street, Rockville, MD 20852. AHCPR Publication No. 94-0614. For copies call 1-800-358-9295.

Additional Information and Services

American Heart Association
7320 Greenville Avenue
Dallas, TX 75231
Phone: (214) 373-6300; Fax: (214) 706-1341
    Publications available.

The Mended Hearts, Inc.
7272 Greenville Avenue
Dallas, TX 75231
Phone: (214) 706-1442

The Coronary Club, Inc.
9500 Euclid Avenue, E-37
Cleveland, OH 44195
Phone: (216) 444-3690

CORONARY ARTERY DISEASE

Other Names
CAD, coronary heart disease, ischemic heart disease, coronary artery insufficiency, angina pectoris, unstable angina, preinfarction angina, variant angina

Prevalence/Incidence in U.S.
Current estimate: 11,200,000
Estimated new cases annually: 350,000
Estimated "heart attacks" annually: 1,500,000
Estimated deaths annually: 547,500
Coronary artery disease is the leading cause of death in the U.S.

Age Group Under 45 years—0.2% of population; 45 to 64 years—6.5% of population; over 65 years—11% of population.

Male-to-Female Ratio Under 45 years—1.5 to 1; 45 to 64 years—3 to 1; 65 to 74 years—1.8 to 1; over 75 years—1 to 1.

Principal Features and Natural History
Coronary artery disease is the all-inclusive term used to designate atherosclerotic disease of the coronary arteries and its significant manifestations: angina pectoris, heart rhythm disturbances, congestive heart failure, and episodes of sudden death. The most familiar feature of CAD is angina pectoris: the development of pain (of varying intensity) in the chest, commonly associated with physical or emotional stress. Anginal pain is caused by a lack of oxygen in heart muscle; it is a sign of deficient blood flow (ischemia) in coronary arteries due to obstruction (atheromatous disease) or constriction (arterial spasm). Atherosclerosis is a chronic, progressive hardening and narrowing of arteries due to the buildup of fatty plaques (atheromas) on their inner walls. When narrowing reaches a critical point, blood flow is impeded, heart muscle is deprived of oxygen, and anginal pain develops. Degeneration and inflammation within atheromas can initiate a blood clot (thrombosis) that completely blocks the coronary artery, causing coronary occlusion—a "heart attack." The heart muscle supplied by the occluded artery is severely damaged; this is referred to as myocardial infarction (heart muscle death). When this occurs suddenly and is associated with severe chest pain, it is referred to as acute myocardial infarction (AMI). When it occurs without pain or other significant symptoms (as during sleep), it is referred to as silent myocardial infarction. During the period of healing after infarction, the damaged heart muscle is replaced by scar tissue, leaving an area of per-

manent weakness in the wall of the heart. This eventually predisposes to heart failure (see the Profile of congestive heart failure in this section).

Classical Angina-of-Effort (Exertional Angina)

A moderate to severe discomfort (pain, pressure, tightness, fullness, squeezing, or burning sensation) usually located deeply behind the breastbone (but may be felt in the jaw, neck, shoulder, arms, upper back, or pit of the stomach). It is characteristically brought on by physical exertion, a large meal, emotional stress, or exposure to cold. It usually lasts one to five minutes and disappears with rest. Many individuals with classical angina learn to recognize the factors that induce anginal pain, and are able to adjust their activities to avoid it. The pattern is predictable, easily managed, and can remain unchanged for long periods of time. This is referred to as "stable angina."

"Unstable" Angina

The development and progression of atheromatous coronary artery disease varies widely and unpredictably among individuals. Symptoms can begin very abruptly and progress rapidly in a short period of time. The pattern of a stable angina can alter quickly without apparent reason; episodes of pain can increase in frequency and severity without provocation. Medications are less effective in preventing and relieving anginal attacks of mounting intensity. This feature of instability signals an ominous progression of arterial disease and increasing risk of occlusion. This is referred to as preinfarction angina—a heart attack in the making. It requires immediate attention to avert acute myocardial infarction (AMI).

Variant (Prinzmetal's) Angina

This is a form of unstable angina. The mechanism responsible for anginal pain is spontaneous spasm (constriction) of a coronary artery, causing ischemia and deficient oxygen supply to heart muscle. It usually occurs at rest, between midnight and 8 A.M. It is unpredictable and unrelated to the situations that provoke effort angina. Variant angina can develop independently, or it can coexist with atheromatous CAD.

Diagnostic Symptoms and Signs

For angina pectoris:

> abrupt development of pain as described above
>
> typical anginal pain is felt in the front of the chest, usually behind the breastbone

ALERT!

Atypical locations of anginal pain are often misinterpreted and not recognized as symptoms of CAD. Unusual sites of anginal pain include:

- facial areas: thought to be neuralgia
- jaws: thought to be a dental problem

- neck: though to be a muscle problem
- shoulder: thought to be bursitis or arthritis
- upper arm: thought to be muscle strain
- lower arm and/or hand: though to be a pinched nerve
- back: thought to be a muscle strain or spine problem
- stomach: thought to be acid indigestion, ulcer, or gallbladder problem

Anginal pain usually subsides with rest and within 15 minutes.

Anginal pain is relieved by nitroglycerin sublingual tablets or spray, usually within 5 to 10 minutes.

If pain is not relieved by three doses of nitroglycerin given five minutes apart, suspect impending myocardial infarction and seek immediate treatment.

For acute myocardial infarction (AMI):

- abrupt development of pain as described above
- pain is characteristically more severe than anginal pain
- pain is often accompanied by other symptoms and signs:
    extreme weakness
    lightheadedness, sense of impending faint
    shortness of breath
    nausea, with or without vomiting
    pale, ashen color
    cold, sweaty skin
    loss of consciousness
- pain persists, is not relieved by rest
- pain is not relieved by nitroglycerin

Diagnostic Tests and Procedures

Electrocardiograms (ECGs, EKGs): resting, with exercise, and serially

Ambulatory dynamic (Holter) ECG monitoring

Echocardiograms

Coronary angiograms

Nuclear imaging studies: technetium angiography; thallium or sestamibi perfusion scans; positron emission tomography (PET scans)

Dipyridamole nuclear perfusion studies

Dobutamine echocardiography

Appropriate serum enzyme levels to determine presence of myocardial infarction

Measurement of cardiac troponin I and T blood levels during anginal syndrome

Diagnostic "Markers" for This Disorder

Specific (and transient) ECG changes during exercise stress testing that confirm ischemic episodes (angina pectoris)

Coronary angiograms that demonstrate measurable arterial stenosis (vessel narrowing or blockage)

Diagnostic elevations of serum enzyme levels (following severe anginal pain) that confirm heart muscle damage (myocardial infarction)

Specific (and lasting) ECG changes (following prolonged episode of anginal pain) that confirm heart muscle damage (myocardial infarction)

Possible Effects of Drugs on Test Results

Beta-blocker drugs (see Appendix 16, Drug Classes) can prevent the exercise-induced increase in heart rate that is necessary for diagnostic interpretations.

The chronic use of digitalis (digoxin) may alter ECG patterns and confuse interpretation.

Similar Conditions That May Confuse Diagnosis

Other conditions that can cause chest pain and shortness of breath include:

pleurodynia ("Devil's grip"): acute intercostal neuralgia due to infection of the muscles between individual ribs

acute pericarditis: infection of the pericardium (envelope that surrounds the heart)

dissecting aortic aneurysm: a tear and separation of tissues in the wall of the aorta (large major artery carrying blood from the heart)

acute pleurisy: infection on the outer covering of the lung

pulmonary embolism: a dislodged fragment (embolus) of a blood clot (thrombus) that is carried by the blood stream to the lung where it obstructs small blood vessels in lung tissue adjacent to the pleura

esophageal spasm: acute squeezing (constriction) of the esophagus (food tube) due to lodged food or drug product—capsule or tablet

hiatal hernia: the protrusion (herniation) of a portion of the stomach through the opening (hiatus) in the diaphragm into the chest cavity

acute indigestion: stomach pain due to inflammation (gastritis), active peptic ulcer, ulcer perforation

gastroesophageal reflux disorder (GERD): "heartburn" due to regurgitation of stomach acids into the lower esophagus

acute gallbladder disorder: gallbladder infection (cholecystitis); gallstones (cholelithiasis)

monosodium glutamate (MSG) syndrome: see Appendix 14

ALERT!

Pain does not always occur during the preinfarction phase of unstable angina. This is especially true in patients who have diabetes or have a transplanted heart. Instead of acute pain, equivalent symptoms and signs of heart muscle ischemia may occur: episodes of shortness of breath at rest, unexpected shortness of breath with light exertion, X-ray findings of heart enlargement or blood vessel prominence (vascular congestion) in the lungs.

Causes

The principal feature of CAD is the segmental narrowing of arterial vessels by atherosclerosis—the formation of atheromas on interior vessel walls. The cause of the initial injury to the vessel wall that leads to the formation of atheromas is not known. The following risk factors contribute to the development and progression of coronary atherosclerosis:

genetic predisposition: family history of CAD in a first degree relative before 55 years of age

sedentary lifestyle: lack of regular aerobic exercise

family history of cholesterol disorders

personal cholesterol disorder: total cholesterol over 240 mg; LDL cholesterol over 160 mg; HDL cholesterol under 35 mg; triglycerides over 400 mg (see Profile of cholesterol disorders in this section)

central (truncal) obesity: 20% or more above normal weight

cigarette smoking

hypertension (uncontrolled)

diabetes mellitus (uncontrolled)

sustained psychological stress

Drugs That Can Cause This Disorder

The following drugs do not cause coronary artery disease per se, but they can affect heart function adversely and induce or intensify angina in susceptible individuals:

amphetamines

beta-blocker drugs (abrupt withdrawal)

bromocriptine

cocaine

epinephrine

ergot preparations

5-fluorouracil

hydralazine

indomethacin

isoetharine

isoproterenol

metaproterenol

methysergide

nifedipine (first dose)

nylidrin

oral contraceptives

phenylpropanolamine

prazosin
terbutaline
thyroid

Goals of Treatment

Can This Disorder Be Cured?

There is no current therapy that can cure atherosclerosis.

Can This Disorder Be Treated Effectively?

Some studies demonstrate modest success in (1) stabilizing or reversing atherosclerosis, and (2) reducing the incidence of myocardial infarction by the aggressive use of drugs that lower lipid blood levels.

Current medical therapies can satisfactorily manage many cases of stable angina.

Current surgical procedures can provide excellent relief of symptoms and significant prolongation of life.

Specific Goals

- Prompt relief of acute anginal attacks
- Prevention of anticipated angina by use of nitroglycerin just before physical activity
- Long-term prevention of angina: reduced frequency, severity, and duration of recurrent anginal episodes
- Prevention of heart rhythm disturbances (arrhythmias)
- Prevention of heart attack (myocardial infarction)
- Prevention of sudden death
- Improved quality of life
- Prolongation of life

Health Professionals Who Participate in Managing This Disorder

Family physicians
General internists
Geriatricians
Cardiologists
Radiologists
Critical care physicians
Cardiac surgeons
Thoracic surgeons
Psychiatrists
Clinical nurse specialists
Critical care nurses
Nurse practitioners
Nurse educators

Pharmacists
Dietitians

Currently Available Therapies for This Disorder

Drug Therapy

Nitrate preparations:
- amyl nitrite inhalant (Aspirols, Vaporole)
- nitroglycerin lingual aerosol (Nitrolingual Spray)
- nitroglycerin sublingual tablets (Nitrostat)
- nitroglycerin buccal tablets (Susadrin)
- nitroglycerin prolonged-action forms (Nitro-Bid, etc.)
- nitroglycerin ointment (Nitrol, etc.)
- nitroglycerin patches (Nitrodisc, Nitro-Dur, etc.)
- isosorbide dinitrate (Isordil, Sorbitrate)
- isosorbide mononitrate (Ismo, Imdur)
- erythrityl tetranitrate (Cardilate)
- pentaerythritol tetranitrate (Peritrate)

Beta-blocker drugs:
- acebutolol (Sectral)
- atenolol (Tenormin)
- betaxolol (Kerlone)
- carteolol (Cartrol)
- labetalol (Normodyne, Trandate)
- metoprolol (Lopressor, Toprol XL)
- nadolol (Corgard)
- penbutolol (Levatol)
- pindolol (Visken)
- propranolol (Inderal)
- timolol (Blocadren)

Calcium-blocker drugs:
- amlodipine (Norvasc)
- bepridil (Vascor)
- diltiazem (Cardizem, Dilacor XR)
- felodipine (Plendil)
- isradipine (DynaCirc)
- nicardipine (Cardene)
- nifedipine (Adalat, Procardia)
- verapamil (Calan, Isoptin, Verelan)

Others:
- aspirin (antiplatelet effect)
- warfarin (anticoagulant effect)
- vitamin E (antioxidant effect)
- morphine, intravenous (pain management in acute myocardial infarction)

Invasive and Surgical Procedures
- Percutaneous transluminal coronary angioplasty (PTCA)
- Implantation of coronary artery stents
- Coronary artery bypass grafting (CABG)
- Implantation of cardiac pacemakers

Management of Therapy

General Measures
- Aerobic exercise, 30–45 minutes three to six times weekly
- Weight reduction if necessary; achieve and maintain normal body weight
- Low-fat, low-cholesterol, high-fiber diet
- Correction of blood lipid disorders
- Total and permanent cessation of cigarette smoking
- Maintenance of normal blood pressure
- Maintenance of normal blood sugar levels
- Aspirin, 80–325 mg daily or every other day
- Vitamin E, 400 IUs daily

For Stable Exertional Angina
- Frequency and severity of angina-of-effort remain at a constant level.
- Episodes are predictable, of short duration, and respond promptly to treatment.
- Nitroglycerin spray or sublingual tablet for relief of acute attacks
- Long-acting nitrates and/or a beta-blocker
- If control is not adequate, a calcium blocker may be added.

For Unstable Angina
- Frequency and severity of angina increase abruptly. Episodes occur unpredictably with exertion and at rest, are of longer duration (15 to 20 minutes), and are less responsive to treatment.
- Unresponsive episodes require hospitalization in a coronary care unit for monitoring and intensive drug therapy to prevent myocardial infarction.
- Intravenous heparin on admission to coronary care unit
- Mild sedation with benzodiazepines (Valium, etc.)
- Intravenous morphine for pain control as needed
- Combined use of nitrates and beta-blocker
- Aspirin, for antiplatelet effect
- Calcium-channel-blocker drugs are not recommended for routine use in unstable angina.

For Variant (Prinzmetal's) Angina
- Anginal attacks primarily at rest
- Nitroglycerin spray or sublingual tablets

- Long-acting nitrates
- A calcium-blocker may be tried cautiously, with close monitoring.
- It is advisable to avoid beta-blockers (unless it is established that both types of angina are present).

Use of Nitroglycerin

- Nitroglycerin is the mainstay of managing angina. Always have a supply of fresh, active tablets available. Keep them in the original dark glass bottle, tightly closed, no cotton added. Do not transfer them to a metal or plastic container. The sublingual tablet will produce a mild stinging sensation under the tongue, flushing of the face, and throbbing in the head. These reactions are normal and indicate that the drug is active and you are having a good response (dilation of blood vessels).
- Use nitroglycerin promptly and as often as necessary, no matter how often. Unless instructed otherwise, do not consciously keep count of the tablets used. If anginal pain persists after taking three successive sublingual tablets (one tablet at 3- to 5-minute intervals for three doses), consult your physician immediately or seek assistance at the nearest hospital emergency room.
- If the lingual spray or sublingual tablet causes weakness, dizziness, or faintness (drop in blood pressure), sit down or lie down until the sensation passes.
- Use the spray or tablet to prevent an attack by taking it just before starting a specific physical activity that is known to induce angina.
- Nitroglycerin ointment may be used at bedtime to prevent angina during sleep. Follow the instructions for application carefully. Do not use your fingers. Do not rub the ointment into the skin.
- Nitroglycerin patches (discs) may induce tolerance to the drug and cause it to be less effective with continuous use. The intermittent use of oral dosage forms may be more effective for long-term treatment. Ask your physician for guidance.
- If you have glaucoma, consult your physician regarding the periodic measurement of your internal eye pressures while using long-term nitrates for angina.
- Following long-term use, nitrates should be discontinued gradually to prevent symptoms of withdrawal.

Use of Beta-Blocker Drugs

- Do not use this type of drug without your physician's knowledge and guidance. Beta-blockers are not recommended for mild angina that is well controlled by nitrates. Their use is generally reserved for severe and unstable angina. If your angina worsens with the use of a beta-blocker drug, notify your physician promptly.
- Beta-blockers are not recommended for variant (Prinzmetal's) vasospastic angina.

- Atenolol (Tenormin) and metoprolol (Lopressor) are preferred for individuals with asthma, emphysema, diabetes, or peripheral circulatory disorders.
- Atenolol (Tenormin) and nadolol (Corgard) are effective with once-daily dosage and tend to cause less depression and insomnia.
- Beta-blocker drugs must not be discontinued suddenly. Abrupt withdrawal can cause severe angina and increase the risk of myocardial infarction.

Use of Calcium-Blocker Drugs
- Provide effective relief when used as single drug therapy in treating chronic stable angina. Can be used initially by individuals who should not use beta-blockers.
- Considered by some authorities to be the drug of choice in treating vasospastic variant (Prinzmetal's) angina.
- Amlodipine, felodipine, isradipine, nicardipine, and nifedipine cause significant reduction of blood pressure and increased heart rate; some authorities recommend giving these calcium blockers in combination with a beta-blocker.
- Calcium blockers are no longer recommended for routine use in treating unstable angina.

Ancillary Drug Treatment (as required)
For anxiety:
- benzodiazepines (Valium, etc.) (see Appendix 16, Drug Classes)
For hypertension:
  see Profile of hypertension in this section
For congestive heart failure:
  see Profile of congestive heart failure in this section
For hyperthyroidism:
- methimazole (Tapazole)
- propylthiouracil
- propranolol (Inderal)
For anemia:
- iron preparations
  Note: Drug selection, dosage, and administration schedule must be determined by the physician for each patient individually.

Current Controversies in Management
The nitrate drugs are well established as effective therapeutic agents for the management of angina and congestive heart failure, two conditions that require long-term drug therapy. Recent studies have shown that the "standard" practice of continuous administration of nitrates can lead to the development of tolerance (see Glossary) and loss of effectiveness. Tolerance is most likely to occur with frequent dosing and the use of

prolonged-action capsules or tablets and the use of transdermal nitroglycerin patches. Continuous treatment with nitrates produces tolerance within 24 hours of the first dose and complete loss of effect when continued for one week or more. The intermittent use of nitrates ("pulse" dosing) causes only partial tolerance and is more effective for long-term protection. Intermittent rather than continuous nitrate dosing is now recommended for treating angina and congestive heart failure. Isosorbide mononitrate (Ismo, Imdur) is now available for this application of the nitrates.

Comments

Current guidelines for the optimal use of nitrates include the following recommendations.

- Take isosorbide dinitrate (Isordil, short-acting form) two or three (but not four) times daily; take at 8:00 A.M. and 1:00 or 3:00 P.M., or at 8:00 A.M., 1:00 P.M., and 5:00 P.M.; no dosing again until the following 8:00 A.M.
- Take the prolonged-action dosage forms of isosorbide dinitrate at 8:00 A.M., only once daily.
- Use the nitroglycerin patch for only 12 hours daily, from 8:00 A.M. to 8:00 P.M.; leave it off during the night.
- Long nitrate-free intervals appear to preserve responsiveness to the drug.

Possible Drug Interactions of Significance

Bepridil and verapamil may *increase* the effects of
- digoxin, by increasing digoxin blood levels.

Cyclosporine *taken concurrently* with
- diltiazem or
- nicardipine or
- verapamil can result in elevations of cyclosporine blood levels and cyclosporine-induced kidney damage.

Special Considerations for Women

Recent studies suggest that estrogen replacement therapy in post-menopausal women with coronary artery disease and established angina can significantly reduce the frequency and intensity of exercise-induced anginal episodes.

Special Considerations for the Elderly

Coronary artery disease is one of the most common disorders found in older persons. It is important that you recognize the variations of anginal pain that can occur (see the category of "Diagnostic Symptoms and Signs" above).

It is also important that you understand that over 50% of older individuals who have a heart attack (myocardial infarction) do not experience the pain of angina to indicate what is happening—they have what is referred to as a "silent" coronary occlusion. Instead of chest pain, they may experience sudden shortness of breath, weakness, confusion, and sense of impending faint. Should you experience an episode of this nature, report it immediately so that appropriate treatment can be provided.

Quality of Life Considerations

Chronic stable angina of a mild to moderate nature is well recognized and easily managed. The patterns of pain are predictable and anticipated episodes of angina can be prevented with the timely use of nitroglycerin. The quality of one's life is not seriously compromised.

However, the development of unstable and progressive angina is soon recognized as an ominous threat of serious proportions. It demands urgent evaluation and aggressive treatment to avert myocardial infarction or sudden death. Some degree of anxiety, apprehension, and fear are unavoidable. The quality of life—physical and psychological well-being— may be altered drastically. The resolution is to seek the best medical advice available to you regarding an optimal course of action. Your quality of life is best served by immediate intensive medicinal therapy to prevent irreversible damage to the heart, followed by definitive procedures to promptly restore adequate blood flow through the system of occluding coronary arteries—coronary angioplasty or coronary artery bypass surgery. Current treatment outcomes are most gratifying. The vast majority of patients so treated are returned to the quality of life they enjoyed prior to the onset of angina.

The Role of Prevention in This Disorder

Primary Prevention

As early as possible, establish a lifestyle that includes the following features:

- regular, moderate, aerobic exercise
- low-fat, low-cholesterol, high-fiber diet
- dietary supplement of vitamin E: 400 IUs daily
- maintain normal weight for sex, age, and body build
- total and permanent abstention from all forms of tobacco
- moderate intake of alcohol: one to two drinks daily; no more than seven drinks per week
- effective avoidance and management of stress
- annual check of blood pressure; effective control of blood pressure if hypertension develops
- annual check for diabetes; strict control of blood sugar if diabetes develops

- measurement of blood lipids every five years, beginning at age 20 years; effective treatment of any lipid disorders that develop

Secondary Prevention

- Adoption of any of the primary preventive measures listed above, as recommended by your physician
- Strict compliance with all medical therapies recommended by your physician
- Consult your physician regarding the preventive use of daily aspirin
- Careful consideration of any surgical procedures recommended by your physician; obtain a second opinion as warranted

Resources

Recommended Reading

Heart and Stroke Facts, American Heart Association, National Center, Dallas, 1994. For a copy call 1-800-AHA-USA1 (1-800-242-8721).

Unstable Angina: Diagnosis and Management, Clinical Practice Guideline Number 10, U.S. Dept. of Health and Human Services, Public Health Service, Agency for Health Care Policy and Research, AHCPR Publication No. 94-0602, 1994. For a copy call 1-800-358-9295.

Living with Angina: A Practical Guide to Dealing with Coronary Artery Disease and Your Doctor, James A. Pantano, M.D. New York: Harper & Row, 1990.

Additional Information and Services

American Heart Association
Council on Arteriosclerosis
7320 Greenville Avenue
Dallas, TX 75231
Phone: (214) 706-1293; Fax: (214) 706-1341
Publications available.

Coronary Club, Inc.
9500 Euclid Avenue
Cleveland, OH 44106
Phone: (216) 444-3690
Local groups: 20. Publications available: "Heartline" monthly, $15 per year.

CROHN'S DISEASE

Other Names Regional enteritis, regional ileitis, granulomatous colitis, inflammatory bowel disease

Prevalence/Incidence in U.S. 1 million (includes 100,000 children); 15,000 new cases annually

Age Group Onset from infancy to 25 years of age; 15–30% have onset before puberty. Peak incidence is from 10 to 25 years of age.

Male-to-Female Ratio Slightly more common in females

Principal Features and Natural History

Crohn's disease is an intermittent to chronic inflammatory disorder that can affect any part of the digestive tract from the mouth to the rectum. The characteristic patterns of involvement include:

  ileocolonic Crohn's disease (40%): affecting the lower small intestine (ileum), portions of the colon, rectum, and anus

  colonic Crohn's disease (30%): inflammatory involvement of any part of the colon

  small bowel Crohn's disease (30%): affecting various regions of the ileum (regional ileitis)

  upper gastrointestinal Crohn's disease (less than 5%): inflammatory disease in the mouth, esophagus, stomach, and duodenum (first 12 inches of the small intestine)

The characteristic features of this disease include intense and persistent inflammation in the lining tissues of affected organs, with ulceration, bleeding, scarring, infection, and occasional perforation.

The onset is usually insidious, but may be rapid and resemble acute appendicitis. Symptoms include loss of appetite, fatigue, fever, loss of weight, abdominal cramps and pain after eating, nausea, vomiting, diarrhea (occasionally bloody), anal sores, and retarded growth in children. There may also be inflammatory disorders in the skin, eyes, mouth, and large joints. Children may experience fever and joint pains before any indications of disease in the intestine or colon. Adults may have a higher incidence of gallstones or kidney stones. This disorder usually recurs throughout life.

Caution: The early manifestations of Crohn's disease may vary. Loss of appetite and weight in young women may lead to the mistaken diagnosis of anorexia nervosa.

Diagnostic Symptoms and Signs

Abdominal and/or rectal pain
Diarrhea, bloody stools
Indigestion, nausea, vomiting
Loss of appetite, weight loss
Fever, fatigue, weakness
Skin rashes and ulcerations
Painful mouth ulcers

Joint pains (usually without swelling)
Impaired growth and development in children

Diagnostic Tests and Procedures
Complete blood cell counts
Red blood cell sedimentation rate: an indicator of inflammation; useful in
monitoring response to treatment
Appropriate blood chemistries, liver and kidney function tests
Stool examinations for pathogenic (disease-causing) bacteria or parasites
Colonoscopy for direct inspection of the colon and to obtain biopsy
specimens
Endoscopy of the upper gastrointestinal tract for direct inspection and to
obtain biopsy specimens
X-ray studies of the upper gastrointestinal tract
CT scans of the abdomen
Ultrasound studies of the abdomen

Diagnostic "Markers" for This Disorder
Biopsy specimens reveal chronic inflammatory changes characteristic of
Crohn's disease.

Similar Conditions That May Confuse Diagnosis
Irritable bowel syndrome
Diverticulitis
Pelvic inflammatory disease
Ulcerative colitis
Peptic ulcer disease
Zollinger-Ellison syndrome
Subacute or chronic bacterial or parasitic infections of the intestinal tract
Drug-induced colitis: an adverse effect of some antibiotics
Celiac disease: gluten sensitivity, nontropical sprue
Colon or rectal cancer

Causes

Established Causes
The definitive cause is unknown at this time.

Theoretical Causes
The clinical and pathological features of Crohn's disease suggest that it
is an autoimmune disorder (see Appendix 5, The Immune System).

Known Risk Factors for Developing This Disorder
Genetic predisposition. There is a familial clustering in 15–20% of cases;
frequent occurrence in twins.
Relative risk is higher in cigarette smokers.

Drugs That Can Cause This Disorder

By altering the normal balance of bacteria in the intestine, several antibiotics can cause a form of enteritis that might resemble Crohn's disease. These include some of the tetracyclines and penicillin and chloramphenicol. Antibiotic-induced enteritis is transient and easily corrected; no permanent damage occurs.

The vitamin A derivative etretinate (Tegison) has been reported to cause Crohn's disease.

In 1993, two cases of acute reactivation of Crohn's disease (in remission) were caused by interleukin-2 therapy for kidney cancer. Both cases required emergency surgery.

Goals of Treatment

Can This Disorder Be Cured?

There is no curative treatment available at this time.

Can This Disorder Be Treated Effectively?

The judicious use of appropriate medications may induce remissions (temporary reduction of disease activity). Surgical resection (removal) of diseased bowel is often followed by development of new disease in adjacent segments.

Specific Goals

- Induction of a remission (suppression of disease activity) during the active phase of the disease
- Relief of symptoms
- Protection of bowel, avoidance of complications
- Maintenance of general nutrition
- Prevention of recurrence of active disease following medical remission or surgery

Health Professionals Who Participate in Managing This Disorder

Family physicians
General internists
Pediatricians
Gastroenterologists
Inflammatory bowel disease specialists
Clinical immunologists
General surgeons
Colon/Rectal surgeons
Psychiatrists
Dietitians/nutritionists

Currently Available Therapies for This Disorder

Drug Therapy

- Cortisonelike steroids, principally prednisone (treatment of choice for induction of remission in active Crohn's disease; not recommended for long-term use)
- Sulfasalazine (Azulfidine)
- 5-aminosalicylic acid (5-ASA): olsalazine (Dipentum), mesalamine (Asacol, Pentasa)
- Metronidazole (Flagyl)
- Azathioprine (Imuran); 6-mercaptopurine (Purinethol)
- Anti-infectives: amoxicillin (Amoxcil, etc.), tetracycline (Achromycin, etc.), ciprofloxacin (Cipro), trimethoprim-sulfamethoxazole (Bactrim, Septra); used when appropriate for bacterial infections of intestine
- Methotrexate, cyclosporine for severe, unresponsive disease
- Antidiarrheals: diphenoxylate (Lomotil), loperamide (Imodium)
- Antispasmodics: belladonna (Donnatal), dicyclomine (Bentyl)

Nondrug Treatment Methods

- Nutritional supplements as required
- Surgical interventions for complications: bowel obstruction, fistula formation, abscesses, bowel perforation

New Drugs in Development for Treating This Disorder

The following agents, already in use for treating other disorders, are currently being evaluated for the treatment of inflammatory bowel disease: oral sodium cromoglycate, sucralfate enemas, clonidine, eicosapentaenoic acid (fish oil).

Management of Therapy

- For initial treatment of mild disease: sulfasalazine
- For moderate to severe disease: prednisone, used concurrently with sulfasalazine
- For acute recurrences: prednisone
- For long-term maintenance: sulfasalazine; avoid use of cortisonelike steroids (prednisone) if possible (see Appendix 6, Long-Term Corticosteroid Therapy)
- For active disease that fails to respond to combined use of sulfasalazine and prednisone: (1) a trial of metronidazole as replacement for sulfasalazine; (2) a trial of azathioprine or 6-mercaptopurine added to sulfasalazine and prednisone programs
- For severe, unresponsive disease: trials of methotrexate or cyclosporine

Use of Sulfasalazine (Azulfidine)

- Used to initiate treatment in active disease. Usually not effective in preventing recurrences; however, it may be tried for long-term maintenance until a better treatment is developed. About 50% effective when used with prednisone.

- Most beneficial in treating Crohn's disease of the ileo-colon and colon; may be effective in treating disease of the small intestine.
- Common adverse effects are headache, nausea, and vomiting; take with or immediately following food.
- Approximately 30% of patients cannot tolerate sulfasalazine because of side effects and adverse idiosyncratic and hypersensitivity reactions. Some of these may be attributed to its sulfapyridine component.

Use of Other Aminosalicylates

- This group of related drugs consists primarily of 5-aminosalicylate (5-ASA), the active component of sulfasalazine; they do not contain sulfapyridine, the other component of sulfasalazine.
- Olsalazine (Dipentum) is used primarily to maintain remission in ulcerative colitis patients who cannot tolerate sulfasalazine. Its role in treating Crohn's disease has not been defined.
- Mesalamine is available in four different dosage forms; each form is designed to release 5-ASA at a specific area of the bowel. Asacol, a delayed-release form, is used primarily to treat mild to moderate active ulcerative colitis. Several studies have shown it to be effective in treating active Crohn's disease and in maintaining remission. Pentasa, a sustained-release form, releases 5-ASA in the small intestine and colon. Although approved only for the treatment of mild to moderate ulcerative colitis, recent studies have found it effective in treating active Crohn's disease and in maintenance therapy when started within three months after the onset of remission. Rowasa suppositories and retention enemas provide local application of 5-ASA in the rectum of patients with mild to moderate ulcerative proctitis. Their role in treating Crohn's disease has not been defined.

Use of Cortisonelike Steroids (Prednisone, etc.)

- Good initial response in treating Crohn's disease of the colon, but the majority relapse within one year. Usually 60% to 70% effective during first 6 months of treatment; if use is extended to 12 months, only 20% to 30% remain in remission. Long-term use for mild disease or to prevent recurrences is usually ineffective and is not advised.
- Used primarily to control worsening symptoms and to suppress acute flare-ups. Continued use until a sustained improvement is recommended. It is advisable to use the lowest effective dose. When possible, an alternate-day dosing schedule is recommended: a single morning dose every 48 hours. When appropriate, the dose should be tapered very slowly over a period of 4 to 12 months.

- Repeated intermittent short courses are preferable to continual long-term use.
- Crohn's disease of the rectum should be treated with steroid suppositories and retention enemas.

Use of Antidiarrheals
- Use very cautiously and as sparingly as possible.
- Excessive use can induce two complications: (1) paralytic (adynamic) ileus, a paralysis of the small intestine that results in a functional obstruction; (2) toxic megacolon, a marked distention of the colon with air, and a danger of perforation.

Use of Adsorbents
- Cholestyramine (Questran) and aluminum hydroxide (Amphojel) can adsorb bile in the intestine and reduce bile-induced diarrhea.
- These adsorbents can also adsorb other drugs being used concurrently. Schedule all dosages to ensure maximal effectiveness—adequate spacing (three to four hours) between adsorbents and other active drugs.

Use of Immunosuppressants
- Azathioprine (Imuran) and 6-mercaptopurine (Purinethol) may be tried when sulfasalazine and prednisone have failed to control the disease after an adequate trial. Either one may be tried as an adjunct to the established treatment program.
- A trial of no less than four to six months of treatment is often necessary to determine effectiveness. The onset of beneficial effects usually occurs after three months of continual treatment.
- These drugs make it possible to reduce the dose of steroids or withdraw them completely in some individuals.
- Discontinuation should be attempted after one year of continual treatment.
- Cyclosporine (Sandimmune) may also have a cortisone-sparing effect. Its onset of action is one to two weeks. Monitor blood pressure and kidney function closely during its use.

Use of Anti-Infectives
- Appropriately selected anti-infectives may be used to treat a diarrhea due to specific bacterial overgrowth (superinfection).
- Antibiotics should not be taken concurrently with sulfasalazine.
- Metronidazole (Flagyl) may be effective in treating ileocolitis and colitis that do not respond to standard therapy. It can be used in combination with aminosalicylates and corticosteroids.

ALERT!
Remember that the chronic use of prednisone or immunosuppressive drugs can mask the usual warning signs of infection: fever, chills, local

inflammation, and pain. Patients who develop complications with infection and have taken prednisone in the past may require stress doses of corticosteroids because of adrenal gland insufficiency.

Ancillary Drug Treatment (as required)

For anemia (common):
- iron preparations, vitamin B_{12}, folic acid (as required)

For malnutrition:
- multiple vitamins and the minerals calcium, magnesium, zinc

For depression:
see the Profile of depression in this section

Note: Drug selection, dosage, and administration schedule must be determined by the physician for each patient individually.

Possible Drug Interactions of Significance

Sulfasalazine may *increase* the effects of
- sulfonylureas and increase the risk of hypoglycemia (see Appendix 16, Drug Classes).

Prednisone *taken concurrently* with
- cyclosporine may increase the blood levels of both drugs; dose reductions of both drugs may be needed.
- oral hypoglycemic drugs (sulfonylureas) or insulin may impair glucose control (see Appendix 16, Drug Classes).

Metronidazole *taken concurrently* with
- birth control pills (oral contraceptives) may impair their effectiveness and result in pregnancy.
- cyclosporine may lead to cyclosporine toxicity.
- lithium may lead to lithium toxicity.
- sulfa drugs (Bactrim, Septra, others) may result in a disulfiramlike reaction (see Glossary).

Note: If you are taking drugs other than those mentioned, consult *The Essential Guide to Prescription Drugs*, or a similar drug reference book for all possible interactions (see Appendix 17, Drug Information Sources).

Special Considerations for Women

Pregnancy

Strict attention must be given to the maintenance of adequate nutrition. This may take the form of special enteral (by mouth) or parenteral (intravenous) food supplements.

The use of metronidazole during pregnancy has been controversial for many years. This drug causes genetic mutations in bacteria and cancer in rodents. Studies of its association with birth defects in humans have yielded contradictory and inconclusive results. Although the FDA Pregnancy Category for this drug is B, the manufacturer and the Center for Disease Control and Prevention (CDC) consider it to be contraindicated during the first trimester (see Appendix 15, FDA Pregnancy Categories).

Azathioprine (Imuran) and 6-mercaptopurine (Purinethol) are both designated Pregnancy Category D drugs. Their safe use during pregnancy is questionable (see Appendix 15, FDA Pregnancy Categories).

Breast-Feeding

Metronidazole is excreted into breast milk. If the drug is taken during nursing, the American Academy of Pediatrics recommends discontinuing breast-feeding for 12–24 hours to allow excretion of the drug.

The Role of Prevention in This Disorder

Primary Prevention

There is no known way to prevent the initial development of Crohn's disease.

Secondary Prevention

Every effort should be made to determine the therapeutic program that is most effective for each patient individually. There is no standard treatment that can be recommended for all patients. If disease activity is not controlled after adequate trials of medical therapy, consideration should be given to surgical resection of unresponsive bowel. This is the only feasible means of preventing life-threatening complications that are the hallmark of this disease.

Resources

Recommended Reading

The Angry Gut: Coping with Colitis and Crohn's Disease, W. Grant Thompson. New York: Plenum Press, 1993.

Additional Information and Services

American Digestive Disease Society
60 East 42nd Street, Room 411
New York, NY 10165

Telecommunications services: Gutline, available to the public every Tuesday evening from 7:30 to 9:00 P.M. Publications available.

Crohn's and Colitis Foundation of America
386 Park Avenue South, 17th Floor
New York, NY 10016
Phone: 1-800-932-2423, (212) 685-3440; Fax: (212) 779-4098

Local groups: 73. Publications available.

DEPRESSION

Other Names

Depressive reaction (reactive depression, secondary depression), depressive illness (biologic depression, major depressive disorder), dysthymia (depressive neurosis), seasonal affective disorder, unipolar mood disorder, depressive phase of manic-depressive disorder

Prevalence/Incidence in U.S.

Approximately 15 million; 5–7% of the general population. One in five will experience depression during their lifetime. One-third of all depressions are severe enough to require medical treatment.

Age Group Can occur at any age. Peak occurrence is between 25 and 44 years of age.

Male-to-Female Ratio 1 male to 2 females; 25% of women and 10% of men will experience depression during their lifetime.

Principal Features and Natural History

Depressive Reaction

A situational (exogenous) reactive depression that represents an understandable adaptive response to a significant loss or stressful life situation; a sense of despondency and distress, comparatively mild to moderate, usually self-limiting with a duration of two weeks to six months.

Depressive Illness

A spontaneous (endogenous) unexplained and seemingly unprovoked depression of moderate to severe degree; characterized by (1) a depressed mood—sadness, dejection, hopelessness, despair; (2) reduced energy level—loss of interest, fatigue, inability to function effectively; (3) negative self-image—sense of inferiority, incompetence, exaggerated guilt. Common features include loss of appetite, broken sleep, early morning awakening, constipation. This type of depression is a true medical illness with a biological cause. Approximately 10–15% of all major depressions are associated with medical disorders such as thyroid dysfunction, neurological diseases, cancer, and others. It may clear spontaneously in 6 to 12 months without treatment, or it may persist for years and require intensive therapy to manage satisfactorily.

Dysthymia

A disorder of mood (depressive neurosis) characterized by a depressed feeling (sad, blue, low, down in the dumps) and loss of interest or pleasure in one's usual activities that has persisted for more than two years.

Although negatively affecting the quality of life, the features are not disabling and not severe enough to meet the criteria for major depression.

Seasonal Affective Disorder

A disorder of mood that correlates with the change of seasons, notably in the winter months when days are shorter and sunlight is less intense. It is characterized by mild to moderate depression, fatigue, drowsiness, and impaired thinking and concentration. Symptoms are frequently relieved by scheduled exposure to therapeutic high-intensity light.

ALERT!

Depression occurring in children and adolescents produces a pattern of symptoms quite different from that seen in adults. Although many parents would consider the features that characterize childhood depression to be "normal at that age," the point to be made is that the symptoms are exaggerated, protracted, and unresponsive to counseling or discipline. The characteristic features of childhood depression include:

- behavioral problems
- anger and hostility
- rebelliousness
- poor scholarship
- deterioration of friendships
- troubled rapport with parents

Diagnostic Symptoms and Signs

Major depressive disorder is characterized by the following symptoms if they have been present almost every day, throughout the day, and lasting at least two weeks:

Diagnostic Symptoms

- Loss of interest in things you used to enjoy, including sex
- Feeling sad, blue, pessimistic, or hopeless
- Feeling worthless or guilty
- Loss of energy, constant fatigue
- Difficulty with thinking, concentrating, remembering, or making decisions
- Feeling restless, anxious, or worried
- Insomnia, broken sleep, or need for excessive sleep
- Changes in appetite: loss of appetite and weight; excessive appetite and weight gain
- Thoughts of death or suicide

Associated Symptoms

- Headaches: increased frequency or severity
- Varied body aches and pains

- Digestive disturbances
- Sexual dysfunction

ALERT!
Thoughts of death or suicide are often a major feature of depression. If you experience such thoughts, recognize them as natural manifestations of serious depression and seek immediate treatment just as you would for any other major illness. Inform your personal physician and explain that you need help urgently. You will be amazed and gratified at how promptly these symptoms will abate with appropriate treatment.

Diagnostic Tests and Procedures
There are no specific tests that establish the diagnosis of depression. Your physician will utilize the following procedures to make the diagnosis:
1. Evaluation of your symptoms (as outlined above)
2. Review of your family history regarding medical and mental disorders
3. Review of your personal history of medical and mental disorders
4. A general physical examination to detect conditions that could contribute to depression
5. Request for pertinent laboratory tests to detect conditions that could be related to depression
6. Request for information regarding all medications you are taking, your alcohol consumption, and substance abuse
7. Questions regarding current stresses in your life that could contribute to depression

Similar Conditions That May Confuse Diagnosis
A significant degree of depression may be a presenting feature of the following disorders:
Addison's disease
Alzheimer's disease
chronic kidney failure (uremia)
Cushing's disease
diabetes mellitus
focal cerebral infarction (stroke)
HIV infection (AIDS)
hypothyroidism, apathetic hyperthyroidism
lupus erythematosus
manic-depressive (bipolar) mood disorder
multiple cerebral infarct dementia ("mini-strokes")
multiple sclerosis
parathyroid disorders
Parkinson's disease

postpartum depression (following childbearing)
premenstrual syndrome
temporal lobe epilepsy
viral hepatitis

Causes

Established Causes

The primary cause of major depressive disorder is unknown.

Theoretical Causes

The actual onset of depressive illness is attributed to a deficiency of certain brain chemicals—the neurotransmitters norepinephrine, dopamine, and/or serotonin. What initiates the deficiency is not known.

Research indicates that in many cases there appears to be a genetic (constitutional) predisposition to depression.

Known Risk Factors for Developing This Disorder

A family history of depression or related mental disorders:
   alcoholism or other substance abuse
   anorexia nervosa
   anxiety disorders
   manic-depressive mood disorder
   obsessive-compulsive disorder

Drugs That Can Cause This Disorder

Drug-induced depressions are more likely to occur in those who are genetically susceptible to depression. The following drugs may precipitate depression:
   alcohol
   amantadine
   amphetamines
   some antineoplastic drugs
   barbiturates
   benzodiazepines (in excess)
   certain beta-blocking drugs
   carbamazepine
   chloral hydrate
   clonidine
   cocaine
   cortisonelike steroids
   cycloserine
   digitalis (toxicity)
   disulfiram
   estrogen

ethambutol
guanethidine
haloperidol
hydralazine
indapamide
indomethacin
levodopa
methyldopa
opiates
oral contraceptives
pentazocine
some phenothiazines
physostigmine
prazosin
procainamide
progesterone
reserpine (and related drugs)
succinimide derivatives
sulfonamides

Note: See Appendix 16, Drug Classes, for individual generic drugs within respective drug classes.

Goals of Treatment

Can This Disorder Be Cured?
Since the primary definitive cause of major depressive disorder is not known, there is no permanently curative therapy.

Can This Disorder Be Treated Effectively?
Currently available therapies can provide excellent results in 80–90% of patients suffering from depression.

Specific Goals
- Alleviation of symptoms
- Termination of depression, restoration of normal mood
- Prevention of recurrence
- Prevention of swing from depression to manic psychosis (in manic-depressive disorder)

Health Professionals Who Participate in Managing This Disorder
Family physicians
General internists
Pediatricians
Geriatricians

Gynecologists
Obstetricians
Neurologists
Neuropsychiatrists
Psychiatrists
Clinical psychologists
Pharmacists
Physician assistants
Nurse practitioners
Psychiatric nurse specialists
Medical social workers

Currently Available Therapies for This Disorder

There are five major types of therapy currently used to treat all forms of depression. These include:

1. Antidepressant drug therapy
2. Psychotherapies
3. Combined drug therapy and psychotherapy
4. Electroconvulsive therapy (ECT)
5. Light therapy

Drug Therapy

SELECTIVE SEROTONIN REUPTAKE INHIBITORS (SSRIs)

- fluoxetine (Prozac)
- paroxetine (Paxil)
- sertraline (Zoloft)

SEROTONIN + NOREPINEPHRINE REUPTAKE INHIBITOR (SNRI)

- venlafaxine (Effexor)

TRICYCLIC ANTIDEPRESSANTS (TCAs)

- amitriptyline (Elavil, Endep)
- clomipramine (Anafranil)
- desipramine (Norpramin, Pertofrane)
- doxepin (Adapin, Sinequan)
- imipramine (Imavate, Janimine, Presamine, Tofranil)
- nortriptyline (Aventyl, Pamelor)
- protriptyline (Vivactil)
- trimipramine (Surmontil)

HETEROCYCLIC ANTIDEPRESSANTS

- amoxapine (Asendin)
- bupropion (Wellbutrin)
- maprotiline (Ludiomil)
- trazodone (Desyrel)

MONOAMINE OXIDASE INHIBITORS (MAOIs)

- isocarboxazid (Marplan)

- phenelzine (Nardil)
- tranylcypromine (Parnate)

OTHER DRUGS

- alprazolam (Xanax)
- lithium (Eskalith, Lithane, Lithobid, Lithotab)
- methylphenidate (Ritalin)

Psychotherapies

- *Behavioral therapy:* intended to modify problematic behavior patterns by systematic alteration of the environment in which the problems arise.
- *Cognitive therapy:* intended to favorably modify a person's ability to adapt by influencing his perceptions, attitudes, beliefs, and patterns of thinking.
- *Interpersonal therapy:* intended to identify, clarify, and resolve interpersonal difficulties, such as role disputes, role transition, social isolation, and prolonged grief reaction.

Electroconvulsive Therapy (ECT)

Formerly referred to as "electric shock therapy," this treatment consists of sending a low-voltage alternating current through portions of the brain to induce a seizure. The patient is appropriately sedated prior to treatment. This procedure is reserved for very severe depressions that are not responsive to drug therapy.

Light Therapy

The use of exposure to carefully controlled high-intensity light that theoretically corrects a seasonal deficiency of sunlight, which is thought to be responsible for the seasonal depression experienced by some individuals.

Management of Therapy

For Depressive Reactions

Reactive depressions are often mild and self-limiting; they usually respond well to supportive psychotherapy. Drug treatment is not necessary for everyone who is depressed. If this type of depression becomes severe or is unreasonably prolonged, a selective serotonin reuptake inhibitor (see SSRIs above) may be tried for four to six weeks to determine its effectiveness.

For Depressive Illness

- Major endogenous depressions are usually very responsive to an appropriate and adequate trial of antidepressant drug therapy. Spontaneous remissions often occur within 6 to 12 months, but recovery can be initiated earlier and greatly accelerated by proper medication. Adequate dosage and a sufficient period of treatment are essential to a successful outcome.

- Treatment is usually started with either (1) a secondary amine tricyclic (TCA) such as nortriptyline, or (2) a new-generation serotonin reuptake inhibitor (SSRI) such as fluoxetine, paroxetine, or sertraline. The tricyclic antidepressants are less expensive but do have a few troublesome side effects. The new SSRI antidepressants are more expensive but are better tolerated and more effective. If response is inadequate after a reasonable trial at maximal dosage, another tricyclic or SSRI antidepressant should be tried. If this fails, a monoamine oxidase inhibitor may be considered. Some cyclic depressions respond better if lithium is added to the antidepressant regimen.
- Not all depressions are recurrent. For a first episode, the antidepressant drug may be gradually reduced and discontinued after three to six months of a stable mood, free of depression.
- For the 50% of depressions that are recurrent, the optimal maintenance dose of the most effective drug should be determined and continued indefinitely.

For Dysthymia

This chronic state of mild depression is considered to be a neurotic personality trait. Careful and thorough psychiatric evaluation is needed to determine optimal therapy. Combination drug therapy and psychotherapy may be necessary. Behavioral and cognitive psychotherapies are being tried. Recommended medications are desipramine, with or without lithium, or fluoxetine.

Use of Selective Serotonin Reuptake Inhibitors (SSRIs)

- These are the drugs of choice for treating mild to moderate depression. They are suitable for outpatient therapy. They are generally better tolerated than the tricyclic antidepressants (TCAs). They are less likely to cause orthostatic hypotension (see Glossary), seizures, blurred vision, dry mouth, constipation, urinary retention, or heart rhythm disturbances.
- The most common adverse effects are headache, tremor, nervousness, agitation, and insomnia. These drugs are more likely to cause sexual dysfunction than the TCAs: inhibited orgasm in both men and women, impaired ejaculation.
- All SSRIs can cause life-threatening reactions if taken concurrently with monoamine oxidase inhibitors (MAOIs). Do not use drugs of these two classes together.

Use of Tricyclic Antidepressants (TCAs)

- These are the drugs of choice when drug treatment is deemed necessary for severe depression. They are also preferred for depressed patients who can benefit from sedation.

- They are 60% to 75% effective in treating major endogenous depressive illness. They may also be effective in treating severe reactive depressions. If one TCA (or equivalent) shows no significant benefit after three weeks of adequate dosage, it is advisable to try another drug of the same or similar class.
- Continual use on a regular schedule for two to five weeks is necessary to determine a drug's effectiveness in relieving depression. Treatment with all antidepressants is necessarily observational; a period of trial and error is unavoidable for both the selection of the best drug and the determination of optimal dosage.
- Periodic measurement of blood levels of the drug can be helpful in determining optimal dosage. During drug trials, and during maintenance treatment later, it is advisable to stay with the same brand (manufacturer) to ensure uniform results.
- Most drugs of this class cause drowsiness, especially during the first several weeks of use. Avoid alcoholic beverages and use extreme caution in driving and engaging in all hazardous activities.
- When the correct total daily dose has been determined, it can usually be taken as a single dose at bedtime.
- Use these drugs cautiously if you have glaucoma, prostatism, or a heart rhythm disorder.
- Avoid rapid withdrawal of TCAs; abrupt discontinuation may cause restlessness, headache, anxiety, insomnia, muscle aches, nausea. It is advisable to withdraw gradually over a period of 10 to 14 days.

Use of Heterocyclic Antidepressants

- Maprotiline (Ludiomil) may act more rapidly than TCAs; it is quite sedating. It is best avoided if you have a seizure disorder.
- Amoxapine (Asendin) is less sedating. It can cause Parkinson-like symptoms, restlessness, and tardive dyskinesia (rarely). Use should not exceed three to four months.
- Trazodone (Desyrel) is also sedating, but it has little or no atropinelike effects. It is very useful in the elderly and for those with glaucoma or prostatism.

Use of Monoamine Oxidase Inhibitors (MAOIs)

- Used to treat biologic endogenous depressions that do not respond to other classes of antidepressants, they are also useful for treating "atypical" and neurotic depressions that are characterized by marked anxiety, phobias, hypochondriasis, excessive eating, and excessive sleeping.
- Continual use on a regular schedule for two to five weeks is necessary to determine effectiveness in relieving depression. If switching from another antidepressant class to a MAOI, allow a "washout" period of 7 to 10 days before starting the MAOI. If switching from a MAOI to an

antidepressant of another class, allow a "washout" period of 14 days before starting the new antidepressant.

- Avoid concurrent use of over-the-counter diet pills, nosedrops, and cold and allergy preparations.
- Avoid foods and beverages that contain tyramine and similar compounds (see Appendix 9, Tyramine-Free Diet).
- MAOIs can cause low blood pressure, overstimulation, insomnia, confusion, nausea, vomiting, diarrhea, and fluid retention. The MAOIs can provoke an abrupt swing from depression to manic psychosis in manic-depressive (bipolar) disorder and MAOIs may activate psychosis in those with schizophrenia.
- Do not discontinue these drugs suddenly. A rebound depression can follow abrupt withdrawal.

Use of Lithium
- Can be 70% effective in stabilizing mood, especially in manic-depressive (bipolar) illness; reduces the frequency and severity of attacks of both mania and depression. Often effective in preventing recurrences of depression in unipolar (depression only) disorders.
- Must be taken in divided doses to avoid stomach irritation and excessively high (toxic) blood levels. Periodic measurements of blood levels are mandatory to maintain effective concentrations and to prevent toxicity. Blood samples should be taken 12 hours after the last dose. Recommended therapeutic blood level range: 0.3–1.3 mEq/L.
- When lithium proves to be effective in preventing recurrence of depression, it is very important to continue maintenance treatment when feeling well and free of depression.
- Mild side effects (not toxicity) include loss of appetite, metallic taste, indigestion, nausea, thirst, fatigue, tremor, fluid retention, acne.
- Early toxic effects include nausea, vomiting, dizziness, unsteadiness, weakness, slurred speech, muscle twitching, and confusion.
- While taking lithium, maintain a high liquid intake, but avoid excessive coffee, tea, and cola drinks.
- Do not restrict your salt intake.
- Use lithium cautiously if you have heart disease, kidney disease, or a thyroid disorder.
- Thyroid and kidney functions should be checked before and during lithium therapy. Lithium can induce hypothyroidism and a loss of kidney concentrating power (excessively dilute urine).

Use of Other Antidepressant Drugs
- Methylphenidate (Ritalin) may be tried for long-term treatment of selected elderly persons with depression.
- Alprazolam (Xanax), a benzodiazepine tranquilizer, may be useful for short-term treatment of minor depression with associated anxiety.

Therapeutic Drug Monitoring (Blood Levels)

Blood level measurements may be useful in monitoring response to the following antidepressant drugs:

Generic Name/Brand Name	Blood Level Range
amitriptyline/Elavil, etc.	120–250 ng/ml
amoxapine/Asendin	200–500 ng/ml
desipramine/Norpramin, Pertofrane	150–300 ng/ml
doxepin/Adapin, Sinequan	100–275 ng/ml
imipramine/Janimine, Tofranil	150–300 ng/ml
lithium/Lithobid, Lithotabs, etc.	0.3–1.3 mEq/L
nortriptyline/Aventyl, Pamelor	50–150 ng/ml
combined with amitriptyline	120–250 ng/ml
protriptyline/Vivactil	70–250 ng/ml

Ancillary Drug Treatment (as required)

For mild anxiety:
• alprazolam (Xanax)

For severe anxiety and agitation:
• thioridazine (Mellaril)
• thiothixene (Navane)

For psychosis:
• amitriptyline and perphenazine (Etrafon, Triavil)

For constipation:
• docusate (Colace, Doxinate, etc.)

Note: Drug selection, dosage, and administration schedule must be determined by the physician for each patient individually.

Important Points to Consider

• Appropriate drug therapy in combination with psychotherapy is effective in treating up to 90% of patients with significant depression.
• In order to determine the effectiveness of treatment, an antidepressant drug must be taken continually in adequate dosage for a period of four to eight weeks.
• If an adequate trial of drug therapy does not yield a satisfactory response, psychotherapy should be considered. Drug therapy and psychotherapy used together are more effective than either method used alone.
• After a satisfactory therapeutic response is obtained, drug treatment should be continued for at least another six to nine months to avoid relapse. Withdrawal of medication must be gradual with tapering dosage over a period of weeks to months and under careful monitoring.
• Drug-induced sexual dysfunction (impaired erection, delayed ejaculation, inhibited orgasm) may be a side effect of most antidepressant drugs.

Possible Drug Interactions of Significance

Because of the number of drugs that may be used to manage this disorder, adequate consideration of the volume and complexity of potential drug interactions is beyond the scope of this book. Consult *The Essential Guide to Prescription Drugs*, or a similar drug reference book for possible interactions of significance (see Appendix 17, Drug Information Sources).

Treatment Outcomes

	Methods of Treatment		
	Drug Therapy	*Psychotherapy*	*Combined Therapy*
OUTCOMES			
Beneficial	50–65%	45–60%	50–65%
Minor risks (side effects)	50%	None	50%
Stopped therapy	3–10%	None	3–10%
Major risks	Less than 1%	None	Less than 1%

Special Considerations for Women

Pregnancy

The following antidepressant drugs are designated Pregnancy Category D (see Appendix 15, FDA Pregnancy Categories):

amitriptyline (Elavil, Endep, Etrafon, Triavil, etc.)
imipramine (Janimine, Tofranil, etc.)
lithium (Lithobid, Lithonate, Lithotabs, etc.)
nortriptyline (Aventyl, Pamelor)

Breast-Feeding

Most antidepressant drugs are secreted in breast milk. Ask your physician for guidance regarding nursing. If antidepressant drug therapy is needed, it is generally considered safest to refrain from breast-feeding.

Special Considerations for the Elderly

Approximately 25% of older adults report symptoms of depression, but only 1% have major depressive disorder. Depression in the elderly is more likely to result from a medical condition or a dementing illness. Potential causes for symptoms that suggest depression include:

abnormally low blood potassium level
alcohol abuse
Alzheimer's disease
cancer
cerebral infarction (stroke)
congestive heart failure
drug-induced dementias
hypochondriasis (preoccupation with imaginary disease)

hypothyroidism, apathetic hyperthyroidism
multiple infarction dementia ("mini-strokes")
Parkinson's disease

True depression in the elderly usually responds well to combination drug therapy and supportive psychotherapy. Drug dosages should be reduced appropriately, and response to therapy must be monitored closely. In the absence of significant organic brain disease, the elderly tolerate electroconvulsive therapy (ECT) well and find it beneficial.

Quality of Life Considerations

Depressions of any type may become recurrent or chronic illnesses. Quite often, they are underdiagnosed and undertreated. Individuals with a major depressive disorder may experience a quality of life significantly worse than the nondepressed person with hypertension, coronary artery disease, diabetes, arthritis, chronic back pain, and numerous other maladies.

It is essential that depressed individuals, their families, friends, and associates all recognize and understand that true depressive states are genuine medical disorders analogous to the diseases mentioned above. Effective therapies are available. All individuals so afflicted should be urged to accept appropriate help and strive to achieve an acceptable quality of life.

Resources

Recommended Reading

Depression Is a Treatable Illness: A Patient's Guide, Department of Health and Human Services, Agency for Health Care Policy and Research, Rockville, MD 20852; Publication No. AHCPR 93-0553, April 1993. For a copy call 1-800-358-9295.

Understanding Depression: A Complete Guide to Its Diagnosis and Treatment, D.F. Klein and P.H. Wender. New York: Oxford University Press, 1993.

How to Heal Depression, H.H. Bloomfield, M.D., and Peter McWilliams. Los Angeles: Prelude Press, 1994. To order a copy call 1-800-LIFE-101.

A delightfully different and effective book.

Additional Information and Services

Depressives Anonymous: Recovery From Depression
329 East 62nd Street
New York, NY 10021
Phone: (212) 689-2600
Publications available.

Emotions Anonymous
P.O. Box 4245

St. Paul, MN 55104-0245
Phone: (612) 647-9712; Fax: (612) 647-1593
Telecommunications services: telephone referrals to local chapters. Regional groups: 48. Local groups: 1,600. Publications available.

National Depressive and Manic-Depressive Association
730 North Franklin Street, Suite 501
Chicago, IL 60610
Phone: 1-800-82-NDMDA, (312) 642-0049; Fax: (312) 642-7243
Offers information, one-to-one support, referrals by telephone. Local groups: 190. Publications, audio- and videotapes available.

National Mental Health Information Center
1020 Prince Street
Alexandria, VA 23314-2971
Phone: 1-800-969-6642

Disease Management Expertise
Depression Awareness, Recognition and Treatment
National Institutes of Health
Room 10-85
5600 Fishers Lane
Rockville, MD 20857
Phone: 1-800-421-4211

DIABETES MELLITUS

Other Names Insulin-dependent diabetes mellitus (IDDM), Type I diabetes; noninsulin-dependent diabetes mellitus (NIDDM), Type II diabetes

Prevalence/Incidence in U.S.
Current estimate: 12 to 15 million; approximately one-half are undiagnosed Type I diabetes: 10%; Type II diabetes: 90%
Estimated new cases annually: 650,000
Estimated deaths annually: 160,000; a major contributor to an additional 300,000

Age Group

Age Group	% of Total
Under 18 years	2%
18 to 44 years	15%
45 to 64 years	44%
65 to 74 years	27%
Over 75 years	12%

Male-to-Female Ratio Type I—same incidence in men and women; Type II—greater incidence in women.

Principal Features and Natural History

Diabetes mellitus is a chronic disorder of carbohydrate, protein, and fat metabolism that renders the body unable to convert foods properly into energy for vital functions. The principal feature of this disorder is the uncontrolled increase in the amount of sugar (glucose) in the blood, the result of insulin deficiency. The key factor in Type I diabetes is the inability of the pancreas to produce sufficient insulin. In Type II diabetes, sufficient insulin may be present but body tissues develop a resistance to its action. There is a disproportionate risk of developing diabetes in American Blacks, Hispanic Americans, Native Americans, Asian Americans, and Pacific Island Americans thought to be due to cultural changes in lifestyle. Factors that contribute to the development of Type II diabetes include inadequate physical activity; high-fat, low-fiber diets; obesity; blood lipid abnormalities; hypertension; and aging.

Another inherent feature of diabetes is the predisposition to develop atherosclerosis (see Glossary) of large and small arteries. This is responsible for the serious complications that are common in late stage diabetes: vascular degeneration in the retina of the eyes and in the brain, heart, kidneys, and lower extremities. In adults, diabetes is the most common cause of new-onset blindness, endstage kidney disease, and lower extremity amputations.

In spite of the advances made in our understanding of diabetes and its proper management, it is still one of the leading causes of serious illness and death in this country. This is due in part to the lack of forceful education by the health care community regarding the importance of rigorous control of blood glucose, and also to the generally poor compliance of many patients in all aspects of treatment.

Type I (10% of All Diabetes)

Also referred to as juvenile-onset diabetes, this form occurs most commonly in children and adolescents with peak onset from 11 to 14 years of age. However, it can begin at any age. Individuals are usually thin or normal in weight (nonobese). It generally requires lifelong insulin for control of blood glucose and for the prevention of acidosis and long-term complications.

Type II (90% of All Diabetes)

Also known as adult-onset diabetes, this form occurs most commonly after 40 years of age with peak onset from 45 to 64 years. Up to 80% of individuals are obese. Usually it does not require lifelong insulin for control and is not prone to development of acidosis. It has always been thought of as a relatively mild disease. However, it is now recognized to be just as formidable as Type I diabetes in its potential to cause long-term vascular complications.

Diagnostic Symptoms and Signs
Excessive hunger (polyphagia)
Excessive thirst (polydipsia)
Excessive urination (polyuria)
Weight loss (in spite of large food intake)
Blurred vision
Numbness and tingling sensation in feet (paresthesia)
Orthostatic hypotension (see Glossary)
Nausea, vomiting, abdominal pain (associated with acidosis)
Fatigue, drowsiness, progressing to coma

Diagnostic Tests and Procedures
Measurements of blood glucose levels; the following values are diagnostic for diabetes:
- Fasting plasma glucose (FPG): over 140 mg/dl on two separate occasions
- Random plasma glucose (RPG): over 200 mg/dl
- Glucose tolerance test (GTT): any timed interval blood sample—30, 60, 90, or 120 minutes (after glucose administration)— that contains over 200 mg/dl indicates diabetes.

Analysis of urine for glucose (glycosuria): glucose (sugar) is not normally present in the urine; when the blood glucose level exceeds 175 mg/dl (the kidney threshold for excreting glucose), it will be present in the urine, indicating diabetes.

Analysis of urine for ketones (acids derived from fats and carbohydrates) not normally present in the urine; the presence of ketones denotes acidosis due to diabetes.

Measurement of glycosylated hemoglobin (glycohemoglobin, glycated hemoglobin, Hb A_{1c}): an indicator of the mean plasma glucose level during the previous 6 to 12 weeks; the following values are used to monitor long-term blood glucose level control:
- Normal range: 4–6%
- Good diabetic control: 7%
- Fair diabetic control: 10%
- Poor diabetic control: 13–20%

Diagnostic "Markers" for This Disorder
The following definitive tests establish the diagnosis of IDDM:
Islet cell autoantibodies (ICAs): positive test result in 80% of new-onset IDDM patients. The islet cells in the pancreas produce insulin and glucagon; autoantibodies destroy the islets, resulting in insulin deficiency—diabetes (see Appendix 5, The Immune System).

Serum C-peptide (an insulin marker): none present within five minutes following test injection of 1 mg of glucagon, indicating the inability of the islet cells to produce insulin.

Similar Conditions That May Confuse Diagnosis
acanthosis nigricans
acromegaly
adverse effects of some medicinal drugs (see below)
chronic pancreatitis
Cushing's syndrome
glucagonoma
pheochromocytoma

Causes

Established Causes
The primary definitive cause of diabetes is not known.

Theoretical Causes
For Type I IDDM: This is currently thought to be an autoimmune disorder, possibly triggered by a viral infection of the pancreas in a susceptible individual. The damaged pancreatic islets produce little or no insulin.

For Type II NIDDM: There appears to be a genetic predisposition for the development of this form of diabetes. Insulin levels may be low, normal, or high; diabetes is due to marked resistance of body tissues to the action of insulin.

Known Risk Factors for Developing This Disorder
Predisposition to autoimmune disorders
Family history of diabetes in parents or siblings
Obesity: 20% or more over ideal weight
History of diabetes only during pregnancy (gestational diabetes)
The presence of syndrome X: concurrent hypertension, blood lipid disorders, premature atherosclerosis, and insulin resistance

Drugs That Can Cause This Disorder
The following drugs may impair the secretion of insulin or induce resistance to insulin:
    beta-adrenergic-blocking drugs
    calcium-channel-blocking drugs
    clonidine
    cortisonelike steroids (glucocorticoids)
    cyclosporine
    estrogen
    ethacrynic acid

furosemide
indomethacin
lithium
nicotinic acid
oral contraceptives
pentamidine
phenothiazines
phenytoin
thiazide diuretics
tricyclic antidepressants

See Appendix 16, Drug Classes, for specific generic drugs within respective drug classes.

Goals of Treatment

Can This Disorder Be Cured?

There is no known curative treatment at this time.

Can This Disorder Be Treated Effectively?

Very effective therapies are available for managing diabetes and preventing complications. These consist of dietary modifications, regular exercise, weight control, and the appropriate use of medications.

Specific Goals

- Normalization of carbohydrate, protein, and fat metabolism insofar as possible; control of blood glucose levels; elimination of acidosis
- Elimination of symptoms; restoration of well-being
- Prevention of hypoglycemia (insulin "shock")
- Prevention of recurrent acidosis
- Promotion of normal growth and development in diabetic children
- Prevention or minimization of late complications
- Achievement of normal life expectancy

Health Professionals Who Participate in Managing This Disorder

Family physicians
General internists
Pediatricians
Geriatricians
Clinical endocrinologists
Diabetes specialists
Ophthalmologists
Optometrists
Neurologists
Nephrologists

Peripheral vascular specialists
Vascular surgeons
Pharmacists
Physician assistants
Nurse practitioners
Dietitians/Nutritionists
Medical social workers

Currently Available Therapies for This Disorder

Nondrug Treatment Methods
- Dietary management
- Weight control
- Exercise programs

Drug Therapy
The following drugs are currently used to regulate plasma glucose levels:
- The insulins: injectable drugs of choice for glucose control
- The sulfonylureas: oral hypoglycemic drugs
  - First generation (1956–1966):
    acetohexamide (Dymelor)
    chlorpropamide (Diabinese)
    tolazamide (Tolinase)
    tolbutamide (Orinase)
  - Second generation (1970–1990):
    glimepiride (Amaryl)
    glipizide (Glucotrol)
    glyburide (DiaBeta, Micronase, Glynase)
- metformin (Glucophage)
- acarbose (Precose)

New Drugs in Development for Treating This Disorder
There are more than 20 new medicines in development to control diabetes and its complications. These include:
- Nicotinamide: studies to determine its ability to interfere with the immune system's attack against islet cells, delaying or preventing Type I IDDM
- Islet cell transplants: encapsulation of insulin-producing cells in semipermeable membranes that can be transplanted into patients without immunosuppressive therapy
- New dosage forms of insulin to be taken orally
- Insulin skin patches to replace syringe and needle

Management of Therapy
- "Good control" consists of the optimal balance of properly selected foods, exercise, and drugs—either insulin and/or a sulfonylurea in cor-

rect dosage. The degree of control is estimated by periodic (but not daily) measurement of blood sugar levels or urine sugar content.

- "Tight control" consists of maintaining a fasting blood sugar between 100 and 140 mg, and a 2-hour (after eating) blood sugar between 140 and 200 mg. These values correspond to a glycosylated hemoglobin of less than 7%. Consideration must be given to the possible benefits of "tight control" versus the possible risks of inducing hypoglycemia.

- "Tight control" is appropriate for the young diabetic who is otherwise healthy, free of coronary artery and cerebral circulatory disease, capable of excellent self-care, and not living alone. It is not appropriate for the elderly, those with circulatory disorders of the brain or heart, those with established complications of longstanding diabetes, and those with other serious disorders.

- Although more expensive and inconvenient, the home monitoring of blood sugar levels is the method of choice for managing diabetic control. An accurate blood glucose monitor is recommended for this purpose.

- The use of urine testing strips for the detection of urine sugar and ketones is a useful and practical alternative to the use of blood sugar strips. Regular testing of urine before meals and at bedtime provides adequate information for the proper adjustment of insulin dosage schedules and the prevention of hypoglycemia and acidosis. Accuracy is improved when the bladder is first emptied and the urine for testing is collected 30 minutes later; the sugar content of this second voiding is more representative of the current blood sugar level.

- If urine testing reveals the repeated presence of ketones, consult your physician promptly.

- The following drugs can cause a *false positive* test result for urine sugar when using Clinitest: aspirin (with doses larger than 2400 mg/day), ascorbic acid (vitamin C), cephalosporins, chloral hydrate, chloramphenicol, isoniazid, levodopa, methyldopa, nalidixic acid, penicillin G, probenecid, streptomycin.

- The following drugs can cause a *false negative* test result for urine sugar when using Diastix or Testape: aspirin (with doses larger than 2400 mg/day), ascorbic acid (vitamin C), levodopa, methyldopa.

- The following drugs can cause a *false positive* test result for urine ketones when using Acetest or Ketostix: aspirin (in moderate to high doses), levodopa, phenazopyridine (Ketostix only).

- Learn to recognize the early indications of hypoglycemia and what to do to correct it. Signs that warn of a developing insulin reaction include hunger, sweating, headache, dizziness, nervousness, trembling, blurred vision, drowsiness, confusion, inability to think, sense of inebriation. At the first indication of impending hypoglycemia, take sugar immediately: five small sugar cubes; or 2 teaspoons or two packets of granulated sugar; or 1 cup of fruit juice; or one candy bar. An alternative treatment is the injection of 1 mg of glucagon, repeated in 5 to 10 minutes if necessary. Glucagon is a pancreatic hormone that increases the level of blood sugar.

- Learn to recognize the early indications of acidosis. These include the slow development of increasing thirst, excessive urination, drowsiness, fatigue, nausea, vomiting, stomach pain.
- The use of beta-blocking drugs (especially in high doses) may predispose to hypoglycemia and mask its symptoms.

For Type I, IDDM

- Insulin is usually a lifelong requirement for control. Sulfonylureas (oral hypoglycemics) are not as effective and are generally not used.
- Insulin requirements will vary continually throughout a lifetime. Therefore, you must learn how to manage your diabetes on a day-by-day basis, modifying insulin types and dosage schedules as necessary, according to the results of regular blood or urine sugar testing.
- For the newly diagnosed diabetic who is not acutely ill and is without complications, the usual American procedure for initiating treatment is to give a single morning dose of 15 to 30 units of an intermediate-acting insulin (NPH or Lente) before breakfast; the dose is then increased by 5 units every 48 hours as required to achieve normal blood sugar levels. The British method is to start with 6 to 10 units of an intermediate-acting insulin given twice daily, before the morning and evening meals. Either method will relieve most symptoms in 90% of cases within four days.
- The optimal schedule of insulin injections for regulating the disordered metabolism is determined by periodic monitoring of blood sugar levels at appropriate times during the 24-hour day. In this way individual patterns of blood sugar fluctuation and response to insulin can be studied so that the most appropriate types and doses of insulin are given in proper relationship to eating.
- A most effective and practical method of providing adequate insulin for the average diabetic is to give a mixture (one injection) of a rapid-acting insulin (Regular) and an intermediate-acting insulin (NPH or Lente) 20 to 30 minutes before the morning and evening meals, just two injections daily. This scheme provides for easy modification of doses of each type of insulin as necessary to obtain smooth control throughout 24 hours.
- During periods of stress—infections, injuries, surgery—insulin requirements will increase. Consult your physician for guidance if you have difficulty in making the necessary adjustments of insulin dosage, food intake, etc.

- Even during periods of fasting, small amounts of insulin are necessary to control blood sugar and prevent acidosis.

For Type II, NIDDM

- Diet is of primary importance and should be tried diligently before starting drugs. Dietary goals are reduction of blood sugar and correction of obesity. Seventy-five percent of cases of Type II diabetes can be controlled by diet alone.
- If an adequate trial of dietary management fails, either sulfonylurea drugs (oral hypoglycemics) or insulin may be added to the treatment program. If the blood sugar is only moderately above normal, a sulfonylurea may be tried. If the blood sugar is quite high and the individual is thin, it is best to initiate drug treatment with insulin. After the blood sugar has been stabilized for three to four weeks, the insulin may be withdrawn and a sulfonylurea may be started to determine its effectiveness. Occasionally, the best control of blood sugar will be achieved by using a combination of insulin and a sulfonylurea drug.
- The major reaction to sulfonylureas is hypoglycemia. It is most likely to occur in the elderly, alcoholics, and those with significant impairment of liver or kidney function. Hypoglycemic reactions occur most frequently with the use of chlorpropamide (Diabinese), the longest acting sulfonylurea.
- If you experience a primary failure (on initial trial) or a secondary failure (after a temporary period of effectiveness) on attempting control with a sulfonylurea, you may need insulin to manage your diabetes successfully.
- Insulin is used primarily to control the levels of blood sugar. It is not required to prevent acidosis except under stressful conditions, such as infections, trauma, or surgery.
- Type II diabetes is often well controlled with a single daily dose of an intermediate-acting insulin. Some individuals with a high degree of insulin resistance may require unusually high doses of insulin to achieve satisfactory control.

Use of Insulins

- Twenty percent of all diabetics require insulin for satisfactory control.
- The peak action times and the duration of action of available insulins vary greatly from person to person. An understanding of these differences is necessary for planning an insulin schedule and adjusting it to control your individual pattern of blood sugar fluctuations during each 24-hour day. Each individual will show variations of absorption from one injection site to another and from day to day. Insulin programs must be tailored to each person individually based on response to trials. All insulin schedules need adjustment from time to time. The following chart illustrates the characteristics of the three principal types of insulin.

Type of Insulin	Peak Action (hours)	Duration (hours)	Hypoglycemia Most Likely to Occur:
Short-Acting			
Lispro (Humalog)	0.5–1	3–4	Before Lunch
Regular	2–4	5–7	Before lunch
Semilente	2–8	12–16	Before lunch
Actrapid	2.5–5	8	Before lunch
Semitard	7	9	Early afternoon
Velosulin	2–5	8	Before lunch
Humulin R	2–5	6–8	Before lunch
Intermediate-Acting			
Lente	8–12	18–28	Late afternoon
NPH	6–12	18–28	Late afternoon
Monotard	7–15	18–24	Late afternoon
Lentard	8–12	16–24	Late afternoon
Insulatard	4–12	16–24	Mid-afternoon
Humulin N	6–12	14–24	Late afternoon
Novolin N	4–12	18–24	Mid-afternoon
Long-Acting			
Protamine Zinc	14–24	24–36	During night–early morning
Ultralente	18–24	32–36	During night–early morning
Ultratard	10–28	24–36	During night–early morning

- Most insulin-dependent diabetics require from 20 to 60 units of insulin daily. If the requirement reaches 200 units/day, a marked degree of insulin resistance has developed. This is best treated with highly purified pork insulin or human insulin.
- Most of the time satisfactory control can be achieved with an intermediate-acting insulin, or with the addition of a short-acting insulin. Regular insulin can be mixed with either Lente or NPH in the same syringe and given as a single injection. The mixture retains the short and intermediate characteristics of action. Long-acting insulins are rarely necessary and are seldom used.
- Hypoglycemia that occurs during the night (excessive insulin effect) causes a "rebound" hyperglycemia that is detected by blood or urine sugar testing the next morning. This is known as the Somogyi effect. The proper adjustment is to reduce the dose of the long-acting insulin taken in the morning or the dose of the intermediate-acting insulin taken before the evening meal; this will prevent the nocturnal hypoglycemia that causes the confusing high blood or urine sugar on arising.
- If a true allergy to insulin develops, or if the fatty tissue under the skin at the sites of insulin injection should disappear (lipoatrophy), change to a form of human insulin.
- If insulin use is to be intermittent (as in some cases of Type II diabetes), it is best to use human insulin to reduce the possibility of developing insulin antibodies that cause insulin resistance.

- Insulin pumps using either Regular or Ultralente insulin have been developed for use in selected individuals. Although they are capable of providing excellent control, their use is quite complex and demanding. They are suitable only for the highly motivated and educated individual who needs and is dedicated to achieving "tight control."

Use of Sulfonylurea (Oral Hypoglycemic) Drugs

- These drugs are used primarily for the treatment of Type II, NIDDM, in those whose diabetes is not adequately controlled by diet and exercise and who cannot or will not take insulin. Currently glipizide (Glucotrol) and glyburide (DiaBeta, Micronase) are most commonly used.

    The best candidates for a trial of sulfonylureas

       are over 50 years old;

       are otherwise healthy;

       are not allergic to "sulfa" drugs;

       have no tendency to develop acidosis;

       have an insulin requirement of less than 30 units/day;

       prefer tablets by mouth to injections.

    Sulfonylureas are not suitable for treating

       Type I, insulin-dependent diabetes;

       the acutely ill diabetic patient with acidosis;

       the diabetic with infection or with injury, or undergoing surgery;

       the diabetic using long-term cortisonelike steroids;

       the pregnant diabetic;

       the diabetic whose blood sugar is over 300 mg.

    Sulfonylureas should be used with caution in treating

       the very old;

       alcoholics;

       those taking multiple drugs;

       those with significantly impaired liver or kidney function;

       those who comply poorly with recommendations.

- Recommended dosage schedules:

	Duration (hours)	Doses/day
Short-Acting		
tolbutamide	6–12	2–3
Intermediate-Acting		
acetohexamide	12–24	1–2
glimepiride	2–24	1
glipizide	18–30	1–2
glyburide	10–30	1–2
tolazamide	10–18	1–2
Long-Acting		
chlorpropamide	60	1

- All sulfonylureas can cause hypoglycemia. Because of its accumulative effects and long period of action, chlorpropamide requires the greatest caution in use; any hypoglycemic reaction is apt to be quite prolonged.
- Sulfonylureas as a group have a high rate of primary failure (40%). A primary failure is an inability to control hyperglycemia after three months of continual treatment with adequate dosage. Secondary failures (25–30%) occur when a sulfonylurea drug loses its effectiveness after an initial period of demonstrated ability to control hyperglycemia.
- During apparently successful long-term use of a sulfonylurea, it is prudent to periodically reduce the dosage and gradually withdraw the drug to determine if its continued use is justified. The success rate of adequate control by long-term use of sulfonylureas is no more than 20–30%.
- There appears to be a change of attitude regarding the concurrent use of sulfonylureas and insulin. Some experts now recommend that if insulin is necessary for adequate control, the sulfonylurea can be continued to advantage at half the maximal dose.

Use of Metformin

This orally administered drug is used to lower blood sugar levels in Type II NIDDM. Its action improves tissue sensitivity to insulin and reduces insulin resistance that is common in this form of diabetes. It is as effective as the sulfonylureas. It can be used alone or in combination with a sulfonylurea drug as necessary to achieve satisfactory control. Contraindications to its use include: impaired liver or kidney function; impaired heart or lung function; severe infections; alcohol abuse; use of intravenous contrast agents for X-ray studies; a history of lactic acidosis.

Use of Acarbose

This orally administered drug may be used in conjunction with insulin or a sulfonylurea drug to lower blood sugar levels that follow a meal. It should not be taken together with metformin. Taken at the beginning of a meal, it impairs the digestion of complex carbohydrates and reduces the absorption of glucose, resulting in lower blood glucose levels. It may cause excessive intestinal gas, cramping, and diarrhea, which diminish with continued use.

Ancillary Drug Treatment (as required)

For yeast infections of skin:
- ciclopirox (Loprox)
- clotrimazole (Lotrimin)
- haloprogin (Halotex)
- miconazole (Micatin)
- nystatin (Mycostatin)

For yeast infections of the vagina:
- clotrimazole (Gyne-Lotrimin, Mycelex-G)
- miconazole (Monistat)

For diabetic diarrhea:
- diphenoxylate (Lomotil)
- loperamide (Imodium)

For peripheral neuritis:
- carbamazepine (Tegretol) and amitriptyline (Elavil) concurrently

For neurogenic bladder:
- bethanechol (Urecholine)

For high blood pressure:
- an ACE inhibitor antihypertensive
  See the Profile of hypertension in this section.

Note: Drug selection, dosage, and administration schedule must be determined by the physician for each patient individually.

Important Points to Consider

- The optimal control of diabetes requires an ongoing balance of diet, exercise, and medication: insulin, a sulfonylurea, acarbose, or metformin. To properly manage the dosage and timing of all drugs, it is necessary to perform regular self-monitoring of blood glucose levels.
- For insulin-dependent patients, blood glucose levels should be measured at least twice daily, before breakfast and supper. For "tight control," testing should be done four times daily, before meals and at bedtime. For those with Type II diabetes, measurements once daily may be sufficient; for those who do not require medication, monitoring three days a week is usually adequate.
- Intensive control of blood glucose levels (three or more insulin injections daily governed by self-monitoring four times daily) can result in a 76% reduction of retinal damage, a 56% reduction in the risk of kidney damage, and a 61% reduction in the risk of nerve damage (late complications of diabetes).
- The use of "tight control" does increase the risk of insulin shock (hypoglycemia) two to three times. Patients should check their blood glucose level for impending hypoglycemia immediately before driving or other dangerous activities.

Possible Drug Interactions of Significance

Because of the number of drugs that may be used to manage this disorder, adequate consideration of the volume and complexity of potential drug interactions is beyond the scope of this book. Consult *The Essential Guide to Prescription Drugs*, or a similar drug reference book for possible interactions of significance (see Appendix 17, Drug Information Sources).

Special Considerations for Women

The use of oral contraceptives by young women with Type I IDDM does not pose an additional risk for the development of early diabetic retinal vascular disease or kidney damage.

Women with Type II NIDDM have a four- to fivefold increased risk for developing cardiovascular disease. When feasible, women should adhere to strict control of blood glucose as consistently as possible to prevent complications.

Pregnancy

- Pregnant women who are at high risk for diabetes should be monitored closely for the development of gestational diabetes by periodic measurement of blood glucose levels.
- Sulfonylurea drugs should not be used to treat gestational diabetes.
- Metformin is designated Pregnancy Category B. However, the manufacturer does not recommend the use of this drug during pregnancy.
- The following drugs are designated Pregnancy Category D and should not be used during pregnancy: acetohexamide, chlorpropamide, tolazamide, tolbutamide (see Appendix 15, FDA Pregnancy Categories).
- Because birth defects have been associated with poorly controlled blood glucose levels during pregnancy, experts recommend that insulin be used exclusively to manage all pregnant diabetics.

Breast-Feeding

Insulin treatment of the mother has no adverse effects on the nursing infant. Breast-feeding may decrease insulin requirements; dosage adjustment may be necessary.

Oral hypoglycemic drugs should not be used during breast-feeding. It is advisable to avoid these drugs or refrain from nursing.

Special Considerations for the Elderly

Every effort should be made to avoid episodes of hypoglycemia in older persons. "Tight" control of blood glucose levels is not advised. Because of their long duration of action, diabinese and glyburide should not be used by the elderly.

Sulfonylurea drugs should be started at 50% of the usual recommended dose for younger individuals.

The Role of Prevention in This Disorder

Primary Prevention

There is no known method for the primary prevention of diabetes at this time.

Individuals with a strong family history of severe diabetes may wish to consider genetic counseling and family planning.

Secondary Prevention

Long-term studies clearly demonstrate that near-normalization of blood glucose levels in Type I IDDM patients can delay the development and progression of retinal vascular disease by 76%, kidney damage by 56%, and peripheral neuritis by 61%.

Resources

Additional Information and Services

American Diabetes Association
National Service Center
P.O. Box 25757
1660 Duke Street
Alexandria, VA 22314
Phone: (703) 549-1500, 1-800-232-3472; Fax: (703) 836-7439
   State groups: 55. Local groups: 800. Publications available.

Joslin Diabetes Center
One Joslin Place
Boston, MA 02215
Phone: (617) 732-2400; Fax: (617) 732-2562
   Publications available.

Juvenile Diabetes Foundation International
432 Park Avenue South, 16th Floor
New York, NY 10016-8013
Phone: 1-800-JDF-CURE, (212) 889-7575
Telecommunications services: Fax: (212) 725-7259
   Local groups: 150. Publications, films, tapes available.

Disease Management Expertise

CURRENT CLINICAL TRIALS

   Diabetes Prevention Trial—Type I:
Operations Coordinating Center
University of Miami School of Medicine
P.O. Box 016960 (D-110)
Miami, FL 33101
Phone: 1-800-425-8361, (305) 243-6146; Fax: (305) 243-4484
   Call or write for detailed information on eligibility and treatment methods to be tested.

   Diabetes Prevention Trial—Type II:
The National Institutes of Health is sponsoring the first nationwide study to determine whether Type II diabetes can be either prevented or delayed in persons who are prone to develop this disease. Twenty-five

medical centers across the country are conducting the study. They are seeking 4,000 participants. For a list of participating medical centers call 1-888-377-5646.

EMPHYSEMA
(em fi SEE ma)

Other Names Classic emphysema, alpha-antitrypsin deficiency emphysema, chronic obstructive pulmonary disease, COPD

Prevalence/Incidence in U.S.
Current estimate: Approximately 2.4 million
Estimated deaths annually: 90,000

Age Group
For late-onset classic emphysema: 55 years and older
For early-onset (alpha-antitrypsin deficiency): 30 to 40 years

Male-to-Female Ratio Approximately 2 to 1

Principal Features and Natural History

For Late-Onset Classic Emphysema
The lungs contain more than 200 million tiny air sacs (alveoli) that perform the vital functions of transferring oxygen from incoming air to the blood and carbon dioxide from the blood to outgoing air. The walls of alveoli consist of very thin and fragile elastic tissue that in some individuals is quite vulnerable to damage by air pollutants: tobacco smoke, ozone, carbon monoxide, particulate matters, etc. As a result of long periods of exposure, alveolar walls are destroyed and significant portions of lung tissue are progressively converted into inelastic, overly inflated cavities. As the elasticity of tissue is lost, the lungs are unable to expand and contract normally. Small bronchial tubes leading to alveoli may collapse, obstructing airflow and trapping air within the lungs. Eventually, irreversible lung damage results in seriously impaired breathing, increased blood pressure within the lungs, and subsequent heart failure (cor pulmonale). The characteristic breathing pattern consists of effortless inhaling but marked impairment in the ability to exhale. Thus the lungs are never completely emptied, significant amounts of oxygen-poor air remain within, and the body's ongoing oxygen needs are never fully met. Breathing becomes an ever-increasing struggle, physical activity is drastically impeded, and the sufferer eventually becomes dependent upon the administration of oxygen, even at rest.

For Early-Onset Alpha-Antitrypsin Deficiency Emphysema

This rare form of emphysema (2% of all emphysema cases) afflicts about 20,000 to 40,000 Americans. Its technical name is "alpha 1-antitrypsin deficiency-related emphysema." It is genetically transmitted and is due to a missing single gene on chromosome number 14. This gene bears the code that directs the liver to produce a protein known as alpha 1-antitrypsin (AAT). This protein is a lung protector: it modulates the action of tissue enzymes that destroy bacteria, remove cellular debris, and, in the process, also damage lung tissue itself. As a result of AAT deficiency, the balance of competing activities is shifted toward lung destruction, and emphysema is inevitable. Tobacco smoke and other air pollutants hasten the process. The only available therapy is AAT replacement using human blood donor plasma. This requires intravenous administration every week for life—a costly and difficult therapy. Since AAT deficiency involves a single gene, it is now feasible to attempt a cure using gene therapy. Animal research is already underway, and clinical trials of human gene therapy for AAT deficiency are likely within the decade (see Appendix 11, Genetic Disorders and Gene Therapy).

Diagnostic Symptoms and Signs
Progressive shortness of breath on exertion
Fatigability, loss of stamina and endurance
Coughing (due to associated chronic bronchitis)
Expanding rib cage ("barrel chest")

Diagnostic Tests and Procedures
X-ray examinations of the lungs
Lung function tests
Arterial blood gas analysis
Blood assay for alpha 1-antitrypsin deficiency

Similar Conditions That May Confuse Diagnosis
Asthmatic bronchitis
Chronic bronchitis (often coexists with emphysema)

Causes

Established Causes
Alpha 1-antitrypsin deficiency.

Known Risk Factors for Developing This Disorder
Cigarette smoking (responsible for 82% of chronic lung disease)
Occupational exposures to noxious dusts and fumes

Air pollutants
Long-term chronic bronchitis

Goals of Treatment

Can This Disorder Be Cured?
Irreversible damage to lungs and heart cannot be cured.

Can This Disorder Be Treated Effectively?
Available drugs can provide some measure of symptomatic relief.

Specific Goals
- Prudent control of coughing and mucus production if present
- Suppression of bacterial infections
- Bronchodilator therapy to ease breathing
- Treatment of congestive heart failure if present

Health Professionals Who Participate in Managing This Disorder
Family physicians
General internists
Geriatricians
Pulmonologists
Behavioral psychologists
Thoracic surgeons
Transplant surgeons
Pharmacists
Physician assistants
Nurse practitioners
Physical therapists
Medical social workers

Currently Available Therapies for This Disorder

Drug Therapy
- albuterol (Proventil, Ventolin)
- metaproterenol (Alupent, Metaprel)
- salmeterol (Serevent)
- theophylline
- ipratropium (Atrovent)
- cortisonelike drugs (corticosteroids)
- anti-infectives (for bacterial infections)
- alpha 1-antitrypsin (if deficient)
- oxygen

Nondrug Treatment Methods
- Pneumococcal and influenzal vaccinations
- Exercise training programs
- Pulmonary rehabilitation programs
- Lung transplantation
- Lung volume reduction

Management of Therapy
Stepped Care Approach (Ziment Routine):

Step 1: For episodic shortness of breath on exertion: metered dose inhaler of beta-agonist bronchodilators.

Step 2: For persistent symptoms due to reversible bronchospasm: metered dose inhaler of ipratropium and beta-agonist bronchodilators.

Step 3: For symptoms that limit exercise, add oral theophylline slow-release preparations or albuterol oral slow-release preparations.

Step 4: For persistent symptoms or nocturnal wheezing, consider use of metered dose inhaler of salmeterol.

Step 5: For asthmatic symptoms or rapid deterioration, add oral prednisone to achieve satisfactory stabilization and determination of minimally effective dose; then switch to metered dose inhaler of aerosol corticosteroid.

Step 6: For further exacerbations or congestive heart failure: anti-infectives as required; digoxin and diuretics as required.

(Adapted from the therapeutic regimen of Dr. Irwin Ziment, with the author's permission.)

Therapeutic Drug Monitoring (Blood Levels)
Recommended blood level range for theophylline: 8–14 mcg/ml.

Ancillary Drug Treatment (as required)
For congestive heart failure:
- diuretics
- digoxin (controversial)

See Profile of congestive heart failure in this section.

Note: Drug selection, dosage, and administration schedule must be determined by the physician for each patient individually.

Possible Drug Interactions of Significance
Because of the number and nature of drugs that may be used to manage this disorder, adequate consideration of the volume and complexity of potential drug interactions is beyond the scope of this book. Consult *The Essential Guide to Prescription Drugs,* or a similar drug reference book for possible interactions of significance (see Appendix 17, Drug Information Sources).

Special Considerations for the Elderly

In older persons with breathing difficulties it is often difficult to distinguish between the possible causes—asthma, chronic bronchitis, or emphysema. Asthma, which is reversible with medication, occurs much more frequently in the elderly than was previously thought. Recent studies have documented that between 15% and 50% of older people may have airway obstruction (COPD) that is reversible. Simple tests of pulmonary function can readily determine this.

Quality of Life Considerations

Progressive respiratory failure eventually leads to severe functional impairment and loss of independence. It is not surprising that many sufferers will experience anxiety, lowered self-esteem, and depression as a result of role reversal and sexual dysfunction. A reasonable degree of rehabilitation is possible with appropriate counseling, exercise programs, good nutrition, avoidance of infections, and intelligent use of medications.

The Role of Prevention in This Disorder

Primary Prevention

- Total and permanent cessation of smoking
- Avoidance of harmful industrial dusts and fumes

Secondary Prevention

- Prompt treatment of intercurrent lung infections
- Maintenance of ideal body weight
- Assurance of good nutrition
- Appropriate exercise as tolerated

Resources

Recommended Reading

Facts About Emphysema, Pamphlet #0301, American Lung Association. For a copy call 1-800-LUNG-USA.

Facts About A1AD Related Emphysema, Pamphlet #0222, American Lung Association. For a copy call 1-800-LUNG-USA.

Around the Clock with C.O.P.D.: Helpful Hints for Respiratory Patients, Pamphlet #1230, American Lung Association. For a copy call 1-800-LUNG-USA.

Additional Information and Services

American Lung Association
1740 Broadway
New York, NY 10019-4374
Phone: 1-800-LUNG-USA, (212) 315-8700; Fax: (212) 265-5642

State groups: 59. Local groups: 72. Publications and videotapes available.

Alpha 1 National Association
1829 Portland Avenue
Minneapolis, MN 55404
Phone: (612) 871-1747

Disease Management Expertise
AAT Deficiency Detection Center
University of Utah
1160 East, 1st South, Suite 109
Salt Lake City, UT 84102
Phone: (801) 328-4254, ext. 202

EPILEPSY

Other Names Seizure disorders, convulsive disorders

Prevalence/Incidence in U.S.
Current estimate: Approximately 2.5 million, 1% of the population
Estimated new cases annually: 125,000

Age Group
24% of epileptics are under 18 years of age; 53% are 18 to 44 years; 18% are 45 to 64 years; 4% are 65 to 74 years; 1% is 75 years and older

Male-to-Female Ratio Incidence is equal

Principal Features and Natural History
True epilepsy is a chronic disorder of the central nervous system characterized by recurring episodes of electrical disturbance within the brain. The principal feature is the occurrence of "seizures" that last from a few seconds to several minutes and require specific medication for prevention and control. Sixty-six percent of epileptic patients require lifelong drug therapy. The principal types of epilepsy include:

Tonic-Clonic Seizures (Grand Mal)
Sudden attacks that begin with an involuntary cry, followed by a loss of consciousness and falling; violent convulsive movements of the head, trunk, and extremities; excessive salivation; and sometimes loss of bladder and/or rectal control. The seizure usually lasts from one to three minutes. The individual awakens spontaneously, is confused and exhausted, and then falls into a deep sleep that lasts several hours. The subject cannot remember the episode.

Absence Seizures (Petit Mal)

These begin between 2 and 12 years of age; 50% go on to develop tonic-clonic seizures by 20 years of age. The seizure consists of a sudden, momentary lapse of awareness lasting several seconds (30 at the most), during which the subject has a blank stare and is oblivious of surroundings. There is no actual loss of consciousness, no fall, and no convulsion. There may be a minor twitching of an eyelid or facial muscle, chewing movements, or a jerk of a hand or arm. Such episodes may recur more than 100 times a day. Following each seizure, the subject resumes normal functioning as though nothing had happened. However, he may be aware that his mind "had gone blank for a few seconds."

Complex Partial Seizures (Psychomotor or Temporal Lobe Epilepsy)

This type comprises 40% of all epilepsies. It consists of sudden alterations of behavior that may involve speech, hearing, memory, and emotional response. Some episodes begin with an "aura" that may take the form of distorted vision, unpleasant odors, visual and auditory hallucinations, or bizarre illusions. The subject may walk about aimlessly, talk irrationally, laugh, or engage in purposeless and inappropriate actions, such as striking at walls in anger or fear. Occasionally he will lose consciousness, fall, and appear to have fainted. Seizures may last a few minutes to several hours. When the seizure ends, the subject is confused and does not recall what has happened.

Diagnostic Symptoms and Signs

Some impairment of consciousness, from brief periods of unawareness to total loss of consciousness

Involuntary muscular activity, from isolated muscle twitching to severe and generalized convulsions

Psychological aberrations, from brief disorientation to psychotic behavior patterns

Various degrees of amnesia following seizures

Diagnostic Tests and Procedures

Electroencephalograms (EEGs) to differentiate partial from generalized seizure patterns

24-hour ambulatory EEG monitoring to detect frequency and nature of abnormal electrical activity in the brain

In-hospital monitoring with continuous videotaping to distinguish epileptic seizures from nonepileptic events

Computed tomography (CT scans) or magnetic resonance imaging (MRI) studies to detect possible causes for seizures

Cerebral angiogram: dye visualization of blood vessels in the brain

Cerebrospinal fluid examinations to detect clues of possible causes for seizures

Screening tests for alcohol or drug abuse

Battery of blood chemistry tests

Similar Conditions That May Confuse Diagnosis

Orthostatic hypotension (see Glossary)

Heart rhythm disturbances with brief, transient cardiac arrest

Sleep disorders: nightmares, narcolepsy, cataplexy

Psychiatric disorders: panic attacks, fugue states, psychogenic seizures

Transient ischemic attacks (TIAs): brief interruptions of blood flow to the brain

Migraine headache variations

Breath-holding episodes of childhood

ALERT!

A normal EEG does not eliminate the possibility of a seizure disorder. An abnormal EEG does not necessarily confirm the diagnosis of a seizure disorder. The diagnosis is based on consistent clinical observations of seizure patterns.

Causes

Established Causes

The definitive cause that initiates epileptic seizures is not known. No apparent cause can be found in up to 70% of persons with seizures.

Theoretical Causes

The actual seizure is due to a sudden, abnormal, and excessive electrical discharge within the brain. Normal electrical impulses of 80/second are suddenly increased to 500/second. Critical alterations in brain chemistry can disturb the equilibrium between excitatory and inhibitory controls and thus provoke electrical disarray.

Known Risk Factors for Developing This Disorder

For primary (cause unknown) epilepsy: genetic predisposition.

For secondary epilepsy: head injuries, bacterial meningitis, malaria, cerebral palsy, mental retardation, brain tumors and cysts, hydrocephalus, stroke, degenerative brain diseases.

Drugs That Can Cause This Disorder

The following drugs have been reported to cause seizures or to aggravate existing epileptic disorders:

amphetamines

antihistamines

chloroquine
cimetidine (with large doses in the elderly)
cycloserine
isoniazid
metronidazole
monoamine oxidase inhibitors (MAOIs)
nalidixic acid
oral contraceptives
phenothiazines
tricyclic antidepressants
vincristine
See Appendix 16, Drug Classes, for specific generic drugs within respective drug classes.

Goals of Treatment

Can This Disorder Be Cured?

There is no known cure for the fundamental defects that cause epilepsy.

Can This Disorder Be Treated Effectively?

Depending upon the type of epilepsy, 50% of patients can achieve complete control of seizures. Another 30% can achieve partial control. Surgical procedures can be very effective in a small selected group of patients whose seizures cannot be controlled by medication.

Specific Goals

- Complete prevention of seizures if possible (or marked reduction in frequency), with no (or minimal) adverse drug effects
- Restoration of ability to function independently
- Promotion of participation in scholastic, occupational, and social activities

Health Professionals Who Participate in Managing This Disorder

Family physicians
General internists
Pediatricians
Neurologists
Neuropsychiatrists
Pharmacists
Physician assistants
Nurse practitioners
Medical social workers

Currently Available Therapies for This Disorder

Drugs Used to Treat This Disorder

In order of preference:

FOR GENERALIZED TONIC-CLONIC SEIZURES (GRAND MAL)

Drugs of choice:

- valproate (Depakote)
- carbamazepine (Tegretol)
- phenytoin (Dilantin)

Alternative drugs:

- lamotrigine (Lamictal)
- primidone (Mysoline)
- phenobarbital (Luminal)

FOR COMPLEX PARTIAL SEIZURES (PSYCHOMOTOR, TEMPORAL LOBE)

Drugs of choice:

- carbamazepine (Tegretol)
- phenytoin (Dilantin)
- valproate (Depakote)

Alternative drugs:

- primidone (Mysoline)
- phenobarbital (Luminal)
- lamotrigine (Lamictal) as adjunct
- gabapentin (Neurontin) as adjunct

FOR ABSENCE SEIZURES (PETIT MAL)

Drugs of choice:

- ethosuximide (Zarontin)
- valproate (Depakote)

Alternative drugs:

- clonazepam (Klonopin)
- lamotrigine (Lamictal)

FOR ATYPICAL ABSENCE, MYOCLONIC, AND ATONIC SEIZURES

Drug of choice:

- valproate (Depakote)

Alternative drugs:

- clonazepam (Klonopin)
- phenobarbital (Luminal)

Management of Therapy

- Each individual who is subject to epilepsy experiences a pattern of seizures that is unique; the onset, frequency, severity, and specific type (or types) of seizures are never exactly the same as those experienced by someone else.
- The drugs used to control epilepsy are selected according to the specific type(s) of seizures the patient experiences.

- Antiepileptic drugs are not curative; they are used to control seizures—to reduce their frequency and severity. Seizures should be prevented whenever possible; repeated, uncontrolled convulsions can cause significant brain damage.
- When the drug of choice is used in adequate dosage to manage a correctly diagnosed type of epilepsy, seizures can be controlled completely in 60% of patients and substantially reduced in another 20%. In every case a period of trial and error is necessary to find the most effective drug, the optimal dose, and the correct timing of use. Dosage schedules are adjusted gradually to achieve the maximum of seizure control with the minimum of drug side effects.
- Complete control of seizures with one drug is the ideal; this is possible in 85% of cases. If one drug does not give adequate control, a second drug may be added. The first drug may be continued or gradually withdrawn, depending upon individual response.
- Because of the wide variation in drug absorption and elimination from person to person, the periodic measurement of drug levels in blood is necessary to determine the optimal dosage for each drug. An attempt is made to establish for each individual that drug level which will ensure freedom from seizures without toxic drug effects. Blood samples for measurement are usually taken just before the morning dose (see "Therapeutic Drug Monitoring" below).
- All antiepileptic drugs have toxic effects when taken in large doses; dosage adjustments are often necessary to prevent toxicity. However, the controllable risks of proper use do not justify withholding treatment in view of the much greater risks resulting from uncontrolled repeated seizures.
- Birth defects are two to three times higher in children whose parents (father or mother) are using antiepileptic drugs, especially phenytoin, trimethadione, and valproic acid. Consult your physician regarding the best course of action for you in managing your epilepsy during pregnancy.
- Do not discontinue any antiepileptic drug suddenly unless advised to do so by your physician. Normally the dosage should be reduced gradually over a period of several weeks. Abrupt withdrawal can cause status epilepticus—a prolonged period of continual seizures without interruption.
- Any consideration of discontinuing antiepileptic medications permanently should be made jointly with your physician. Such consideration can be made for absence seizures (petit mal) after a period of two to three years without a seizure. For other types of epilepsy, a period of three to five years is advisable. Seizures tend to return in 20% to 50% of cases after stopping medication. Any attempt to withdraw medication must be done very gradually over a period of several months.

Use of Phenytoin

- Used to control all types of epilepsy except absence seizures. When the daily maintenance requirement has been established, it may be taken in a single dose.
- A drug blood level within the therapeutic range correlates well with a decrease in seizure frequency and relative freedom from toxic effects. Indications of early toxicity include rapid involuntary eye movements (nystagmus), dizziness, unsteadiness, lethargy, and slurred speech.
- Due to variation of absorbability among available products, it is advisable to stay with the same brand to gain and maintain control.
- Possible adverse effects include a measleslike rash within the first two weeks, excessive growth of hair (5%), and enlargement of the gums (30%).
- If another drug is added for concurrent use, any significant interaction will usually occur within six weeks.

Use of Phenobarbital

- Used to control all types of epilepsy except absence seizures. Should be taken twice a day with the largest dose at bedtime.
- Should be used with caution if liver or kidney function is impaired.
- More sedative than phenytoin and carbamazepine, but relatively free of long-term adverse effects.
- Indications of early toxicity include drowsiness, unsteadiness, and impaired thinking.

Use of Primidone

- Closely related to phenobarbital. Used to control all types of epilepsy except absence seizures. Must be taken in divided doses because of its sedative effect.
- Indications of early toxicity are the same of those for phenobarbital.

Use of Ethosuximide

- Used to control absence seizures and some myoclonic seizures. About 75% effective in reducing the frequency of absence seizures when used in adequate dosage.
- Indications of early toxicity include headache, drowsiness, and dizziness.

Use of Valproate

- Used primarily to control both simple and complex absence seizures. Also used adjunctively to control all other types of epilepsy. It may control both absence and tonic-clonic seizures in the same individual. Multiple doses are necessary to maintain 24-hour control.
- Should be avoided in presence of liver disease.
- A possible side effect is weight gain.
- Close monitoring for indications of liver toxicity is advised. If used concurrently with other antiepileptic drugs, the periodic measurement

of blood levels of all drugs being used is necessary to ensure adequate dosage and prevent toxicity.

Use of Carbamazepine

- Used to control both tonic-clonic seizures and partial complex seizures (psychomotor epilepsy). Should be taken with food to improve absorption.
- Should be avoided in presence of liver disease or impaired liver function. Indications of early toxicity include double vision, blurred vision, dizziness, unsteadiness, and tremor.
- Routine, periodic, complete blood counts are mandatory to detect early bone marrow toxicity.

Use of Gabapentin

- Used adjunctively to treat refractory partial seizures in adults, with or without secondary generalization.
- Does not interact unfavorably with other antiepileptic drugs.
- The most frequent adverse effects are mild to moderate drowsiness, fatigue, dizziness, and impaired muscle coordination.

Use of Lamotrigine

- Used adjunctively to treat refractory partial seizures in adults.
- The most common adverse effects are mild headache, dizziness, double vision, nausea, and rash; these usually resolve without discontinuation of the drug.

Therapeutic Drug Monitoring (Blood Levels)

Antiepileptic Drug	Recommended Range
carbamazepine (Tegretol)	5–10 mcg/ml
clonazepam (Klonopin)	10–50 ng/ml
ethosuximide (Zarontin)	40–100 mcg/ml
mephobarbital (Mebaral)	1–7 mcg/ml
methsuximide (Celontin)	up to 1.0 mcg/ml
phenobarbital (Luminal)	10–25 mcg/ml
phenytoin (Dilantin)	10–20 mcg/ml
primidone (Mysoline)	6–12 mcg/ml
trimethadione (Tridione)	10–30 mcg/ml
valproic acid (Depakene)	50–100 mcg/ml

Ancillary Drug Treatment (as required)

For increased seizures before or after menstruation:
- acetazolamide (Diamox)

For anxiety:
- benzodiazepines (Tranxene, Valium, etc.)

For depression:
    see Profile of depression in this section

Note: Drug selection, dosage, and administration schedule must be determined by the physician for each patient individually.

ALERT!

Recently some popular news programs have featured stories about "seizure dogs"—canines trained to alert their epileptic owners of an impending seizure. Analogous to "seeing-eye dogs" for the blind, seizure dogs are intended to provide a measure of safety for those with epilepsy. This author's attempts to confirm that dogs can be trained to perform this service were unsuccessful. Epilepsy information specialists explain that reports concerning seizure dogs are promoted by kennels that are selling them, but that there is no scientific evidence to support the authenticity of the claims. Potential buyers are advised to be skeptical until proof is available.

Possible Drug Interactions of Significance

Because of the number of drugs that may be used to manage this disorder, adequate consideration of the volume and complexity of potential drug interactions is beyond the scope of this book. Consult *The Essential Guide to Prescription Drugs*, or a similar drug reference book for possible interactions of significance (see Appendix 17, Drug Information Sources).

Special Considerations for Women

The following drugs may *reduce* the effectiveness of oral contraceptives, thereby increasing the risk of becoming pregnant:

- barbiturates (phenobarbital, etc.)
- carbamazepine (Tegretol)
- griseofulvin (Fulvicin, etc.)
- penicillins (ampicillin, penicillin V, etc.)
- phenytoin (Dilantin)
- primidone (Mysoline)
- rifampin (Rifidin, Rimactane)
- tetracyclines

See Appendix 16, Drug Classes, for the specific generic drugs in respective drug classes.

Pregnancy

It is most important that you discuss the issue of pregnancy with your physician, preferably *before* you become pregnant. The following questions deserve serious consideration:

- Although 92% of women taking antiepileptic drugs during pregnancy give birth to normal infants, these drugs may increase the risk of birth defects. Should you attempt to discontinue antiepileptic drugs before pregnancy? If so, when and how? What are the chances of your seizures returning?

- Is the risk of seizures during pregnancy potentially more harmful to the fetus than the risk of drug-induced birth defects?
- Is the risk of seizures during pregnancy potentially more hazardous for you than the risk of drug-induced birth defects for the fetus?
- If it is necessary for you to continue to take antiepileptic medication during pregnancy, which drug poses the least risk for you and the fetus?

Breast-Feeding

Most antiepileptic drugs are secreted in breast milk. Consult your physician regarding the advisability of nursing.

Special Considerations for the Elderly

Approximately 90% of older persons who experience new-onset seizures are found to have an identifiable organic brain disorder as the cause. The most common findings include strokes, tumors, and Alzheimer's disease. If antiepileptic drugs are necessary, it is advisable to begin treatment with small doses and to increase dosage slowly as tolerated.

Quality of Life Considerations

Epilepsy often has a catastrophic impact on all important aspects of the patient's life. Due to lack of understanding by family, friends, and society at large, those who experience seizures may find themselves isolated and excluded from normal human relationships, educational opportunities, and gainful employment. Until education of the public achieves appropriate insight and acceptance of this disorder, those so afflicted must do all in their power to maintain a seizure-free state and to demonstrate that they can live a normal, enjoyable, and productive life.

The Role of Prevention in This Disorder

Primary Prevention

The principal methods of primary prevention available at this time are genetic counseling and family planning.

The avoidance of head injury will reduce the incidence of secondary epilepsy.

Secondary Prevention

The frequency and severity of seizures can be significantly reduced by:
- complying fully with the treatment program recommended by your physician, especially the proper use of antiepileptic drugs
- total abstinence from alcohol and drug abuse
- avoidance of known seizure "triggers:" flashing lights, provocative sounds, video games, intense exercise, emotional stress, lack of sleep

Resources

Recommended Reading

Seizures and Epilepsy in Childhood: A Guide for Parents, J.M. Freeman, E.P.G. Vining, and D.J. Pillas. Baltimore: Johns Hopkins Press, 1993.

Brainstorms: Epilepsy in Our Words, S.C. Schachter, M.D. New York: Raven Press, 1993.

Additional Information and Services

American Epilepsy Society
638 Prospect Avenue
Hartford, CT 06105-4298
Phone: (203) 232-4825
Telecommunications services: Fax: (203) 232-0819
Publications available.

Epilepsy Concern Service Group
1282 Wynnewood Drive
West Palm Beach, FL 33417
Phone: (407) 683-0044
Telecommunications services: Fax: (407) 881-5085
Promotes formation of self-help groups. Publications and telephone referrals available.

Epilepsy Foundation of America
4351 Garden City Drive
Landover, MD 20785
Phone: 1-800-EFA-1000, (301) 459-3700
Telecommunications services: Fax: (301) 577-2684
Provides a low-cost pharmacy program for members. Publications and audiovisual materials available.

Disease Management Expertise

National Institutes of Health
National Institute of Neurological and Communicative Disorders and Stroke
9000 Rockville Pike
Building 10, Room 5C205
Epilepsy Branch
Bethesda, MD 20892
Phone: (301) 496-1505

GLAUCOMA

Other Names Primary glaucoma, secondary glaucoma, open-angle glaucoma, closed-angle glaucoma

Prevalence/Incidence in U.S.

Current estimate: 3 million known, an estimated 1 million undiagnosed. 1.3% of the white population over 40 years of age; 4.7% of the black population over 40 years of age. By age 80, 10% of the population has glaucoma.

Age Group

Age Group	% of Total
Under 18 years	1%
18 to 44 years	7%
45 to 64 years	30%
65 to 74 years	31%
75 years and over	31%

Male-to-Female Ratio

Under 45 years—same incidence in men and women; 45 to 64 years—more common in men; 65 years and over—more common in women

Principal Features and Natural History

The glaucomas are a group of chronic eye disorders that are currently the third leading cause of blindness among white Americans and the leading cause of blindness among black Americans. The cardinal feature of glaucoma is progressive destruction of the optic nerve that leads to irreversible loss of vision. Although abnormally high internal eye pressure is responsible for the majority of cases, some individuals with normal internal eye pressure develop glaucomatous changes in the optic nerve. The reasons for this are not apparent.

The glaucomas are classified according to their principal features:
Cause:
  Primary glaucoma—cause is unknown
  Secondary glaucoma—cause is apparent
Eye structure:
  Open-angle—drainage canal open
  Closed-angle—drainage canal closed
Current status:
  Acute—abrupt onset, rapid progression
  Chronic—insidious onset, slow progression

Chronic Open-Angle (Simple, Wide-Angle) Glaucoma

This primary glaucoma is the most common type found in adults. It usually begins after 30 years of age, but may occur rarely in children and young adults. The rise in internal eye pressure begins without symptoms and continues to increase gradually. Constant compression of the optic nerve in the back of the eye causes irreversible damage to nerve fibers. The resulting loss of vision is insidious and slowly progressive. Usually both eyes are affected. If not detected and treated, characteristic symptoms eventually develop. These include blurring of vision, frequent need for change of glasses, occasional headache, colored halos seen around electric lights, and impaired visual adaptation to the dark.

Acute/Chronic Closed-Angle (Narrow-Angle) Glaucoma

This type of primary glaucoma usually occurs after 60 years of age. The acute attack begins in one eye; the rise in internal eye pressure is sudden and dramatic. Within a few hours the patient experiences severe headache, throbbing eye pain, blurred vision, halos around lights, tearing, swollen eyelids, nausea, and vomiting. Initially, the episode may be misdiagnosed as an acute abdominal disorder, such as gallbladder disease. Attacks of lesser severity can recur in chronic fashion.

Secondary Glaucoma

The rise in internal eye pressure is a consequence of injury or a preexistent condition, such as an eye infection (uveitis), eye tumor, enlarged cataract, or long-term treatment with cortisonelike drugs. Headache, halos, and blurred vision occur in proportion to the degree and duration of increased pressure on the optic nerve.

Diagnostic Symptoms and Signs

With early glaucoma: none
With advanced glaucoma: blurred vision, loss of peripheral vision ("tunnel" vision), halos seen around lights, decreased night vision
Need for change in glasses

Diagnostic Tests and Procedures

Visual acuity: permanent change and loss of vision
Tonometry: increased internal eye (intraocular) pressure above 21 mm Hg (millimeters of mercury). This may not occur in some cases.
Visual field examinations: permanent loss of peripheral vision
Ophthalmoscopic examination: abnormal depression (cupping) of optic nerve head, usually due to chronic compression
Gonioscopy: inspection of the outflow canal for internal eye fluid (aqueous humor); inspection of the angle between the cornea and iris to determine if it is open or closed
Visual image analysis: to detect changes in the optic nerve before the loss of vision; used to evaluate glaucoma that occurs with normal or low intraocular pressure

Diagnostic "Markers" for This Disorder

Characteristic degeneration of the optic nerve found on ophthalmoscopic examination
Characteristic decrease in visual fields

ALERT!

Glaucoma can develop in the presence of normal intraocular pressure (IOP). An increased IOP reading is not essential to the diagnosis of glaucoma.

Causes

Established Causes

The definitive cause that initiates degeneration of the optic nerve in primary glaucoma is not known.

Theoretical Causes

The normal internal eye pressure is 10 to 21 mm Hg. Increased pressure is due to an imbalance between production and drainage of the liquid (aqueous humor) in the front portion of the eye; obstruction to normal drainage is the main mechanism. The primary types of glaucoma occur in individuals with hereditary predisposition, but specific initiating causes responsible for the rise in pressure are not known.

Known Risk Factors for Developing This Disorder

Genetic predisposition: the prevalence of glaucoma is 40% among first-
   degree relatives
Age: the incidence is significantly higher after 60 years of age
Concurrent conditions: myopia, diabetes mellitus, excessive alcohol consumption
Secondary types of glaucoma are associated with other eye disorders:
   uveitis, tumors, cataracts, hemorrhage, injury. "Steroid responders"
   develop increased pressure after one to eight weeks of using cortisonelike steroids.

Drugs That Can Cause This Disorder

The following drugs do not cause true, permanent glaucoma, but they can increase intraocular pressure and possibly precipitate an attack of acute closed-angle glaucoma or aggravate chronic open-angle glaucoma:
   amyl nitrite
   atropine and atropinelike drugs (anticholinergics)
   cortisonelike drugs (corticosteroids)
   epinephrine
   isosorbide dinitrate
   nitroglycerin
   phenylephrine
   tolazoline
   tricyclic antidepressants
   See Appendix 16, Drug Classes, for specific generic drugs within respective drug classes.

Goals of Treatment

Can This Disorder Be Cured?

Since the definitive cause of glaucoma is unknown, no curative treatment is available. Optic nerve damage cannot be repaired. Lost vision cannot be restored.

Can This Disorder Be Treated Effectively?

Medicinal and surgical therapies currently available are very effective in controlling intraocular pressure and preserving vision.

Specific Goals

- Early detection of elevated intraocular pressure and/or significant changes in the optic nerve
- Gradual reduction and long-term normalization of intraocular pressure in primary, chronic, open-angle glaucoma
- Prompt reduction of intraocular pressure in acute closed-angle glaucoma; stabilization of eye status in preparation for corrective eye surgery
- Prevention of optic nerve damage; preservation of vision

Health Professionals Who Participate in Managing This Disorder

Family physicians
General internists
Pediatricians
Geriatricians
Ophthalmologists
Glaucoma specialists
Optometrists
Pharmacists
Physician assistants
Nurse practitioners
Medical social workers

Currently Available Therapies for This Disorder

Drug Therapy

Eyedrops/inserts (for local effects):

- betaxolol (Betoptic)
- carbachol (Carbacel, Isopto Carbachol)
- carteolol (Ocupress)
- demecarium (Humorsol)
- dipivefrin (DPE, Propine)
- dorzolamide (Trusopt)

- echothiophate (Phospholine)
- epinephrine (Epifrin, Epitrate, Glaucon, Lyophrin)
- latanoprost (Xalatan)
- levobunolol (Betagan)
- metipranolol (Optipranolol)
- phenylephrine (Neo-Synephrine, Ocusol)
- pilocarpine solution (Almocarpine, Isoptocarpine, etc.)
- pilocarpine gel
- pilocarpine inserts (Ocuserts Pilo-20, Pilo-40)
- timolol (Timoptic)

Internal medications (for systemic effects):

- acetazolamide (Diamox)
- glycerine (Glyrol, Osmoglyn)
- methazolamide (Neptazane)

Surgical procedures:

- Argon laser trabeculoplasty to create openings for the flow of aqueous humor
- Trabeculectomy to create a bypass for the drainage of aqueous humor
- Implantation of a tube-shunt to divert aqueous humor to a reservoir
- Ablation (surgical removal) of the ciliary body within the eye—the site of aqueous humor production

Management of Therapy

- Drug treatment cannot cure glaucoma, but it can control it.
- Factors that can increase intraocular pressure and reduce the effectiveness of drugs include emotional stress (anger, fear, worry); heavy physical exertion; straining with defecation; tight collars, belts, and girdles; upper respiratory infections.
- Periodic measurement of intraocular pressure is strongly advised during long-term use of cortisonelike steroid drugs, especially eyedrops and ointments.
- Soft contact lenses can act as a drug reservoir for pilocarpine (when administered in eyedrop solutions).
- Some individuals cannot use pilocarpine Ocuserts successfully; some cannot retain them in the eye, and the loss may be unnoticed; some cannot tolerate the foreign-body sensation.
- Pilocarpine is the pupil-constricting (miotic) drug of choice for use in the elderly. The stinging sensation felt on initial use usually disappears with continued application. Some blurring of distant vision is unavoidable.
- Timolol (a beta-blocker) is as effective as pilocarpine in treating open-angle and secondary glaucoma; twice daily dosage (every 12 hours) is usually sufficient; it should be used very cautiously in those with asthma, slow heart rates, or borderline congestive heart failure.

- Epinephrine may be used concurrently with pilocarpine (or other miotic drugs) for greater effectiveness in reducing intraocular pressure; it is important that the pilocarpine be used first and be allowed to act for five minutes before using epinephrine. It should not be used in the presence of high blood pressure (hypertension). Discolored solutions of epinephrine should not be used.
- Acetazolamide is usually reserved for glaucoma that is unresponsive to eyedrops alone. Effectiveness is improved when both are used concurrently.

For Chronic Open-Angle Glaucoma
- Eyedrops: pilocarpine, timolol, carbachol, epinephrine, dipivefrin, demecarium
- Internal medications: acetazolamide
- Most cases are controlled by eyedrops alone.
- Treatment is started with the weakest strength; the most effective strength and dosage schedule are determined by trial and error.
- Acetazolamide is not used routinely; it is added after an adequate trial of eyedrops fails to maintain normal intraocular pressure.

For Acute Closed-Angle Glaucoma (Acute Attack)
- Eyedrops: pilocarpine, timolol
- Internal medications: glycerine and water mixture, acetazolamide
- The initial treatment is designed to lower intraocular pressure as rapidly as possible to prevent irreversible damage to the optic nerve. Eyedrops and internal medications are used concurrently. The combination can reduce the pressure rapidly and abort the acute attack.
- The ultimate treatment for this condition is surgical.

For Chronic, Recurrent Episodes of Subacute Closed-Angle Glaucoma
- Eyedrops: pilocarpine and timolol concurrently
- Internal medications: glycerine and water; acetazolamide is used only during the acute phase, not long-term
- The ultimate treatment is surgical.

For Secondary Glaucoma
- Eyedrops: atropine, cortisonelike steroids
- Internal medications: cortisonelike steroids, acetazolamide
- When appropriate, corrective treatment is directed at the primary eye disorder that is causing increased intraocular pressure.

For Cortisone-Induced Glaucoma
- Discontinue all cortisonelike steroids if possible
- Eyedrops: pilocarpine, timolol, demecarium
- Internal medications: acetazolamide

Ancillary Drug Treatment (as required)

For itching, burning, redness of eyes:

- naphazoline (Naphcon, Privine, Vasoclear)
- tetrahydralazine (Visine)

Note: Drug selection, dosage, and administration schedule must be determined by the physician for each patient individually.

Possible Drug Interactions of Significance

Because of the number of drugs that may be used to manage this disorder, adequate consideration of the volume and complexity of potential drug interactions is beyond the scope of this book. Consult *The Essential Guide to Prescription Drugs*, or a similar drug reference book for possible interactions of significance (see Appendix 17, Drug Information Sources).

Special Considerations for Women

Pregnancy

Acetazolamide is designated Pregnancy Category C. However, animal studies revealed limb and skeletal defects in mice and rats. It is advisable to avoid this drug completely during the first three months of pregnancy (see Appendix 15, FDA Pregnancy Categories).

Breast-Feeding

The American Academy of Pediatrics considers acetazolamide to be compatible with breast-feeding.

Special Considerations for the Elderly

Acetazolamide should be used in small doses and with caution. Large doses may cause weakness, confusion, nausea, and numbness in the extremities. If you are also taking digoxin, you may need a high-potassium diet or potassium supplements. Ask your physician for guidance (see Appendix 10, High-Potassium Foods).

Quality of Life Considerations

Normal aging unavoidably reduces the quality of life. Do not compound this by ignoring the possibility of age-related glaucoma and loss of vision. Obtain a thorough eye examination annually that includes appropriate tests for glaucoma. Lost vision cannot be recovered.

The Role of Prevention in This Disorder

Primary Prevention

There is no way to prevent the development of primary glaucoma in a genetically susceptible individual.

Secondary Prevention

Early detection and prompt treatment of glaucomatous changes in the optic nerve can prevent significant loss of vision.

Resources

Recommended Reading

Understanding and Living with Glaucoma: A Reference Guide for Patients and Their Families, L.A. Whitmore. The Foundation for Glaucoma Research, 1992.

Additional Information and Services

Foundation for Glaucoma Research
490 Post Street, Suite 830
San Francisco, CA 94102
Phone: 1-800-826-6693, (415) 986 3162; Fax: (415) 986-3763

Quarterly newsletter and patient guide available. Also offers telephone-based peer support network for glaucoma patients.

National Society to Prevent Blindness
500 East Remington Road
Schaumburg, IL 60173
Phone: 1-800-331-2020, (708) 843-2020; Fax: (708) 843-8458

Answers questions about vision problems. Provides publications and films on specific problems and conditions.

Disease Management Expertise

National Institutes of Health
National Eye Institute
Building 31, Room 6A32
31 Center Drive, MSC 2510
Bethesda, MD 20892-2510
Phone: (301) 496-5248

GOUT

Other Names Gouty arthritis, podagra, hyperuricemia

Prevalence/Incidence in U.S.

Approximately 2.3 million, 2.8% of males in middle age
Hyperuricemia occurs in 5–10% of the population; 1–2% will have gout manifestations during a lifetime.

Age Group

Age Group	% of Total
Under 18 years	<1%
18 to 44 years	14%
45 to 64 years	45%
65 to 74 years	22%
75 years and over	18%

Male-to-Female Ratio Approximately 95% in men, 5% in women

Principal Features and Natural History

Gout is the most common form of acute inflammatory arthritis in men over 40 years of age. The term gout refers to a group of related disorders that have a single underlying feature—abnormally high blood levels of uric acid (hyperuricemia). The normal ranges for uric acid are 4.3 to 8.0 mg/dl for men and 2.3 to 6.0 mg/dl for women. Any value above the upper limit of normal indicates hyperuricemia and potential for gouty arthritis. Hyperuricemia develops when the body overproduces uric acid (10–15% of gout patients), or the kidneys underexcrete uric acid (80–90% of gout patients). Both mechanisms occur in some individuals.

The natural history of gout consists of four stages: (1) hyperuricemia without symptoms, (2) acute gouty arthritis, (3) symptom-free intervals between acute attacks, and (4) chronic tophaceous gout with smoldering joint pain, stiffness, and impaired function.

During the early years of primary (genetic) gout, hyperuricemia may exist without any symptoms to indicate its presence. During their lifetime, a small minority of individuals with hyperuricemia will experience recurrent acute attacks of severe joint pain with swelling and inflammation (usually one joint in an upper or lower limb). Gouty arthritis of the big toe (podagra) is a universal symbol of this disorder, occurring in 90% of patients. Some will experience episodes of urate kidney stones, serious impairment of kidney function, or the development of tophi—localized deposits of urate crystals in the skin, on earlobes, or on tendons near joints (tophaceous gout).

Diagnostic Symptoms and Signs

For stage 2 gout:
- sudden attacks (often nocturnal) of severe pain, swelling, and inflammation in a single joint, usually in a lower extremity
- other joint involvement (in decreasing order of frequency): the instep, ankle, heel, knee, wrist, finger, elbow
- fatigue, fever, chills, headache, loss of appetite

For stage 4 gout:
- recurrent episodes of joint pain and swelling, resulting in tissue damage and loss of function
- tophi formation (deposition of urate crystals in connective tissues)

Diagnostic Tests and Procedures

Measurement of blood uric acid level

Measurement of 24-hour urine excretion of uric acid to identify "overexcretors" and "underexcretors"

Aspiration of joint (synovial) fluid or tophi content for crystal analysis

X-ray studies of involved joints for diagnostic changes

Diagnostic "Markers" for This Disorder

Specific needle-shaped urate crystals found in joint fluid

Elevated blood uric acid level

Similar Conditions That May Confuse Diagnosis

Calcium pyrophosphate deposition disease (CPPD), referred to as "pseudo-gout"

Joint infections (septic arthritis)

Rheumatoid arthritis

Reiter's syndrome

Acute bursitis, knee or elbow

Causes

Established Causes

The definitive cause of hyperuricemia is unknown.

Theoretical Causes

Primary gout is thought to be due to an inherited defect in the metabolism of purines—endproducts of protein digestion. In approximately 10% of cases the defect results in an overproduction of uric acid; in 90% the defect is responsible for decreased excretion of uric acid by the kidneys. Either defect causes hyperuricemia. When tissue fluids cannot dissolve excessive levels of urate (due to saturation), urate crystals are deposited in joints (acute arthritis), kidneys (kidney damage and stone formation), and soft tissues (tophi formation).

Known Risk Factors for Developing This Disorder

Family history of gout

Male gender

Over 40 years of age

Obesity

Alcohol abuse

Hypertension
Impaired kidney function
Leukemias, lymphomas

Provocative Factors That Can "Trigger" Acute Gout
Repeated joint injuries
Excessive alcohol or "rich food" binges
Surgical procedures
Serious medical illnesses

Drugs That Can Cause This Disorder

The following drugs can raise the blood level of uric acid and precipitate acute gouty arthritis in susceptible individuals:

acetazolamide
antineoplastic drugs
aspirin (less than 2 grams/day)
cyclosporine
ethacrynic acid
ethambutol
furosemide
levodopa
nicotinic acid
pyrazinamide
thiazide diuretics
triamterene

Goals of Treatment

Can This Disorder Be Cured?
The fundamental genetic flaw responsible for hyperuricemia cannot be removed.

Can This Disorder Be Treated Effectively?
Currently available drug therapies can effectively relieve the pain of acute gouty arthritis and control blood levels of uric acid.

Specific Goals
• Prompt relief of symptoms of acute attack of gouty arthritis
• Maintenance of blood uric acid level below 8 mg/dl
• Prevention of recurrent attacks of acute arthritis, kidney stone formation, kidney damage, and tophi formation
• Dissolution of existing tophi

Health Professionals Who Participate in Managing This Disorder

Family physicians
General internists

Rheumatologists
Pharmacists
Physician assistants
Nurse practitioners
Dietitians

Currently Available Therapies for This Disorder

Drug Therapy
For reducing blood and tissue levels of uric acid:
- allopurinol (Lopurin, Zyloprim)
- probenecid (Benemid)
- sulfinpyrazone (Anturane)

For treating and preventing acute attacks of arthritis:
- colchicine
- diclofenac (Voltaren)
- fenoprofen (Nalfon)
- flurbiprofen (Ansaid)
- ibuprofen (Advil, Motrin, Nuprin, Rufen)
- indomethacin (Indocin)
- ketoprofen (Orudis)
- meclofenamate (Meclomen)
- naproxen (Naprosyn)
- phenylbutazone (Azolid, Butazolidin)
- piroxicam (Feldene)
- prednisone (Deltasone, Meticorten, Orasone, etc.)
- sulindac (Clinoril)
- tolmetin (Tolectin)

Nondrug Treatment Methods
- Dietary modification: If initial blood uric acid levels are unusually high, a low-purine diet is advisable until medication requirements are determined. Long-term purine restriction is impractical and of questionable value.
- Activities: Avoid excessive use of affected joints until symptoms are relieved.

Management of Therapy
- Only 20% of individuals with hyperuricemia will develop manifestations of gout during their lifetime. At present there is no way of identifying those who will.
- Gouty arthritis is the most responsive to treatment and the most easily controlled of all types of arthritis.
- The patient and physician together should determine by trial and error which drug is most effective and acceptable for treating acute attacks of gouty arthritis.

- After the acute attack of arthritis has subsided, minor symptoms may persist for two to three months. If maintenance treatment with antigout drugs is started, it is advisable to use low-dose colchicine concurrently to prevent recurrent flare-ups.
- Measurement of the amount of uric acid in a 24-hour collection of urine can identify the overproducer of uric acid (greater than 800 mg) and the underexcretor (less than 800 mg). The overproducer is best treated with allopurinol; the underexcretor is best treated with probenecid or sulfinpyrazone.
- Authorities differ on whether and when to initiate long-term treatment for hyperuricemia.

  Conservative opinion: initiate drug therapy only after two or more episodes of gouty arthritis or kidney stone within a year. Many first attacks are not followed by recurrent episodes. Withholding long-term treatment avoids the risks of adverse drug reactions.

  Aggressive opinion: initiate drug therapy after the first episode of gouty arthritis or kidney stone to prevent recurrent attacks and reduce the risks of kidney damage and tophi formation.
- Hyperuricemia is often present for 20 years or more before the first attack; bone, cartilage, and kidney damage may already have occurred. The risks of untreated hyperuricemia are thought to exceed the risks of long-term drug therapy. The prudent physician will consider the pros and cons of each case individually and make the decision jointly with the patient.
- Once long-term treatment is started with allopurinol and/or probenecid or sulfinpyrazone, it should be maintained for life. Start–stop treatment has no lasting benefit and may precipitate acute attacks. Low-dose colchicine should be taken preventively until the uric acid blood level is stabilized below 8.0 mg/dl and there have been no acute attacks for 6 to 12 months.
- Acute attacks of gouty arthritis can be precipitated by injury, surgery, systemic infections, and severe medical illnesses. Colchicine may be used preventively to minimize acute episodes of arthritis when such events occur.
- Patients with kidney stones should use allopurinol to treat hyperuricemia; probenecid and sulfinpyrazone should be avoided because they increase the uric acid content of urine.
- Do not take aspirin (or other salicylates) in doses of less than 2 grams while taking probenecid or sulfinpyrazone. Small doses of aspirin raise the blood level of uric acid; large doses of aspirin lower the blood level of uric acid.
- Avoid fasting to lose weight; fasting can raise the blood level of uric acid. Treat obesity by long-term reduction of food intake and gradual loss of weight.

- While taking antigout drugs on a regular basis, drink 2 to 3 quarts of liquids daily to ensure a copious flow of dilute urine.

Use of Allopurinol

- Used to lower the blood level of uric acid by reducing its formation. Of no value in treating the acute attack and should not be started until all symptoms of acute arthritis have subsided, but it is the drug of choice for individuals who
  - are overproducers of uric acid (more than 800 mg/24-hour urine excretion);
  - are over 60 years of age;
  - have impaired kidney function;
  - are subject to kidney stones;
  - have tophi formations;
  - are allergic or overly sensitive to probenecid or sulfinpyrazone.
- The total daily requirement may be taken in a single dose. Once started, a commitment should be made to a lifetime of continual use. May be combined with all other antigout drugs as appropriate for increased effectiveness. Serious toxicity is extremely rare.
- Recommended for use prior to and during chemotherapy or irradiation therapy for selected cancers to counteract resulting hyperuricemia.

Use of Colchicine

- Used to treat acute attacks of gouty arthritis. It does not lower the blood level of uric acid.
- For the quickest response and best results, treatment should be started as soon as possible after the onset of symptoms. If started within the first 12 hours, colchicine gives effective relief of acute arthritis in 90% of cases.
- The long-term use of low-dose colchicine is very effective in preventing recurrent acute attacks of gouty arthritis.
- Its use is recommended during the early months of maintenance therapy with allopurinol and/or probenecid or sulfinpyrazone to prevent flare-ups of acute arthritis.
- Should be used with caution and reduced dosage in the presence of liver disease or impaired liver function.
- Colchicine is destroyed by exposure to light. Be sure your supply is fresh and fully effective.

Use of Nonsteroidal Anti-Inflammatory Drugs

- Now considered by many authorities to be the drug(s) of choice for treating acute attacks of gouty arthritis. They relieve pain and inflammation, but do not lower the blood level of uric acid. When given promptly and in adequate dosage, these drugs usually provide relief within 6 to 12 hours and complete recovery in three days.

- Should be taken with food to prevent stomach irritation and indigestion.
- Should be avoided in the presence of active peptic ulcer disease.
- Should be used with caution in hypertension and congestive heart failure.

See Appendix 8, Nonsteroidal Anti-Inflammatory Drugs: A Guide to Selection for Therapy.

Use of Prednisone (or Similar Cortisonelike Steroids)

- Used to abort acute attacks of gouty arthritis. Not recommended for frequently repeated or long-term use. Relieves inflammation, swelling, and pain, but does not lower the blood level of uric acid.
- Should be used only after adequate trials of all other appropriate drugs have failed to relieve the acute attack. "Rebound" attacks are common following withdrawal of steroid medications.

Use of Probenecid or Sulfinpyrazone

- Used to lower the blood level of uric acid by increasing its excretion in the urine. Of no value in treating the acute attack and should not be started until acute arthritis has subsided; it is best suited for individuals who
  - are underexcretors of uric acid (less than 800 mg/24-hour urine excretion);
  - are under 60 years of age;
  - have good kidney function;
  - have no history of kidney stones.
- Should not be used by those who
  - are overproducers of uric acid (more than 800 mg/24-hour urine excretion);
  - have impaired kidney function and low urine volume;
  - are subject to kidney stones.
- It is advisable to begin treatment with small doses to avoid precipitating an acute attack of arthritis.
- Should be taken in 2 to 4 doses/day.
- If the tolerance of either drug is limited, the two drugs can be taken concurrently in reduced dosage.
- Ensure a high intake of liquids (up to 3 quarts daily). Effectiveness is improved by the concurrent use of sodium bicarbonate or potassium citrate.

Ancillary Drug Treatment (as required)

For mild pain:
- acetaminophen (Tylenol, etc.). Do not use aspirin or other salicylates.

For severe pain:
- codeine or meperidine (Demerol)

For diarrhea due to colchicine:
- paregoric or loperimide (Imodium)

For high blood pressure:
see Profile of hypertension in this section

For "secondary" gout due to chemotherapy for leukemia, lymphoma, multiple myeloma, polycythemia:
- allopurinol (Zyloprim)

Note: Drug selection, dosage, and administration schedule must be determined by the physician for each patient individually.

Possible Drug Interactions of Significance

Because of the number of drugs that may be used to manage this disorder, adequate consideration of the volume and complexity of potential drug interactions is beyond the scope of this book. Consult *The Essential Guide to Prescription Drugs,* or a similar drug reference book for possible interactions of significance (see Appendix 17, Drug Information Sources).

Special Considerations for the Elderly

Pseudogout (calcium pyrophosphate deposition disease) is a common cause of joint pain in the elderly and resembles true gout in some respects. It characteristically involves the knees and wrists more commonly than other joints. The correct diagnosis is made by detecting calcium pyrophosphate crystals (rather than uric acid crystals) in joint fluid. It is advisable to confirm the specific diagnosis because treatment and prognosis differ somewhat between the two disorders.

The Role of Prevention in This Disorder

Primary Prevention

No method is known to deter the development of genetically induced hyperuricemia.

Secondary Prevention

Once the diagnosis of hyperuricemia is established, episodes of acute gouty arthritis and long-term complications can be prevented by appropriate medications and periodic monitoring of blood uric acid levels.

Resources

Additional Information and Services

Arthritis Foundation
1314 Spring Street, NW
Atlanta, GA 30309
Phone: (404) 872-7100, 1-800-283-7800; Fax: (404) 872-0457
Local groups: 71. Publications available.

Disease Management Expertise
See Appendix 13, Arthritis and Musculoskeletal Disease Centers.

HYPERTENSION

Other Names Arterial hypertension, essential hypertension, primary hypertension, secondary hypertension, high blood pressure

Prevalence/Incidence in U.S.
Current estimate: approximately 50 million; 15% of adult white population; 25% of adult black population
Estimated deaths annually: 36,000

Age Group

Age Group	% of Total
Under 18 years	<1%
18 to 44 years	21%
45 to 64 years	41%
65 to 74 years	23%
75 years and over	14%

Male-to-Female Ratio
Under 45 years—same incidence in men and women; 45 to 64 years—slightly more common in women; 65 years and over—more common in women (2 to 1)

Principal Features and Natural History
Hypertension is the most common chronic disorder in the United States. It is also the most common reason for visits to physicians' offices and the most common indication for the use of prescription drugs. Hypertension is a major contributing factor to the first and third leading causes of death among Americans, namely heart disease and stroke. The risks for serious illness and death are directly related to the degree and duration of elevated blood pressure.

During the early years of hypertension there are usually no symptoms to indicate its presence, hence its reputation as "the silent killer." Brief periods of sudden elevation of blood pressure above usual levels may cause transient throbbing headaches and/or dizziness. After years of untreated high blood pressure, manifestations of "target organ" disease may occur: stroke (blood clot or hemorrhage in the brain), impaired vision (retinal hemorrhage and deterioration), heart attack (myocardial infarction), congestive heart failure, and chronic kidney failure (uremia).

The very significant morbidity and mortality attributable to hypertension are truly regrettable. We now have sufficient understanding of this disorder to detect it in early stages of development, manage it effectively, and significantly blunt its predictable consequences.

Diagnostic Symptoms and Signs

The following symptoms *may* or *may not* be due to hypertension. However, if you experience any of them, have your blood pressure checked promptly.

frequent headaches

recurring spells of dizziness

unusual changes in vision

chest pains, with or without exertion

leg muscle cramps while walking

numbness or weakness occurring in the face or extremities

slurred speech

impaired thinking or concentration

swelling of the feet or ankles

Diagnostic Tests and Procedures

Blood pressure measurements, after five minutes rest, in lying, sitting, and standing positions, and in both arms initially to detect a significant difference

Ambulatory blood pressure monitoring to clarify blood pressure status and to correlate symptoms and blood pressure recordings. One study revealed that 20% of patients diagnosed as having mild hypertension were shown to have normal blood pressure with ambulatory monitoring.

Ophthalmoscopic examination of the retinal blood vessels

Electrocardiogram to evaluate heart rhythm and status of heart muscle

Echocardiogram to detect heart enlargement

Battery of relevant blood chemistries

24-hour urine collection for diagnostic urine analysis

Sonograms of the kidneys

Radioactive kidney scans

Computed tomography (CT scan) of the adrenal glands

Diagnostic "Markers" for This Disorder

Blood pressure readings of 140/90 or higher on three separate occasions

Optimal conditions for blood pressure measurement:

- the subject is relaxed, comfortable, and free of anxiety and pain;
- he has not smoked or consumed caffeine within 30 minutes before examination;
- he has rested for 5 minutes before measurement;
- he is comfortably seated during measurement.

ALERT!
The diagnosis of hypertension should never be made on the basis of a single measurement.

Possible Effects of Drugs on Test Results
Some over-the-counter drug products can cause transient elevations of blood pressure. The ingredients of some cold remedies and appetite control preparations can increase the blood pressure significantly in sensitive individuals. Inform your physician if you are taking any drug products of this nature.

See also the section "Drugs That Can Cause This Disorder" below.

Similar Conditions That May Confuse Diagnosis
Chronic kidney disorders
Constriction of kidney artery
Aldosteronism
Cushing's disease
Pheochromocytoma
Hyperthyroidism

Causes

Established Causes
In primary (essential) hypertension (95% of all hypertension), no specific cause is apparent.

Secondary hypertension (5% of all hypertension) is due to a demonstrable (and sometimes curable) cause: narrowing of the main artery to one or both kidneys, chronic kidney disease, adrenaline- or renin-producing tumors, coarctation (constriction) of the aorta.

Theoretical Causes
There is a definite hereditary (genetic) predisposition; 80% of hypertensive individuals have a close relative with high blood pressure. The basic mechanisms that initiate hypertension are thought to be due to alterations of the regulatory functions of sodium and calcium in vascular tissues.

Known Risk Factors for Developing This Disorder
Family history of hypertension
Obesity
Excessive salt intake (in salt-sensitive individuals)
Sedentary lifestyle
Excessive alcohol consumption: more than 1–2 ounces daily
Tobacco smoking
Sustained psychological stress

Chronic lipid disorders
Diabetes mellitus
Chronic kidney disease

Drugs That Can Cause This Disorder

The following drugs (or drug combinations) can cause significant elevations of blood pressure:

amphetamines and related drugs
carbenoxolone
cyclosporine
ephedrine
ergot preparations
licorice
nonsteroidal anti-inflammatory drugs (NSAIDs)
oral contraceptives
phenylephrine
phenylpropanolamine
pseudoephedrine
tricyclic antidepressants taken concurrently with appetite suppressants, decongestants, or antihistamines

See Appendix 16, Drug Classes, for specific generic drugs within respective drug classes.

Goals of Treatment

Can This Disorder Be Cured?

Primary (essential) hypertension cannot be cured by any therapy currently available.

Some types of secondary hypertension can be cured by surgical correction of the principal cause: adrenaline-producing tumors, constricted kidney artery, etc.

Can This Disorder Be Treated Effectively?

Mild hypertension can be controlled quite well by appropriate modifications of lifestyle and without medication.

There are numerous medications currently available that are very effective in controlling moderate to severe hypertension.

Specific Goals

- Maintenance of blood pressure below 140/90, or as close as possible to this level with an acceptable program of drug therapy (minimal drug side effects and expense)
- Prevention or postponement of "target organ" damage in the brain, retina, heart, major blood vessels, and kidneys

Health Professionals Who Participate in Managing This Disorder

Family physicians
General internists
Obstetricians
Geriatricians
Cardiologists
Ophthalmologists
Optometrists
Nephrologists
Endocrinologists
Neurologists
Vascular surgeons
Pharmacists
Physician assistants
Nurse practitioners
Dietitians/Nutritionists
Clinical psychologists

Currently Available Therapies for This Disorder

Nondrug Treatment Methods

- Dietary modifications: sodium restriction to 2 grams or less daily (a no-salt-added diet)
- Dietary supplements of calcium, magnesium, and potassium if deficiencies are shown to exist
- Weight control: maintain ideal weight for sex, age, and body build
- Alcohol consumption: limit to 1 ounce daily
- Exercise: 15–20 minutes of moderate aerobic exercise daily
- Total and permanent cessation of smoking
- Relaxation and stress reduction programs as appropriate

Drug Therapy

The following classes of antihypertensive drugs are currently used to treat hypertension:

Alpha-adrenergic-blocking drugs:
- doxazosin (Cardura)
- prazosin (Minipres)
- terazosin (Hytrin)

Alpha/beta-adrenergic-blocking drugs:
- labetalol (Normodyne, Trandate)

Angiotensin-converting enzyme (ACE) inhibitors:
- benazepril (Lotensin)
- captopril (Capoten)
- enalapril (Vasotec)

- fosinopril (Monopril)
- lisinopril (Prinivil, Zestril)
- moexipril (Univasc)
- perindopril (Aceon)
- quinapril (Accupril)
- ramipril (Altace)

Angiotensin-receptor blocker:
- losartan (Cozaar)

Beta-adrenergic-blocking drugs:
- acebutolol (Sectral) with intrinsic sympathomimetic activity (ISA)
- atenolol (Tenormin) without ISA
- betaxolol (Kerlone) without ISA
- bisoprolol (Zebeta) without ISA
- carteolol (Cartrol) with ISA
- metoprolol (Lopressor) without ISA
- nadolol (Corgard) without ISA
- penbutolol (Levatol) with ISA
- pindolol (Visken) with ISA
- propranolol (Inderal) without ISA
- timolol (Blocadren) without ISA

Calcium-channel-blocking drugs:
- amlodipine (Norvasc)
- diltiazem (Cardizem)
- felodipine (Plendil)
- isradipine (DynaCirc)
- nicardipine (Cardene)
- nifedipine (Procardia)
- nisoldipine (Sular)
- verapamil (Calan, Isoptin)

Centrally acting drugs (in the brain):
- clonidine (Catapres)
- guanabenz (Wytensin)
- guanfacine (Tenex)
- methyldopa (Aldomet)

Direct vasodilators:
- hydralazine (Apresoline)
- minoxidil (Loniten)

Diuretics:
- thiazides (see Appendix 16, Drug Classes)
- chlorthalidone (Hygroton)
- quinethazone (Hydromox)
- metolazone (Diulo, Zaroxolyn)
- indapamide (Lozol)
- bumetanide (Bumex)

- furosemide (Lasix)
- torsemide (Demadex)
- potassium-saving diuretics: amiloride (Midamor), spironolactone (Aldactone), triamterene (Dyrenium)

Peripherally acting drugs (in peripheral blood vessels):
- guanadrel (Hylorel)
- guanethidine (Ismelin)
- reserpine (Serpasil)

Management of Therapy

- Although hypertension is difficult to define precisely, blood pressure is considered to be abnormally high if the systolic level is 140 or above or the diastolic level is 90 or above.
- Hypertension may be classified as follows:

Category	Systolic BP	Diastolic BP
Normal	<130	<85
High normal	130–139	85–89
Hypertension		
Stage 1	140–159 or	90–99
Stage 2	160–179 or	100–109
Stage 3	180–209 or	110–119
Stage 4	210 & above or	120 & above

- Most men who develop primary hypertension will have a diastolic pressure of 90 or above by age 35, most women by age 40 to 45.
- An adequate program of drug therapy for hypertension will postpone serious disability and death for most hypertensive individuals.
- The selection of antihypertensive drugs for initial treatment is based upon the range of the abnormally high pressures recorded on repeated measurements *and* the status of the "target organs" (brain, heart, kidneys, and blood vessels) at the time hypertension is discovered.
- Tranquilizers and sedatives are not effective for lowering elevated blood pressure and should not be relied upon as primary treatment for hypertension.
- Obtain a blood pressure measuring instrument (preferably an aneroid manometer, arm cuff, and stethoscope) and ask your physician to teach you how to take your own blood pressure. Measurements of blood pressure made at home (or at work) are far more representative of your actual day-by-day pressures than are readings made in the physician's office. By taking your own blood pressure at home, at work, and at varying times and under different circumstances, you can create a record that clearly reflects your response to the antihypertensive drugs prescribed for you.

- Avoid isometric exercises—bodybuilding, weight lifting, or push-ups; these raise the blood pressure significantly. Consult your physician regarding the advisability of isotonic (acrobic) exercises—walking, bicycling, swimming.
- Consumption of more than 2 ounces of alcohol daily can raise the blood pressure. One ounce of alcohol is present in 2 ounces of 100-proof whiskey, in 8 ounces of wine, or in 24 ounces of beer.
- Five percent of oral contraceptive users will develop a diastolic blood pressure of over 90. If this occurs, the contraceptive pill should be discontinued for six months and the blood pressure monitored. Women with this sensitivity should use an alternative method of contraception.
- In Type I diabetes, thiazides are well tolerated, but beta-blockers may mask the symptoms of hypoglycemia. In Type II diabetes, thiazides are best avoided; small doses of furosemide or spironolactone are preferable. Beta-blockers can impair insulin release.
- After blood pressure has been well controlled for a year, consideration may be given to a "step-down" reduction of both drug dosage and the number of drugs used. The blood pressure response to the gradual withdrawal of drugs must be monitored very carefully. A recent study showed that 28% of the group of hypertensives studied had normal blood pressure one year after discontinuing all antihypertensive medication. Your physician can determine if and when you meet the criteria for attempting to discontinue your program of drug treatment.

Treatment of Hypertension According to Severity

For Stage 1 hypertension (140–159/90–99):
- Reduce excessive weight.
- Reduce salt intake moderately. No-salt-added diet.
- Reduce stress in daily living.
- Avoid excessive consumption of alcohol. Limit to 1 ounce daily.
- Stop smoking.
- Avoid isometric exercise.
- Increase isotonic exercise.
- Defer drug treatment for three to six months to determine effectiveness of above measures.

For Stage 2 hypertension (160–179/100–109) (80% of all hypertensives):
- Comply with all Stage 1 measures to modify lifestyle.
- If response is not adequate, drug treatment should be started: It is advisable to use a single drug initially—commonly a thiazide diuretic or a beta-blocker. Some authorities prefer a trial of a calcium-channel blocker or an ACE inhibitor for initiating treatment.

For Stage 3 hypertension (180–209/110–119):
- It is not likely that a single drug will control this degree of hypertension. Two approaches are currently favored: (1) a combination of a

thiazide diuretic and a beta-blocker; or (2) a combination of an ACE inhibitor and diuretic or a calcium-channel blocker and diuretic.

For Stage 4 hypertension (210+/120+):

- Adequate control will probably require treatment with two or three drugs. When multiple drugs are used, smaller doses of individual drugs are often effective and better tolerated. A trial-and-error approach is often necessary to determine the most effective and acceptable combination of drugs.

Use of Diuretics

- Used as Stage 1 or Stage 2 drugs, diuretics are most appropriate for treating hypertensives who are black or elderly, those with congestive heart failure or kidney failure, and those who cannot use a beta-blocker drug.
- A thiazide diuretic is the initial drug tried in many cases. It is effective in a single dose taken in the morning. While using thiazide diuretics, it is advisable to observe for loss of potassium (10% of users), increased blood level of uric acid (66% of users), and increased blood sugar level.
- Spironolactone and triamterene are as effective as thiazides in reducing blood pressure; they are used to prevent potassium loss. The most practical and reliable way to prevent a significant decline in the potassium blood level is to use a potassium-saving diuretic—amiloride, spironolactone, or triamterene. The use of high-potassium foods is often unreliable. Compliance with the long-term use of oral potassium supplements is very poor.
- The more potent diuretics furosemide and ethacrynic acid are no more effective than the thiazides for reducing blood pressure.
- It is advisable to discontinue the use of diuretics gradually to prevent fluid retention (edema) after withdrawal.

Use of Beta-Adrenergic-Blocking Drugs

- Used to initiate treatment, beta-blockers are most appropriate for treating hypertensives who are young; those who have an overactive heart (fast rate, palpitation, premature beats); and those with gout, migraine headaches, and angina (coronary artery disease). It is advisable to avoid beta-blockers if you have asthma, emphysema, or a history of heart block or congestive heart failure.
- These drugs characteristically cause fatigue and lethargy. Propranolol and metoprolol may cause emotional depression. When propranolol is used alone, 10% of users can experience an increase in blood pressure. It is advisable to use a diuretic prior to starting propranolol in sensitive individuals.
- Sudden discontinuation of beta-blockers should be avoided, especially in the presence of coronary artery disease. Abrupt withdrawal can

cause rapid heart rate, palpitation, and intensification of angina; myocardial infarction (heart attack) has been reported.

Use of Labetalol (an Alpha- and Beta-Adrenergic-Blocker)
- This drug may be effective when the beta-blockers have failed to control blood pressure. It functions primarily as a vasodilator in the elderly, with no significant alteration of heart function.
- It should be avoided in presence of asthma, emphysema, heart block, and congestive heart failure.

Use of Angiotensin-Converting Enzyme (ACE) Inhibitors
- These may be used to initiate treatment or to supplement other drugs in treating any stage of hypertension. Full effectiveness of these drugs may not be apparent until after several weeks of continual use.
- To prevent an excessive drop in blood pressure initially, any diuretic in use should be discontinued five to seven days before starting an ACE inhibitor. After the dose is stabilized, a thiazide diuretic may enhance antihypertensive effectiveness.
- Captopril should be taken one hour before eating, two to three times daily, for maximal effectiveness. Enalapril may be taken once or twice daily without regard to eating.
- These drugs may increase the blood potassium level. Do not use any commercial salt substitute (most of which contain potassium) without first consulting your physician.

Use of Calcium-Channel-Blocking Drugs
- These drugs are approved by the U.S. Food and Drug Administration (FDA) for use in the management of angina (coronary artery disease) and hypertension. They are effective antihypertensives and are being used as such by many physicians. These drugs should be used with caution if a beta-blocker drug is being used concurrently. A dosage of three to four times daily is required. They may be used to initiate treatment or to supplement other drugs in treating any stage of hypertension.
- They are especially useful in treating the elderly individual with isolated systolic hypertension.
- Observe for fluid retention. Effectiveness may be improved if a thiazide diuretic is taken concurrently.

Use of Alpha-Adrenergic-Blocking Drugs
- In 10% of users, these drugs can provoke an idiosyncratic reaction that results in a sudden extreme drop in blood pressure following the first dose. It is advisable to begin treatment with a bedtime dose and to arise cautiously the next morning in anticipation of possible orthostatic hypotension (see Glossary).

- These drugs can cause fluid retention and can aggravate angina. It is best used in conjunction with a diuretic and a beta-blocker.
- Do not use these drugs concurrently with hydralazine or guanethidine because of the potential for additive postural hypotension.
- A rapid loss of effectiveness can limit the long-term usefulness of these drugs.

Use of Clonidine
- This drug characteristically causes drowsiness, fatigue, and dry mouth. It may also cause mental depression.
- This drug should not be discontinued abruptly. Sudden withdrawal can cause a severe rebound hypertension with higher blood pressure than prior to treatment. It is advisable to withdraw it over two to four days. After discontinuation of clonidine, the start of a beta-blocker drug should be delayed for 48 hours.

Use of Methyldopa
- This drug usually causes lethargy and fatigue at the beginning of treatment. These side effects often subside with continued use. It may also cause mental depression.
- This drug causes salt and water retention; a diuretic should be taken concurrently.
- If any of the following adverse effects develop, this drug should be discontinued: mental depression, drug fever, breast enlargement, milk production, indications of liver toxicity (loss of appetite, nausea, jaundice).
- Sudden discontinuation of this drug can cause agitation, insomnia, rapid heart rate, and intensification of angina.

Use of Hydralazine
- This drug is rarely used alone. It can cause fluid retention and should be used concurrently with a diuretic.
- This drug characteristically increases heart activity, which can be counteracted by the concurrent use of a beta-blocker drug.
- It should be used cautiously in the presence of angina (coronary artery disease).
- Approximately 13% of users may develop a reaction that resembles lupus erythematosus. Report promptly the appearance of a rash or the development of joint symptoms of any kind.

Use of Minoxidil
- This drug is a potent, long-acting vasodilator. Its use is usually restricted to treating those whose blood pressure cannot be controlled by conventional treatment with other drugs.

- It is generally used concurrently with a diuretic and a beta-blocker drug.
- Observe for excessive growth of hair.

Use of Guanethidine

- This is the most potent antihypertensive drug in general use. It is usually reserved to treat the most severe cases of hypertension and those that have been difficult to control. It causes marked orthostatic hypotension. Users should avoid prolonged sitting (without moving the legs) and prolonged standing (without walking around); these are conducive to excessive drops in blood pressure and resultant fainting. Users should also arise cautiously in the morning to avoid fainting shortly after getting out of bed.
- This drug causes salt and water retention and should be taken concurrently with a diuretic.
- Tricyclic antidepressants can reduce this drug's antihypertensive effectiveness.

Use of Reserpine

- The daily dose should be limited to 0.25 mg or less.
- Avoid completely if you have a history of depression.
- This drug can cause salt and water retention; a diuretic should be used concurrently.
- Do not use this drug concurrently with methyldopa; the combination can cause marked sedation, excessive dreaming, and sexual impotence.
- Observe for the following possible adverse effects: drowsiness, lethargy, depression (can be very insidious), nightmares, nasal congestion, acid indigestion (possible ulcer), diarrhea, impotence, Parkinson-like syndrome.

Ancillary Drug Treatment (as required)

For thiazide-induced gout:
- allopurinol (Zyloprim)
- probenecid (Benemid)

For drug-induced fluid retention:
- bumetanide (Bumex)

For guanethidine-induced diarrhea:
- diphenoxylate (Lomotil)
- loperamide (Imodium)

For tension headache:
- acetaminophen (Tylenol, etc.)

For migraine headache (short-term use):
- ibuprofen (Motrin, Advil, Nuprin)
- oxycodone (Percodan)
  Avoid ergotamine preparations.

For musculoskeletal pain, arthritis (long-term use):
• sulindac (Clinoril)

Note: Drug selection, dosage, and administration schedule must be determined by the physician for each patient individually.

Current Controversies in Drug Management

The earlier "stepped-care" approach to treating hypertension recommended the use of a thiazide diuretic as the drug of choice to initiate therapy. If an adequate trial with thiazide therapy failed to lower blood pressure sufficiently, other drugs of the various classes listed above were added in a somewhat arbitrary and rigid fashion. Although the guidelines provided by a standardized approach were beneficial in promoting rational therapy, new information about the older drugs and the availability of many new and more effective drugs call for a reappraisal of drug selection for managing hypertension.

Recent review of thiazide drug performance discloses that (1) although they are effective in mild hypertension, they have not decreased the incidence of heart attacks; (2) they can cause loss of potassium and/or magnesium and thereby contribute to the development of dangerous heart rhythm disorders; and (3) they cause a 10% increase in LDL cholesterol blood levels and may increase the risk of coronary artery disease. Some authorities no longer consider thiazides to be the drugs of choice for initiating treatment; they also recommend that thiazides be used in the lowest effective dose to reduce the potential risks of long-term therapy.

Current recommendations call for a greater emphasis on individualization of drug management. This includes wider flexibility in selecting drugs for starting treatment and in substituting and deleting drugs as individual monitoring dictates. Several drug classes are admirably suited for initiating treatment and provide a broad spectrum of features that permit tailoring the drug to the individual characteristics of the patient.

It is important to note that at the time of this writing there is no general consensus as to the "preferred way" to treat hypertension. This is not surprising. Given the diverse nature of hypertensive patients and the myriad selection of antihypertensive drugs, the best match of patient and drug must be determined individually by the treating physician. The October 1994 issue of the *American Journal of Hypertension* published the views of seven experts on the drug therapy of hypertension. All use treatment regimens that are different from the "official" guidelines recommended by the Joint National Committee on High Blood Pressure in its fifth report issued in 1994. Critics of the recommendations point out that the most recently approved classes of drugs make it possible to not only lower the patient's blood pressure but to improve his quality of life at the same time. Work closely with your physician to determine the selection of drugs that is most beneficial for you.

Suggestions Regarding Drug Selection

Patient Characteristics	Drugs of Choice (see Drug Classes listed above)
Young patient	ACE inhibitor alpha-adrenergic-blocker centrally acting drug
Elderly patient	alpha-adrenergic-blocker centrally acting drug calcium-channel blocker
Black patient	alpha-adrenergic-blocker centrally acting drug calcium-channel blocker
White patient	ACE inhibitor alpha-adrenergic-blocker centrally acting drug calcium-channel blocker
Pregnancy	hydralazine methyldopa
Menopause	centrally acting drug
Sexual dysfunction	ACE inhibitor alpha-adrenergic-blocker calcium channel blocker
Obesity	ACE inhibitor alpha-adrenergic-blocker centrally acting drug
Nonsteroidal anti-inflammatory drugs (NSAIDs)	calcium-channel blocker centrally acting drug
Migraine headaches	beta-blocker without ISA centrally acting drug calcium-channel blocker
Depression	ACE inhibitor alpha-adrenergic-blocker calcium-channel blocker
Glaucoma	beta-adrenergic-blocker centrally acting drug diuretic
Angina, obstructive	beta-blocker without ISA calcium-channel blocker
Angina, vasospastic	calcium-channel blocker
Asthma, emphysema	alpha-adrenergic-blocker centrally acting drug calcium-channel blocker
Peptic ulcer disease	centrally acting drug calcium-channel blocker
Kidney insufficiency	ACE inhibitor alpha-adrenergic-blocker centrally acting drug calcium-channel blocker

Diabetes mellitus	ACE inhibitor
	alpha-adrenergic-blocker
	centrally acting drug
	calcium-channel blocker
Blood lipid disorders	alpha-adrenergic-blocker
	centrally acting drug
	calcium-channel blocker
Hyperuricemia/Gout	ACE inhibitor
	alpha-adrenergic-blocker
	centrally acting drug
	calcium-channel blocker

Possible Drug Interactions of Significance

Because of the number of drugs that may be used to manage this disorder, adequate consideration of the volume and complexity of potential drug interactions is beyond the scope of this book. Consult *The Essential Guide to Prescription Drugs*, or a similar drug reference book for possible interactions of significance (see Appendix 17, Drug Information Sources).

Special Considerations for Women

Oral contraceptives are the most frequent reversible cause of secondary hypertension. About 5% of women in their mid-30s and older have a two- to sixfold increased risk of developing hypertension while using oral contraceptives. Periodic measurement of blood pressure is advised. If discontinuation of OCs is warranted, blood pressure usually returns to normal within three months.

Postmenopausal estrogen replacement therapy (ERT) is usually associated with a decrease in blood pressure. A small number of women may show a rise in blood pressure, so periodic monitoring is advised. However, ERT is not contraindicated in hypertension.

Pregnancy

Approximately 2% of pregnant women have chronic hypertension. Mild hypertension (140/90 to 150/100) is not a contraindication to pregnancy, and the prognosis for mother and fetus is generally good. Antihypertensive drug therapy should be discontinued before conception or as soon as pregnancy is confirmed. Women with preexisting moderate hypertension (150/90 to 180/110) are generally advised to discontinue diuretics and to begin methyldopa therapy. This may be supplemented with hydralazine if necessary. If severe hypertension (above 180/110) develops, the prognosis for both mother and fetus is poor. Critical decisions must be made jointly by parents and physicians regarding the need to terminate pregnancy.

About 5% of women who are pregnant for the first time and have preexisting hypertension are at increased risk for developing preeclampsia between the 20th week of pregnancy and the end of the first week following delivery. Preeclampsia is characterized by an increase of 30 mm in systolic pressure or 15 mm in diastolic pressure, swelling of the face or hands (fluid retention), and the presence of albumin (protein) in the urine. The cause of this development is unknown. If unresponsive to treatment, preeclampsia can progress to eclampsia, a state of coma with or without convulsive seizures. Preeclampsia may threaten the health and life of the mother and fetus, forcing premature delivery. Close monitoring of blood pressure should begin as soon as pregnancy is confirmed.

Drug Use During Pregnancy

It is generally agreed that no drug should be taken during pregnancy unless it is clearly needed to protect the mother's health and well-being. Of the many drugs in common use, 124 are designated Pregnancy Category D and 35 are designated Pregnancy Category X. Among these are numerous antihypertensive drugs that are widely prescribed. Determine the Pregnancy Category of all drugs you are advised to take for any condition under treatment (see Appendix 15, FDA Pregnancy Categories).

Breast-Feeding

Consult your obstetrician and pediatrician regarding the advisability of nursing and the concurrent use of any medication.

Special Considerations for the Elderly

The elderly individual with hypertension must approach antihypertensive drug therapy very cautiously. Goals of drug treatment are more liberal; reduction of pressures to 140–160/95–100 are usually adequate. This can usually be achieved with small doses of a diuretic.

For isolated systolic hypertension (160+/85–90):

- This is usually found in the elderly. Cautious and conservative drug treatment is recommended for those over age 60.
- Reduction of isolated systolic hypertension in older persons reduces the occurrence of stroke.
- A calcium-channel-blocking drug is effective and well tolerated for treating this type of hypertension. Initial doses should be about half those used in younger individuals.
- It is best to avoid drugs that are more prone to cause orthostatic hypotension.
- If a diuretic is used, it is advisable to monitor for dehydration and potassium loss.

Quality of Life Considerations

All antihypertensive drugs have side effects and possible adverse effects. Most of these are relatively mild and easily tolerated. The most troublesome adverse effect for many is the impairment of sexual function. This varies greatly from drug to drug and among individual users. Pay close attention to all drug-induced effects and work closely with your physician to find the drug that has the best balance of therapeutic effectiveness and acceptable side effects. Do not be reluctant to raise the issue of sexual function. Many physicians are hesitant to explore this aspect of therapy.

Studies have shown that the angiotensin-converting enzyme inhibitor captopril significantly improves the sexual quality of life in both women and men.

The Role of Prevention in This Disorder

Primary Prevention
- Maintain normal weight for sex, age, and body build.
- Restrict use of salt: avoid salty foods, no added salt.
- Take supplements of calcium, magnesium, and potassium if deficiency is verified.
- Maintain a program of regular, moderate, aerobic exercise.
- Limit alcohol consumption to 1 ounce daily.
- Abstain totally from tobacco smoking.
- Avoid sustained psychological or physical stress.

Secondary Prevention
- Full compliance with all recommendations for primary prevention
- Full compliance with the antihypertensive therapy program recommended by your physician
- Self-monitoring of your blood pressure on a regular basis
- Regular periodic follow-up visits to your physician for evaluation of your progress, adjustment of medications as appropriate, and monitoring of "target organ" status

Resources

Recommended Reading
The ABCs of Antihypertensive Therapy, Franz H. Messerli. New York: Raven Press, 1994.

Additional Information and Services
Citizens for Public Action on High Blood Pressure and Cholesterol
7200 Wisconsin Avenue, Suite 1002
Bethesda, MD 20814
Phone: (301) 907-7790; Fax: (301) 907-7792
    Publications available.

National Institute of Hypertension Studies
Institute of Hypertension School of Research

295 Mt. Vernon
Detroit, MI 48202
Phone: (313) 872-0505
   Publications available.

Disease Management Expertise
The Joint National Committee on Detection, Evaluation and Treatment of
High Blood Pressure
National Heart, Lung and Blood Institute
National Institutes of Health
Box 120/80
Bethesda, MD 20892
Phone: (301) 496-4000

HYPOTHYROIDISM

Other Names Hypometabolism, myxedema, primary hypothyroidism,
secondary hypothyroidism, subclinical hypothyroidism

Prevalence/Incidence in U.S.
Overt hypothyroidism: 3 to 4.5% of the general population
Subclinical hypothyroidism: 5% of the general population
Infantile hypothyroidism (cretinism): 1 in 5,000 newborn infants

Age Group
Juvenile hypothyroidism: under 18 years—2% of total incidence. Adult
hypothyroidism: percentage of total incidence by age: 18 to 44 years—
34%; 45 to 64 years—40%; 65 years and over—24%.

Male-to-Female Ratio More common in women—5 to 1

Principal Features and Natural History
Hypothyroidism spans a wide spectrum from very mild thyroid hormone
deficiency (subclinical hypothyroidism) with few nonspecific symptoms
to severe deficiency (myxedema) that can be fatal if not treated adequately. The most common form of hypothyroidism is the mild to moderate hormone deficiency seen primarily in women age 20 to 65 years. The
onset is usually insidious and the early symptoms are so vague that medical attention is rarely sought. With progression of the deficiency, the individual gradually becomes aware of lethargy, fatigability, intolerance of
cold, weight gain (with no increased food intake), loss of hair, vague
muscle and joint pains, and irregular menstruation. The skin may become
dry and scaly, the face may appear puffy (fluid retention), the speech

slows, the voice becomes hoarse, and the pattern of activity becomes sluggish. Hypothyroidism in the elderly can cause mental changes: confusion, paranoia, depression, and dementia.

Subclinical hypothyroidism is a very mild or borderline state of thyroid hormone deficiency that requires confirmation by laboratory testing. It is relatively common, especially in the elderly, but often goes undetected because the symptoms are so vague or mild that neither the patient nor the physician suspects thyroid deficiency. Definitive thyroid testing is usually not performed until the condition progresses to recognizable hypothyroidism.

Hypothyroidism is a known contributor to the development of atherosclerosis, including atherosclerotic heart disease. Currently available diagnostic tests are highly reliable for detecting chronic thyroid deficiency in its early stages. Currently available synthetic thyroxine effectively corrects this hormone deficiency. Patients and physicians alike should utilize this opportunity to practice meaningful prevention.

Diagnostic Symptoms and Signs

Weakness, fatigue, lethargy
Intolerance to cold environment
Impaired thinking, concentration, and memory
Hearing loss
Constipation
Muscle aches and cramps
Joint pains (without inflammation or swelling)
Modest weight gain (without increased food intake)
Decreased perspiration
Menstrual irregularity
Dry, coarse skin
Loss of scalp and body hair
Swelling of face and extremities
Huskiness of voice
Subnormal body temperature
Slow heart rate
Decreased systolic blood pressure
Increased diastolic blood pressure
Sluggish reflexes
Enlargement of thyroid gland (goiter)

Diagnostic Tests and Procedures

Measurements of thyroid-stimulating hormone (TSH) in blood by ultra-
sensitive assay
Measurements of total or free thyroxine (T-4) in blood
Measurements of total or free triiodothyronine (T-3) in blood

Measurements of reverse triiodothyronine (rT-3) in blood
Measurements of T-3 resin uptake
Measurement of 24-hour radioactive I^{131} uptake by thyroid gland
Demonstration of thyroid peroxidase antibodies in blood
Pertinent blood cell counts and blood chemistries, including blood lipid
  profile

Diagnostic "Markers" for This Disorder

The combination of a low total T-4 (normal range: 5.0–12.5 ng/dl) or free
T-4 (normal range: 0.7–2.0 ng/dl) *and* a high TSH (normal range:
0.4–10.0 mIU/L) is diagnostic of primary hypothyroidism.

Possible Effects of Drugs on Test Results

The following drugs can cause a low total T-4 test result in the presence
of normal thyroid gland function:
  cortisonelike drugs (adrenocorticosteroids)
  phenobarbital
  phenytoin
  salicylates (aspirin, sodium salicylate, etc.)
  testosterone

Causes

Primary hypothyroidism can be due to (1) a congenital defect in thyroid
gland development or function; (2) Hashimoto's thyroiditis, an "autoimmune" impairment of thyroid hormone production (45% of cases); (3) a
lack of iodine in the food or water supply; or (4) intentional thyroid
gland suppression by the administration of radioactive iodine or by surgical removal of thyroid tissue (35% of cases).

Secondary hypothyroidism is due to inadequate stimulation of thyroid
gland function from the hypothalamus (in the brain) or from the pituitary gland (the "master" gland that regulates most hormone-producing
glands). The causes of these stimulation failures is not known.

Drugs That Can Cause This Disorder

The following drugs can impair the normal production of thyroid hormones and induce varying degrees of hypothyroidism:
  amiodarone
  cyclophosphamide
  disulfiram (questionable)
  ethionamide
  iodine compounds (iodides)
  lithium
  methimazole
  pentazocine

phenylbutazone
propylthiouracil
sulfonylurea antidiabetic drugs
See Appendix 16, Drug Classes, for specific generic drugs within respective drug classes.

Goals of Treatment

Can This Disorder Be Cured?

Hypothyroidism is a state of hormone deficiency. Hormone replacement therapy provides a cure.

Can This Disorder Be Treated Effectively?

Appropriate thyroid function tests can determine the degree of hormone deficiency and serve as a guide to dosage of hormone replacement.

Specific Goals

- Adequate replacement of thyroxine: restoration of normal blood levels of T-4 and thyroid-stimulating hormone (TSH)
- Relief of symptoms associated with deficiency of thyroid hormones (hypothyroidism, cretinism, myxedema)
- Periodic monitoring of thyroid function status to avoid overdosing or underdosing of thyroxine

Health Professionals Who Participate in Managing This Disorder

Family physicians
General internists
Pediatricians
Geriatricians
Clinical endocrinologists
Thyroidologists
Pharmacists
Physician assistants
Nurse practitioners

Currently Available Therapies for This Disorder

Drug Therapy

- synthetic levothyroxine (T-4) (Synthroid, Levothroid)
- synthetic liothyronine (T-3) (Cytomel)
- synthetic liotrix (combinations of T-4 and T-3) (Euthroid, Thyrolar)
- thyroid extract (animal origin) (Desiccated thyroid Armour)
- thyroglobulin (animal origin) (Proloid)

Management of Therapy

- Primary hypothyroidism is diagnosed by finding the blood level of the principal thyroid hormone—thyroxine (T-4)—below the normal range and the blood level of the pituitary hormone—thyroid-stimulating hormone (TSH)—above the normal range.

- Once the diagnosis of true primary hypothyroidism is established, treatment for life is generally thought to be necessary. However, periodic evaluation is advisable to determine the need for continual thyroid hormone replacement.

- Individuals taking replacement thyroid hormones should be monitored every 6 to 12 months by measurements of T-4 and TSH along with evaluation of general well-being.

- Until thyroid deficiency is adequately corrected, the patient may be overly sensitive to drugs that depress brain function—sedatives, tranquilizers, hypnotics, narcotic analgesics, or general anesthetics.

- In treating hypothyroidism of infancy, it is advisable to avoid formula feedings that contain soybean extract; they can prevent the absorption of thyroxine and perpetuate cretinism.

- Anxious, thin individuals usually require smaller doses of maintenance thyroxine than lethargic, obese individuals. Significant reduction in weight (correction of obesity) is usually followed by reduction in the daily requirement of maintenance thyroxine.

- The use of thyroid hormones for weight reduction in the presence of normal thyroid function (no hormone deficiency) is unjustified and dangerous.

- Hypothyroidism causes an increase in bone mass. Thyroid replacement therapy can result in a significant loss of bone (osteoporosis) in the lumbar vertebrae (spine). Consult your physician regarding the advisability of taking supplements of calcium and vitamin D during thyroid hormone replacement (see the Profile of osteoporosis in this section).

Use of Levothyroxine

- Hypothyroidism is best treated with a synthetic preparation of levothyroxine. This provides replacement that approximates most closely the normal status of thyroid hormones in circulating blood.

- Young, basically healthy individuals with hypothyroidism may take thyroxine in full dosage—1 microgram per pound of body weight daily. This usually achieves normal blood levels of T-4 and TSH. Older individuals, with incipient or established heart disease, should initiate thyroxine treatment with small doses that can be increased gradually over two to three months. This reduces the risk of precipitating disturbances of heart function, such as angina and abnormal heart rhythm. Should chest pain or palpitation develop, discontinue thyroxine and inform your physician promptly.

- Thyroxine should be taken in the morning on an empty stomach to ensure maximal absorption and uniform effectiveness. Observe for possible seasonal variation in your response to thyroxine replacement therapy. Some individuals may need less in warm months and more in cold months. If the winter dose of thyroxine is somewhat excessive for summer requirements, you may develop nervousness, insomnia, headaches, intolerance of heat, and loss of weight. Consult your physician if you think seasonal dosage adjustment is necessary.
- Cholestyramine and colestipol can reduce absorption of thyroxine and liothyronine; for best results, take thyroxine (and/or liothyronine) first, preferably in the morning and fasting, five hours before the first daily dose of either cholestyramine or colestipol.
- Long-term thyroxine therapy may lead to premature bone loss in the lower spine or upper femur (thigh bone) in women. Periodic monitoring of thyroxine blood levels is advised to detect excessive dosage.
- Do not purchase thyroxine tablets in large quantities (such as 500 to 1,000). Thyroxine products can lose up to 6% of their potency per year. It is advisable to obtain a three to six months' supply (100 to 200 tablets) to ensure full-strength medication.

ALERT!

It is advisable to initiate treatment with an established brand of thyroxine (such as Synthroid) and to obtain the same brand each time prescriptions are refilled. Generic versions of thyroxine have been found to vary in potency and uniformity.

Ancillary Drug Treatment (as required)

For anemia:
- iron preparations
- vitamin B-12 (if appropriate for type of anemia)

For constipation:
- docusate (Colace, Doxinate, etc.)
- docusate with casanthranol (Peri-Colace, etc.)

For muscle or joint ache/pain:
- aspirin
- acetaminophen (Tylenol, Panadol, etc.)
- ibuprofen (Advil, Nuprin, etc.)

Note: Drug selection, dosage, and administration schedule must be determined by the physician for each patient individually.

Possible Drug Interactions of Significance

Levothyroxine may *increase* the effects of
- warfarin (Coumadin) and increase the risk of bleeding; reduced warfarin dosage may be necessary; prothrombin times should be monitored closely.

Levothyroxine may *decrease* the effects of
- digoxin (Lanoxin) during treatment of hypothyroidism; a larger dose of digoxin may be required.

Levothyroxine *taken concurrently* with
- all antidiabetic drugs (insulin and sulfonylureas) may require increase in their dosages to properly control blood sugar levels.
- tricyclic antidepressants may enhance the activity of both drugs; monitor for signs of overdosage.

The following drugs may *decrease* the effects of levothyroxine:
- antacids may reduce absorption of levothyroxine.
- carbamazepine (Tegretol) may hasten elimination of levothyroxine.
- cholestyramine (Cuemid, Questran) and colestipol (Colestid) may reduce absorption of levothyroxine; separate the intake of lipid-lowering drugs and levothyroxine by five hours.
- iron salts may reduce absorption of levothyroxine.
- lovastatin (Mevacor) may reduce absorption of levothyroxine.
- phenytoin (Dilantin) may hasten elimination of levothyroxine.
- rifampin (Rifadin, Rimactane) may hasten elimination of levothyroxine.

See Appendix 16, Drug Classes, for specific generic drugs within respective drug classes.

Special Considerations for Women

Pregnancy

Studies of pregnant women being treated for primary hypothyroidism demonstrate that the need for thyroxine increases during pregnancy. The average woman with primary hypothyroidism needs a 25–50% increase in her T-4 dose during pregnancy to maintain the TSH within the normal range. It is advisable to monitor thyroid function every two months and after delivery, and to adjust thyroxine dosage as needed to maintain normal TSH blood levels.

Breast-Feeding

Thyroxine is secreted in breast milk in minimal amounts. Breast-feeding is considered safe.

Special Considerations for the Elderly

Hypothyroidism of mild to moderate degree is found in 6–10% of women and 2–3% of men over 65 years of age.

Subclinical hypothyroidism is estimated to be as high as 15% in healthy women over 60 years of age. This can slowly progress to overt hypothyroidism.

Dosage requirements of thyroxine in older persons is often 25% less than in the young. Dosage should be adjusted to maintain TSH within the normal range.

Hypothyroidism in the elderly can produce a pattern of symptoms somewhat different from that seen in younger individuals. Impairment of central nervous system functions can result in apathy, memory loss, inability to think abstractly, confusion, incoordination, and seizures. An erroneous diagnosis of depression and/or dementia may be considered. Appropriate thyroid hormone replacement therapy can produce swift and dramatic improvement.

Quality of Life Considerations

This can be the key to motivating the person with subclinical hypothyroidism to seek clarification from his personal physician. This condition is the nebulous "gray area"—not fully well and not truly ill. Symptoms are vague, difficult to describe, and not clearly diagnostic: unreasonable fatigability, lack of stamina and endurance, sluggish thinking, increased need for rest and sleep, decreased sexual function. Many physicians are not interested in pursuing indeterminate disorders. Actually, the issue of subclinical hypothyroidism is quite easy to resolve. If you are the patient seeking an answer, ask your physician to provide a sensitive TSH and a T-4 measurement for you. If the test results are normal or near normal (within "normal" ranges), and not, in the physician's judgment, diagnostic of subclinical hypothyroidism, ask him to consider giving you a 3- to 4-month therapeutic trial of thyroxine. He can determine the feasibility of this and provide appropriate dosage and instructions. The results of the experiment will be your subjective response to thyroxine. If you were experiencing subclinical hypothyroidism, the gradual improvement of your symptoms will be genuine, convincing, and lasting—considerably beyond any potential placebo effect. It is very possible that you will find the improvement in your quality of life fully justifies your efforts to seek the answer.

It is important to understand that every individual has an endogenous "set point" that dictates his optimal blood level of thyroxine (T-4). The "normal ranges" of TSH and T-4 are probably too wide and imprecise to identify individual parameters for subclinical hypothyroidism.

Resources

Recommended Reading

The Thyroid Book: What Goes Wrong and How to Treat It, Martin I. Surks, M.D. Yonkers, NY: Consumer Reports Books, 1993.

Additional Information and Services

American Thyroid Association
Endocrine-Metabolic Service
Walter Reed Army Medical Center

Washington, DC 20307-5001
Phone: (202) 882-7717, 1-800-542-6687; Fax: (202) 882-7813
Maintains professional membership directory for geographical referrals.

Thyroid Foundation of America
Box RD, Ruth Sleeper Hall RSL350
40 Parkman Street
Boston, MA 02114-2698

LUNG CANCER

Other Names Bronchogenic carcinoma, carcinoma of lung, large-cell carcinoma, oat-cell carcinoma, small-cell carcinoma

Prevalence/Incidence in U.S.
Approximately 170,000 new cases annually
The most common cancer in men (22%) and in women (20%)
The most common cause of cancer deaths in men (35%) and in women (30%)

Age Group Most common between 45 and 70 years of age

Male-to-Female Ratio 10 men to 7 women

Principal Features and Natural History
There are four major types of *primary* lung cancer, based upon the cell structure of the tumor.

Adenocarcinoma
This type begins in the outer portions of the lungs, invades the outer covering of the lung (pleura) in 50% of cases, and spreads through the bloodstream to other tissues throughout the body (metastasis, see Glossary). It is the most common type of lung cancer in women, and also the predominant tumor in nonsmokers.

Squamous Cell Cancer (Epidermoid)
This is the most common type of lung cancer (40%). It usually begins in the larger bronchial tubes (air passages) and spreads directly into adjacent tissues and regional lymph nodes. It occurs most frequently in men, predominantly in smokers. Metastatic spread to other organs is common.

Undifferentiated Large-Cell Cancer
This type usually begins along the outer edges of the lungs, frequently invading the pleura and regional lymph nodes. It also spreads through the bloodstream to distant organs and tissues.

Undifferentiated Small-Cell (Oat-Cell) Cancer

This type usually begins in the medium-sized and smaller bronchial tubes, extending along the bronchial lining and invading adjacent tissues. It also spreads through the bloodstream earlier than the other types, most commonly invading the bone marrow. It is a more aggressive type of cancer, usually widespread before symptoms appear, and is more resistant to treatment. It also occurs more frequently in smokers.

The usual pattern of metastasis of *primary* lung cancers involves the brain, liver, adrenal glands, and bone. Such spread may occur early and produce symptoms at these remote sites before the appearance of chest symptoms.

Many forms of *secondary* lung cancer occur; these are metastases that have spread via the bloodstream from primary cancers in other organs and tissues: breast, colon, prostate, kidney, thyroid, stomach, cervix, rectum, testicle, bone, and melanoma.

The average survival time for untreated lung cancer is eight months following diagnosis.

The five-year survival rate for resectable tumors (10–35% of all types) is less than 10%.

Diagnostic Symptoms and Signs

Most primary lung cancers involve the bronchial tubes; this causes a persistent cough that worsens with time. The resulting sputum may gradually increase in quantity and become blood-streaked. A narrowed bronchial tube may cause wheezing and can eventually produce blockage that predisposes to infection (pneumonia or lung abscess) with fever, loss of appetite, and chest pain. Late manifestations include progressive weakness, shortness of breath, and weight loss.

Some lung cancers can produce a perplexing pattern of symptoms and/or signs that occur in body areas and systems other than the chest and lungs; these are referred to as "extrapulmonary paraneoplastic manifestations." They are remote effects of primary tumor activity and not the direct result of metastases. These include enlargement ("clubbing") of the ends of fingers and toes, altered mentality, impaired stance and gait, myasthenialike muscle weakness, Cushing's syndrome, breast enlargement, hyperthyroidism, skin pigmentation, thrombophlebitis, etc. They may be the first sign of tumor occurrence or an indication of tumor recurrence.

Diagnostic Tests and Procedures

Conventional chest X-ray examinations
Tomographic X-ray studies of specific lung areas
Computed axial tomography (CAT, CT scans) of lungs, brain, liver, adrenal glands (sites of possible metastases)

Magnetic resonance imaging (MRI) of brain and spinal cord for possible
    metastases
Radionuclide scans for bone metastases
Cytologic studies of sputum and pleural fluid
Needle aspirations of tumors through the chest wall
Tissue biopsy examinations of lung and lymph nodes
Bronchoscopic examination: direct visualization, specimen retrieval by
    washing, brushing, and biopsy of specific areas
Mediastinoscopy: using a scope to directly visualize the interior of the
    chest cavity between the lungs for detection of tumor and biopsy of
    lymph nodes
Thoracoscopy: using a scope (inserted through the chest wall) to exam-
    ine specific areas inside the chest cavity and to retrieve biopsy speci-
    mens for study
Exploratory thoracotomy: surgical exploration of chest cavity for detec-
    tion and evaluation of tumor

Diagnostic "Markers" for This Disorder

Precise markers include definitive pathological confirmation of cancer on
examination of cells obtained from sputum, bronchial washings and
brushings, and tissue biopsy specimens.

Suggestive markers include the various paraneoplastic manifestations
of lung cancer referred to above: finger and toe "clubbing," Cushing's
syndrome, polymyositis, thrombophlebitis, etc.

Similar Conditions That May Confuse Diagnosis

Foreign bodies within the lung, some forms of pneumonia, tuberculosis,
fungal infections of the lung (coccidioidomycosis, histoplasmosis), and a
few autoimmune disorders can cause similar symptoms, signs, and X-ray
findings suggestive of lung cancer.

Causes

Established Causes

Cigarette smoking causes 90% of cases in men and 70% in women.

Occupational exposures cause 15% of cases in men and 5% in
women:
    asbestos
    radiation
    radon
    arsenic
    chromates
    nickel
    chloromethyl ethers

mustard gas

coke oven emissions

Note: Cigarette smoking and occupational exposures may coexist.

Theoretical Causes

Current research provides evidence that cancer-causing agents (viruses, chemicals, ionizing radiation) contribute to the initiation and progression of malignancy by damaging cellular DNA, activating cellular oncogenes (see Glossary), and producing growth factors that stimulate uncontrolled tissue proliferation.

Known Risk Factors for Developing This Disorder

Tobacco smoking, exposure to cancer-causing chemicals and radiation.

Drugs That Can Cause This Disorder

There are no reports of drugs that are causally related to lung cancer.

Goals of Treatment

Can This Disorder Be Cured?

If detected early and treated aggressively, a symptom-free "remission" can be achieved in some cases of lung cancer. If follow-up examinations reveal no evident recurrence of disease activity, these periods may be referred to as "three-year cures," "five-year cures," etc.

Can This Disorder Be Treated Effectively?

- Can symptoms be relieved?
  - Cough can be controlled with antitussive medications.
  - Infections can be controlled with anti-infective drugs.
  - Pain can be relieved with appropriate analgesics.
  - Many symptoms due to the primary tumor may be relieved by successful surgical excision and/or radiotherapy.
- Can the mechanism(s) of the disorder be:
  - Controlled? Partially, for a limited time, dependent upon the nature of the tumor and its "stage" (extent of spread) when treatment is started.
  - Arrested? Occasionally, depending upon the "sensitivity" of the cancer cells to radiation therapy and/or chemotherapy.
  - Reversed? Yes, if the primary tumor is removed surgically before significant spread occurs, and adjuvant radiation therapy and chemotherapy are successful.

Specific Goals

- Early detection and accurate diagnosis: determining the type of cancer and stage of progression
- Relief of symptoms by medication

- Prompt initiation of optimal treatment plan: surgery, radiation, chemotherapy

Health Professionals Who Participate in Managing This Disorder
Family physicians
General internists
Radiologists
Pulmonologists
Thoracic surgeons
Pathologists
Medical oncologists (chemotherapists)
Surgical oncologists
Radiation oncologists (radiotherapists)
Nurse oncologists
Psychologists
Pharmacists
Dietitians
Medical social workers

Currently Available Therapies for This Disorder
Nondrug Treatment Methods
- Surgical removal of tumor: segmental or wedge resection of the por-
  tion of lung tissue that contains the tumor; lobectomy (removal of one
  lobe of a lung), pneumonectomy (removal of an entire lung)
- Radiation therapy
- Cryosurgery: destruction of tumor by freezing
- Photodynamic therapy: destruction of cancer cells by laser light and
  substances that are sensitive to light

Drug Therapy
The following drugs are used in cancer chemotherapy:
- carboplatin (Paraplatin)
- cisplatin (Platinol)
- cyclophosphamide (Cytoxan)
- doxorubicin (Adriamycin)
- etoposide (VePesid)
- 5-fluorouracil
- ifosfamide
- lomustine
- methotrexate
- mitomycin C (Mutamycin)
- vinblastine (Velban)
- vincristine (Oncovin)

New Drugs in Development for Treating This Disorder

Taxol is currently approved in the United States for treating ovarian cancer. Current studies have demonstrated that taxol can produce significant clinical improvement in treating squamous cell carcinoma of the lung. Taxotere and other compounds closely related to taxol are expected to show significant clinical effectiveness, used alone and in combination with other anticancer drugs.

Management of Therapy

- The first essential requirement for planning the treatment of any cancer is a precise pathological diagnosis: the tissue of origin (histology and cytology), and the estimated degree (grade) of malignancy. The pathologist makes these determinations by examining cell and tissue samples (biopsies) of the tumor. The second essential requirement for planning treatment is determining the basic characteristics of the primary tumor and the extent of spread (metastasis) from its point of origin. This process is called "staging."

- One commonly used method for staging major cancers uses the designations T for (primary) tumor, N for (lymph) node involvement, and M for (distant) metastasis—the TNM system. Tests performed to establish the diagnosis and overall status of the cancer provide the information used to characterize the nature of the disease to be treated. By assigning a value to T, N, and M, the "stage" of the patient's cancer is determined:

Stage I

A small tumor, local invasion only	TI
No regional lymph node involvement	N0
No distant metastasis	M0

Stage II

A larger tumor, moderate local spread	T2
Local regional lymph node involvement	NI
No distant metastasis	M0

Stage III

Any size tumor, extensive local spread	T3
More distant lymph node involvement	N3
No distant metastasis	M0

Stage IV

Any size tumor, invasion of adjacent organs	T4
Any lymph node involvement	N2–3
Distant metastasis	MI

- Once the exact type of cancer and its stage are established, an appropriate treatment plan can be initiated. In addition, an attempt at prognosis is possible, should the patient and/or family wish to consider this.

Treatment of Non-Small-Cell Lung Cancer

Approximately 75% of all lung cancers are non-small-cell types: adenocarcinoma, large-cell, and squamous-cell carcinoma. The preferred treatment for stage I and stage II tumors is surgical resection; 20–30% of tumors are resectable at the time of diagnosis. If resection is impossible, curative radiotherapy is attempted. The three-year survival for stage I/II is 43%.

Stage III is treated with radiotherapy to delay the onset of symptoms or to improve the comfort and function of the patient. The three-year survival for stage III is 13%.

All symptomatic manifestations of stage IV disease are treated with palliative radiotherapy. Chemotherapy, using single or multiple drugs, is used when appropriate; limited response occurs in only 10–20% of cases. The three-year survival for stage IV is 5%.

Treatment of Small-Cell Lung Cancer

This type comprises 25% of lung cancers. It is a very aggressive malignancy, usually spreading widely (extensive stage) before detection. Surgical removal of the primary tumor is rarely necessary or beneficial. Chemotherapy, using drugs in combination, is the treatment of choice for all stages of this cancer. Cisplatin is the most effective drug; it is used in combination with other drugs and with radiation.

If the disease is in the limited stage (involving only one lung), radiation of the primary tumor site and regional lymph nodes improves control and survival. The three-year survival of limited disease is 40%. The three-year survival of extensive disease is 10%. It is estimated that 10% of patients with limited small-cell cancer can be cured by treatment that combines chemotherapy and radiotherapy.

If a complete remission is achieved, preventive radiation of the cranium may be performed to abort progression of metastases in the brain.

Ancillary Drug Treatment (as required)

For anxiety:
- buspirone (Buspar)
- diazepam (Valium)

For pain:
see Appendix 3, Cancer Pain Management

For infection:
- appropriate anti-infective drugs determined by culture and sensitivity testing

For nausea and vomiting:

see Appendix 4, Management of Nausea and Vomiting Associated with Cancer Chemotherapy

For depression:

see Profile on depression in this section

Note: Drug selection, dosage, and administration schedule must be determined by the physician for each patient individually.

Special Considerations for Women

Pregnancy

Lung cancer is a rare occurrence during pregnancy. Decisions regarding treatment must consider: (1) the potential for significant injury to the fetus by chemotherapy and/or radiation therapy; (2) risk to the mother if treatment is withheld; (3) the advisability of therapeutic abortion.

Chemotherapy

Four of the drugs used to treat lung cancer can seriously damage the fetus if given during the first three months (first trimester) of pregnancy; if used during the last six months (second and third trimesters), the risk of fetal injury is negligible. If possible, the following drugs should be avoided during the first trimester: 5-fluorouracil (5-FU), methotrexate, vinblastine, vincristine.

The use of doxorubicin appears to be safe throughout pregnancy. Studies show that this drug does not cross the placenta; it is not found in fetal tissues.

There is a single case report of the use of capsulation during the first trimester without injury to the fetus.

In general, the use of single anticancer drugs and combination chemotherapy (two or more drugs used concurrently) during the first trimester causes fetal malformations in 16% of pregnancies. The use of single-drug or combination chemotherapy during the second and third trimesters does not increase the risk of birth defects.

Chemotherapy during the second and third trimesters can cause abortion, retarded fetal growth, premature birth, and low birth weight.

Radiation Therapy

The small size of the radiation dose used for conventional *diagnostic* X-ray studies of the mother causes negligible risk to the fetus. With proper shielding of the fetus, *diagnostic* X-rays of the chest, skull, neck, upper spine, and extremities are considered safe for diagnosis and initial staging. This includes the use of computed tomography (CAT, CT scanning).

Before *therapeutic* radiation of the abdomen is started, pregnancy status must be determined. The significantly higher radiation doses used for therapy at any time during pregnancy can result in abortion, birth defects, and permanent damage to the fetal brain. If radiation therapy during pregnancy involves only the head, neck, chest, or extremities of the mother, there is no risk to the properly shielded fetus.

Special Considerations for the Elderly

Lung cancer patients over 70 years of age who have acceptable heart and lung function (and reasonably satisfactory general health) should be considered candidates for potentially curative surgery.

The Role of Prevention in This Disorder

Primary Prevention

- Total avoidance of tobacco smoking
- Avoidance of exposure to cancer-causing chemicals in industrial settings
- Avoidance of excessive radiation to the chest

Secondary Prevention

- Prompt detection and treatment of primary cancers elsewhere in the body that are potential sources of metastases to the lungs
- Radiation of the cranium in selected cases to abort brain metastases

Resources

Recommended Reading

The Cancer Patient's Handbook: Everything You Need to Know About Today's Care and Treatment, Mary-Ellen Siegel, M.S.W. Walker and Company, New York, 1986.

Additional Information and Services

The Cancer Information Service
Phone: 1-800-422-6237, 1-800-4-CANCER
Questions answered in English or Spanish.

American Cancer Society (ACS)
1599 Clifton Road, NE
Atlanta, GA 30329
Phone: 1-800-ACS-2345

American Lung Association
1740 Broadway
New York, NY 10019
Phone: (212) 315-8700

Disease Management Expertise

See Appendix 2, Part One: The National Cancer Institute (NCI) Designated Cancer Centers, and Part Two: Clinical Trials.

LUPUS ERYTHEMATOSUS

Other Names Lupus, LE, cutaneous lupus erythematosus, CLE, systemic lupus erythematosus, SLE, disseminated lupus erythematosus

Prevalence/Incidence in U.S.
Current estimate: approximately 1 million
Estimated new cases annually: 16,000

Age Group Onset usually occurs between 15 and 45 years of age. However, lupus can occur in young children and older adults.

Male-to-Female Ratio 90% of cases occur in women; 60% of these are black.

Principal Features and Natural History
This chronic, inflammatory disease of connective tissues is so beastly in its manifestations it was named for the wolf (lupus). Current understanding of its fundamental nature clearly establishes it as a classical autoimmune disorder (see Appendix 5, The Immune System). It occurs worldwide. In the United States the incidence is higher in black Americans, Native Americans, and some Asian Americans than in whites.

There are two relatively distinct forms of lupus: (1) cutaneous lupus erythematosus, a mild form that is confined primarily to the skin and tissues of the mouth; and (2) systemic lupus erythematosus, a severe form that can affect virtually every organ in the body. Both forms of lupus are chronic disorders characterized by unpredictable fluctuations in disease activity (flares and remissions).

Cutaneous Lupus Erythematosus (CLE)
This form of lupus can occur as the only manifestation of the disorder or it can be an integral part of the more serious disseminated form—systemic lupus erythematosus. About 5–10% of cases that begin as the cutaneous form will eventually develop systemic lupus. Cutaneous lupus causes discrete patches of inflammation and scaling on the face, ears, neck, upper trunk, and arms that can result in scarring. The skin changes are aggravated by exposure to sunlight in 40% of patients. Mouth ulcers occur in some cases. Loss of scalp hair may be extensive and permanent. Lupus specialists now classify the varieties of skin rashes and lesions that can occur into acute, subacute, and chronic cutaneous LE subgroups. With early diagnosis and prompt treatment, this form of lupus responds well to cortisonelike creams and ointments and, if necessary, the use of antimalarial drugs by mouth.

Systemic Lupus Erythematosus (SLE)

This more severe form of lupus can affect any organ or system in the body and mimic many other diseases. The tissues most commonly involved include joints, kidneys, brain, heart, blood vessels, lungs, and blood-forming organs. Activity of this disease and resulting organ damage can range from mild to life-threatening. The early symptoms of lupus are usually vague and nonspecific: low-grade fever; weakness; fatigue; loss of appetite and weight; skin rashes; joint pains involving the hands, wrists, elbows, knees, or ankles. Joints may seem stiff on arising and may ultimately become red and swollen. The correct diagnosis may not be made for months or years. As the disorder progresses, involvement of the heart and lungs can cause chest pain and shortness of breath. There may be lowered resistance to infections and abnormal bleeding or bruising. Tissue damage within the nervous system can cause significant alterations of mood and behavior; seizures resembling epilepsy occur infrequently. Kidney damage is quite common in lupus, but symptoms of this may not be apparent until advanced stages are reached. Presently no curative treatment is known. However, symptom relief and acceptable stabilization of organ damage can be achieved in many cases by the skillful use of four classes of effective drugs. If the correct diagnosis is made early, the 10-year survival is over 95%. This can be achieved now without the use of large doses of cortisonelike (corticosteroid) drugs.

Diagnostic Symptoms and Signs

Fatigue, low-grade fever
Loss of appetite and weight
Multiple joint pains, with or without swelling (90%)
Painful ulcers in nose or mouth
Skin rashes on face, scalp, ears, neck, upper trunk, or arms
"Butterfly" rash across nose and cheeks (30%)
Loss of scalp hair can be the first sign of disease activity
Swollen lymph glands
Raynaud's phenomenon (30%) (see Glossary)
Chest pains, shortness of breath, and cough due to heart and/or lung involvement
Psychotic behavior, seizures, paralysis in extremities due to central nervous system involvement

Diagnostic Tests and Procedures

Complete blood cell counts
Red blood cell sedimentation rate (see Glossary)
Demonstration of lupus erythematosus (LE) cells in blood
Urine analysis

Demonstration of specific antibodies in blood:
- antinuclear antibodies (ANA). Positive in over 95% of patients with SLE.
- anti-double-stranded-DNA antibodies (AntidsDNA)
- antiphospholipid antibodies (lupus anticoagulant)

Electrocardiogram
Kidney biopsy
MRI of brain

Similar Conditions That May Confuse Diagnosis
Autoimmune hemolytic anemia
Autoimmune hepatitis
Autoimmune thyroiditis
Biliary cirrhosis
Chronic viral hepatitis
Diabetes mellitus
Graves' disease
Lymphomas
Mixed connective tissue disease
Multiple sclerosis
Porphyria
Psoriasis
Pulmonary fibrosis
Rheumatoid arthritis
Scleroderma
Sjögren's syndrome
Subacute bacterial endocarditis

ALERT!
Not all persons with a positive antinuclear antibody (ANA) test result have systemic lupus erythematosus. All of the disorders listed above can be associated with a positive ANA.

SLE can cause a false positive result in screening tests for AIDS or syphilis. When this occurs, a more specific confirmatory test for AIDS or syphilis will yield a true negative result.

Causes
Although some of the mechanisms responsible for tissue damage are partially understood, the true fundamental cause of lupus is not known. Lupus is a disorder of the body's immune system, the protective system that produces antibodies designed to destroy infective agents (bacteria, viruses, etc.) that invade the body. By unknown means, the immune system is provoked to produce antibodies specifically designed to attack normal tissues of the host. For this reason, lupus is classified as an

"autoimmune" disease. The destructive interaction between specific anti-bodies and respective tissues is responsible for the inflammatory reactions and organ damage that characterize lupus. Studies to date indicate that multiple factors contribute to the induction of lupus. Among these is genetic predisposition: approximately 30% of identical twin pairs will develop lupus; 1 in 20 children born to a parent with lupus will develop SLE. It is well established that some cases of lupus are caused by the use of certain medicinal drugs (see below).

Drugs That Can Cause This Disorder

It has been estimated that 15,000 to 20,000 cases of drug-related lupus occur annually in the United States. More than 50 medications have been thought to be responsible for inducing lupus. A careful analysis of these reports permits their division into three groups: (1) proof of causation is definite; (2) drug causation is very possible; (3) drug causation is unlikely or rarely possible.

Group I: Drug Association Definite

chlorpromazine
hydralazine
isoniazid
methyldopa
procainamide

Group II: Drug Association Very Possible

acebutolol
atenolol
captopril
carbamazepine
ethosuximide
hydrazine
labetalol
levodopa
lithium carbonate
mephytoin
methimazole
methylthiouracil
metoprolol
nitrofurantoin
oxyprenolol
penicillamine
phenylbutazone
phenytoin
practolol
primidone

propylthiouracil
quinidine
trimethadione

Group III: Drug Association Unlikely or Rare

acecainide
allopurinol
aminosalicylic acid
benzylpenicillin
chlorthalidone
chlorprothixene
estrogens
gold salts
griseofulvin
methysergide
minoxidil
nomifensine
propafenone
psoralen
reserpine
streptomycin
sulfasalazine
sulfonamides
tetracycline
tolazamide

Goals of Treatment

Can This Disorder Be Cured?

There is no curative treatment available at this time.

Can This Disorder Be Treated Effectively?

In many cases, currently available medications can relieve symptoms, suppress disease activity, and achieve a favorable quality and duration of life.

Specific Goals

FOR CUTANEOUS LE

- To improve the patient's appearance
- To prevent the development of further skin deformities
- To determine that the lupus disorder is limited to the skin and is not a manifestation of systemic LE

FOR SYSTEMIC LE

- To achieve and maintain optimal control of disease activity
- To provide maximal symptomatic relief consistent with safe drug use
- To prevent or limit organ damage as much as possible

- To determine the selection of drugs and dosage schedules that will provide maximal benefits with minimal risks
- To monitor the course of the disorder and the response to drug therapy so that appropriate adjustments can be made as required

Health Professionals Who Participate in Managing This Disorder

Family physicians
General internists
Pediatricians
Rheumatologists
Dermatologists
Neurologists
Nephrologists
Hematologists
Cardiologists
Pulmonologists
Clinical immunologists
Ophthalmologists
Optometrists
Diagnostic radiologists
Orthopedic surgeons
Pharmacists
Physician assistants
Nurse practitioners
Physical therapists
Dietitians/Nutritionists

Currently Available Therapies for This Disorder

Nondrug Treatment Methods

- Dietary modifications: sodium restriction to control hypertension; fat and cholesterol restriction to manage blood lipid disorders
- Physical therapy for management and rehabilitation of musculoskeletal problems
- Plasmapheresis: the removal of immune complexes from blood plasma as a treatment for thrombocytopenic purpura

Drug Therapy

NONSTEROIDAL ANTI-INFLAMMATORY DRUGS (NSAIDs)

See Appendix 8, Nonsteroidal Anti-Inflammatory Drugs: A Guide to Selection for Therapy.

ANTIMALARIAL DRUGS

- chloroquine (Aralen)
- hydroxychloroquine (Plaquenil)
- quinacrine (Atabrine)

CORTISONELIKE DRUGS (CORTICOSTEROIDS)

Cortisonelike creams and ointments for cutaneous LE:

- flucinolone (Synalar)
- fluocinonide (Lidex)
- hydrocortisone
- triamcinolone (Kenalog)

Cortisonelike drugs for oral administration:

- hydrocortisone
- prednisolone (Delta-Cortef, etc.)
- prednisone (Deltasone, Meticorten, etc.)
- methylprednisolone (Medrol)

IMMUNOSUPPRESSIVE DRUGS

- azathioprine (Imuran)
- chlorambucil (Leukeran)
- cyclophosphamide (Cytoxan)
- cyclosporine (Sandimmune)
- methotrexate

New Drugs in Development for Treating This Disorder

- A new corticosteroid derivative, deflazort, is believed to cause less bone loss than prednisone and similar drugs now commonly used. Deflazort equals prednisone as an anti-inflammatory drug for the long-term treatment of SLE; it may well provide equal therapeutic benefit but with significantly reduced risk of causing osteoporosis (bone loss) and osteonecrosis (bone death) during extended use.
- A major component of fish oil (notably salmon and mackerel) identified as eicosapentaenoic acid (EPA), a form of omega-3 fatty acid, has been shown to have significant anti-inflammatory effects. This may prove to be beneficial in treating inflammatory disorders such as lupus. Studies in mice show that EPA protects against the development of lupus nephritis and that it is relatively nontoxic.

Management of Therapy

- Currently available treatments for lupus have significantly improved the prognosis for both CLE and SLE. Eighty to ninety percent of all SLE patients now live more than 10 years and many live a normal life span.
- Treatment programs must be planned according to the extent and severity of disease activity. Lupus characteristically fluctuates between episodes of increased activity (flares) and periods of decreased activity (remissions). This requires close monitoring by both patient and physician so that appropriate adjustments of medications can be made in a timely manner.
- Approximately 25% of patients have mild lupus that can be controlled with aspirin, NSAIDs (aspirin substitutes), and/or an antimalarial drug.

Another 70% have a more severe form of lupus that usually responds to prednisone or related steroid drugs. A small percent have serious multiple organ disease that requires immunosuppressant drugs for control.

- Marked sensitivity of the skin to sunlight is a prominent feature of lupus. Exposure to the sun (and tanning booths) can initiate and intensify skin lesions of CLE. The regular use of sunscreen lotions or creams is mandatory; the sunscreen chosen should have a sun protective factor (SPF) of 30 or higher.

Use of Local (Topical) Cortisonelike Drugs

- Creams and ointments containing a cortisonelike drug are beneficial but must be applied regularly to prevent thinning, depigmentation, and scarring of the skin. It is advisable to use the least potent preparation that proves to be effective for each patient.
- Lupus lesions on the face should be treated with a low- to mid-potency preparation such as hydrocortisone or desonide. Those on the trunk and extremities may be treated with a high-potency preparation such as Lidex or Synalar.
- Lesions that do not respond to applications of creams or ointments can be injected with triamcinolone.

Use of Antimalarial Drugs

- If lupus skin lesions are not adequately controlled by topical applications (as above), an antimalarial drug should be added to the treatment program. The antimalarial drug of choice is hydroxychloroquine. It is thought to be safer but less effective than chloroquine. If hydroxychloroquine is not effective, cholorquine may be substituted for it, or quinacrine may be added.
- After lupus skin lesions have responded adequately to antimalarial drugs, the dosage should be gradually reduced to the smallest effective maintenance level. Low-dose, long-term therapy with antimalarials is considered to be quite safe.
- The three antimalarial drugs used to treat lupus can infrequently cause damage to the cornea and/or retina of the eye. A complete eye examination should be performed *before* an antimalarial drug is started and *every three to six months* during its use. The drug should be stopped if any evidence of eye damage is found.
- In treating overweight individuals, antimalarial dosage should be carefully determined on the basis of ideal body weight.
- Antimalarial drugs are also effective in treating some features of SLE: fever, fatigue, arthritis, muscle aches, chest pains. A trial of 8 to 12 weeks may be necessary to determine the effectiveness of antimalarial drugs.

Use of Nonsteroidal Anti-Inflammatory Drugs (NSAIDs)

- This group of drugs is the first line of treatment for the symptoms of SLE. Fever, joint and muscle pain, arthritis, and serositis (involvement of heart and lung surfaces) can often be managed by these drugs alone. Aspirin (plain, buffered, sustained-release, or enteric-coated) may be tried first in moderate to large doses (3 to 4 grams per day). A blood salicylate level of 20 to 30 mg/dl is recommended unless satisfactory results are obtained with lower levels.
- If aspirin is not tolerated or is ineffective, one of the NSAID aspirin substitutes may be tried. There are now 21 different NSAIDs available. There is no way of determining in advance which NSAID will be most effective or acceptable for any given patient. A period of trial and error is unavoidable. Physicians will favor one drug or another within the group based upon their experience. For reasons not understood, there are marked differences in response among patients to all NSAIDs. The selected NSAID should be tried for at least two weeks at maximal dose in order to judge effectiveness and acceptance.
- Like aspirin, all NSAIDs may cause gastrointestinal irritation or microscopic ulceration and bleeding in susceptible individuals. Patients with a history of peptic ulcer disease should consult their physicians regarding the need for medications to prevent gastrointestinal ulceration.
- Patients with a history of liver disease or pancreatitis are well advised to avoid the use of sulindac.
- The long-term use of NSAIDs requires periodic evaluation of kidney function for evidence of drug-induced kidney damage. This is especially true in the presence of SLE.
- The following NSAIDs should be avoided in the treatment of SLE: ibuprofen, sulindac, tolmetin. They have been associated with the development of drug-induced meningitis.
- See Appendix 8: Nonsteroidal Anti-Inflammatory Drugs.

Use of Cortisonelike Drugs (Corticosteroids) Systemically

- The drugs of this class possess the most potent anti-inflammatory action available, hence their value in treating the more serious manifestations of SLE. Corticosteroids are the first drugs used to treat SLE organ involvement: pleurisy and pericarditis that are unresponsive to indomethacin, interstitial pneumonia, hemolytic anemia, blood platelet destruction, lupus nephritis (kidney damage), brain and peripheral nervous system tissues.
- Prednisone is the drug most commonly used. It is the drug of choice among the short-acting steroids, which are preferable for most severe SLE involvements. Long-acting steroids are best avoided in treating SLE. Prednisone is usually started with high doses to achieve rapid suppression of disease activity. As improvement occurs, the dose is gradually reduced until the lowest maintenance dose is determined. In

some instances it is possible to use alternate-day dosing. However, activity "flares" on the off days may require return to daily dosing.

- The risks of significant adverse effects that accompany long-term use of prednisone require that maintenance doses be kept as low as possible (see Appendix 6, Long-Term Corticosteroid Therapy).

Use of Immunosuppressive Drugs

- When SLE disease activity reaches life-threatening proportions and corticosteroids in maximal doses are inadequate for control, drugs that are capable of suppressing the abnormal "autoimmune" mechanisms are used. In addition to reducing the degree of disease activity, they also permit the continued use of corticosteroids in smaller (less risky) dosage.
- Because of the serious toxicities associated with these drugs, their use is restricted to the following situations:
  - life-threatening disease that is unresponsive to optimal trials of prednisone
  - active major organ disease that is unresponsive to optimal trials of prednisone
  - active major organ disease that recurs when prednisone dosage is reduced and requires unacceptably high maintenance doses of prednisone
  - intolerable prednisone toxicity in a patient who requires prednisone to suppress disease activity
  - active major organ disease in a patient who has significant contraindications to the use of high-dose prednisone
  - certain active organ disease that has been shown to respond more satisfactorily to the combined use of immunosuppressive drugs and prednisone
- Cyclophosphamide appears to reduce the degree of deterioration of kidney function in the patient with lupus nephritis; however, this drug has marked potential for serious toxic effects. Cyclophosphamide also has potential for suppressing SLE activity in the lung, the brain and peripheral nervous system, and blood-forming organs.
- Azathioprine has been used to treat SLE for over 20 years. It is thought to be effective in treating resistant CLE (discoid lupus) that fails to respond to antimalarial drugs. It is also beneficial in some cases of lupus nephritis. It is not recommended as the first immunosuppressive drug to be tried in life-threatening disease or in organ damage involving the brain, lung, or blood-forming tissues.
- Methotrexate has been used less frequently in treating SLE, but some dramatic improvements have been reported. In patients who become resistant to azathioprine after 10 to 15 months of treatment, a plan of alternate use of azathioprine and methotrexate has proved to be effective in some cases.

Therapeutic Drug Monitoring (Blood Levels)

Long-term use of methotrexate may require periodic drug monitoring. The therapeutic blood level range is up to 0.1 mcmol/L.

Ancillary Drug Treatment (as required)

For intercurrent infections:
- specific anti-infectives based on culture and sensitivity testing as appropriate

For organic brain syndrome with psychosis:
- neuroleptics: haloperidol (Haldol), thiothixene (Navane)

For organic brain syndrome with seizures:
- anticonvulsants; see Profile of epilepsy in this section

For migraine headache:
  see Profile of migraine headache in this section

For hypertension:
  see Profile of hypertension in this section

For Raynaud's phenomenon:
- calcium channel blockers: diltiazem (Cardizem), nifedipine (Procardia)

For hemolytic anemia or blood platelet destruction:
- danazol (Danocrine), as adjunct to prednisone

Note: Drug selection, dosage, and administration schedule must be determined by the physician for each patient individually.

Current Controversies in Drug Management

Lupus nephritis, the kidney disease associated with SLE, is the major cause of morbidity and mortality in this disorder. It is also one of the more difficult aspects of SLE to manage satisfactorily. One prominent disagreement has focused on the relative merits of high-dose versus low-dose prednisone treatment, with or without other drugs. The consensus that seems to have emerged from several studies in diverse settings is that long-term high-dose prednisone modifies the disease course more favorably than low-dose prednisone treatment regimens.

Possible Drug Interactions of Significance

Because of the number of drugs that may be used to manage this disorder, adequate consideration of the volume and complexity of potential drug interactions is beyond the scope of this book. Consult *The Essential Guide to Prescription Drugs*, or a similar drug reference book for possible interactions of significance (see Appendix 17, Drug Information Sources).

Special Considerations for Women

A barrier method of contraception is advised. If oral contraceptives are used, those with the lowest dose of estrogen are recommended.

It is known that estrogen replacement therapy (ERT) can exacerbate SLE in women who have the disease. The Nurses' Health Study currently in progress has recently reported that ERT doubles the risk of SLE developing in women with no prior history of the disorder. The longer the use of ERT, the greater the risk.

Pregnancy

If feasible, it is best to plan pregnancy after SLE has been in remission for four to six months. Pregnancy during periods of SLE activity is associated with substantial risk of intensifying the disease and damaging the fetus.

Hydroxychloroquine, azathioprine, chlorambucil, and cyclophosphamide are all designated Pregnancy Category D. Methotrexate is designated Pregnancy Category X (see Appendix 15, FDA Pregnancy Categories).

Breast-Feeding

All antimalarial and immunosuppressive drugs used to treat SLE are secreted in breast milk. If drug therapy is necessary, refrain from nursing.

Special Considerations for the Elderly

As with numerous other disorders, the manifestations of SLE in older persons may differ somewhat from those in the young. It is not unusual for a correct diagnosis of SLE to be delayed for three to four years in older patients. If your symptoms are similar to those noted above, ask your physician to consider the possibility of SLE. Features that should arouse suspicion include fever, weight loss, arthritis, skin eruptions, and pneumonia.

The Role of Prevention in This Disorder

Primary Prevention

There is no method currently known to prevent the initial development of SLE in individuals who are genetically predisposed to autoimmune disorders.

Secondary Prevention

Early diagnosis and aggressive drug therapy are the keys to controlling SLE and preventing progressive organ damage.

Resources

Recommended Reading

The Lupus Book: A Guide for Patients and Their Families, Daniel J. Wallace, M.D. New York: Oxford University Press, 1995.

The Lupus Handbook for Women, Robin Dibner and Carol Colman. New York: Fireside, 1994.

Additional Information and Services

The American Lupus Society
3914 Del Amo Blvd, Suite 922

Torrance, CA 90503
Phone: 1-800-331-1802, (310) 542-8891
  Publications available.

Lupus Foundation of America
4 Research Place, Suite 180
Rockville, MD 20850-3226
Phone: (301) 670-9292, 1-800-558-0121; Fax: (301) 670-9486
  Local groups: 108 chapters in 48 states; 38 international associates in
18 countries. Publications available: *Lupus News*, official newsletter.

Disease Management Expertise

SPECIALIZED CENTERS OF RESEARCH IN SYSTEMIC LUPUS ERYTHEMATOSUS
Keith B. Elkon, M.D., Director
The Hospital for Special Surgery
535 70th Street
New York, NY 10021
Phone: (212) 606-1074; Fax: (212) 717-1192

Philip L. Cohen, M.D., Director
University of North Carolina at Chapel Hill
Thurston Arthritis Center, CB# 7280
Chapel Hill, NC 27599-7280
Phone: (919) 966-0568; Fax: (919) 966-1739

LYME DISEASE

Other Names Erythema chronicum migrans, ECM, erythema migrans,
EM, Lyme borreliosis

Prevalence/Incidence in U.S.

Current estimate: approximately 65,000 cases reported to date
Estimated new cases annually: 11,603 in 1995
Present in all of the lower 48 states; most common in the northeast
  (Maine to Maryland), southeast (Texas to Florida), north-central (espe-
  cially Wisconsin and Minnesota), and western regions (especially
  northern California and Oregon)
Occurs most commonly from April through November

Age Group Occurs in all age groups, from 2 years to 70 years; the
mean age is 30 years

Male-to-Female Ratio Male cases: 47%; female cases: 53%

Principal Features and Natural History

Lyme disease, the most common tick-borne disease in the United States, is an infection that may involve several systems of the body, causing a variety of symptoms. It can occur in acute and chronic forms and is often difficult to recognize, mimicking numerous other disorders. The disease pattern was first reported in 1883 in Europe and is now known to occur worldwide. In 1975 a cluster of children in Old Lyme, Connecticut, became ill with what at first appeared to be juvenile rheumatoid arthritis. Further investigation revealed the symptoms to be due to a specific infection now known as Lyme disease—a serious disorder that can cause painful, chronic disability in humans and animals. To better understand the nature of this infection and its management, the course of illness is defined according to its stages.

Early Infection: Stage 1

Following the bite of an infected tick, approximately 70% of individuals develop a localized skin rash (erythema migrans) at the site of the bite. This usually appears within a week (but may be delayed for three to four weeks) and may burn or itch. If treatment is not started at this time, the area of rash may gradually expand to a diameter of several inches; the skin at the outer edge may appear swollen. A characteristic feature of the rash is a gradual clearing in the center to create a "bull's-eye" (target) effect. Without treatment, the rash will usually fade in a month; with treatment, it will clear in a few days. This initial stage of infection is confined to the skin (localized) and may be accompanied by mild flu-like symptoms. From 8–17% of Lyme-infected patients may have a flu-like illness without erythema migrans. A significant number of infected individuals (30%) may have no rash or other symptoms during this stage.

Early Infection: Stage 2

If untreated, the bacteria spread to other parts of the body within days or weeks (disseminated infection) causing a variety of symptoms. These may include scattered body rashes (50% of cases), marked fatigue, intense headache, neck stiffness, or joint and muscle pains that are intermittent and migratory. After several weeks or months, 15–20% of infected individuals will develop symptoms of nervous system involvement: drowsiness, mood change, memory loss, meningitis, facial muscle paralysis, or peripheral neuritis (see Glossary). These neurologic symptoms may last several weeks or months, or they may become intermittent or chronic. During the first several weeks of disseminated infection, 4–8% of patients will experience transient disturbances of heart rhythm or infection of the heart muscle. These symptoms are usually brief (three days to six weeks). On an average of six months (range of two weeks to two years) after the onset of infection, 60% of patients will experience brief attacks of arthritis usually involving the large joints, most commonly the knee.

Late Infection: Stage 3

If Lyme bacteria are not completely eradicated from the body after a year (persistent infection), the late manifestations of chronic infection may become apparent. These can include (1) recurrent episodes of arthritis (during the second and third years after the onset of infection) which may last for several months to several years; (2) intermittent peripheral neuritis with numbness, tingling, and/or pain in the extremities; (3) a chronic dermatitis consisting of bluish-red areas of discoloration on an extremity that progress to inflammation and deterioration of the skin. Once rare but now more common, late manifestations of chronic Lyme infection can include progressive disease of both the central and peripheral nervous system. Inflammation of the brain (encephalitis) can cause excessive drowsiness, impaired thinking and memory, seizures, paralyses, and dementia.

Diagnostic Symptoms and Signs

The only diagnostic sign of Lyme disease is the characteristic erythema migrans—the "bull's-eye" rash that may develop at the site of a tick bite. This is round or oval, from 2 to 6 inches in diameter, with a slightly raised, reddish border, and a progressive clearing in the center as the outer edge expands.

All other symptoms and signs that occur during any stage of the disease are not specific for Lyme disease and are commonly associated with numerous other disorders.

Diagnostic Tests and Procedures

Complete blood cell counts

Immunofluorescence assay (IFA) to detect specific antibodies to the causative organism (*Borrelia burgdorferi*)

Enzyme-linked immunosorbent assay (ELISA) to detect antibodies

Western blot assay to detect antibodies

Bacterial cultures of blood, cerebrospinal fluid, and of skin biopsies taken from the site of erythema migrans

Polymerase chain reaction (PCR) assay to detect specific DNA (deoxyribonucleic acid) of *B. burgdorferi* in blood or body tissues

Diagnostic "Markers" for This Disorder

A positive blood or tissue culture: demonstration of *B. burgdorferi*. (This is very difficult to obtain and is not a practical routine procedure.)

A positive PCR assay that detects *B. burgdorferi* DNA. (This test is specific for Lyme infection and has replaced procedures to culture the organism.)

Similar Conditions That May Confuse Diagnosis
Chronic fatigue syndrome
Drug eruptions
Ehrlichiosis
Erythema multiforme
Fibromyalgia syndrome
Insect bites
Multiple sclerosis
Polymyalgia rheumatica
Rat-bite fever
Rheumatoid arthritis
Rocky Mountain spotted fever
Scleroderma
Secondary syphilis
Systemic lupus erythematosus
Tinea corporis (ringworm)
Viral or bacterial meningitis
Viral myocarditis

ALERT!
Approximately 10% of patients with Lyme disease in southern New England are also infected with babesiosis—two concurrent active infections. The causative organisms for both diseases can be present in the same tick and transmitted with a single bite. The severity and duration of illness in patients with both infections are greater than in patients with either infection alone. When moderate to severe Lyme disease is diagnosed, the possibility of concurrent babesiosis infection should be considered so appropriate therapies can be given.

Causes
Lyme disease is caused by a corkscrew-shaped bacterium called *Borrelia burgdorferi* that enters the body via the bite of an infected tick. There are six species of ticks in the United States that are known to transmit Lyme disease: the deer tick, the American dog tick, the black-legged tick, the western black-legged tick, the Lone Star tick, and the Pacific coast tick. Insects other than ticks, such as the deer fly and mosquito, are suspected to be possible vectors. Field mice are thought to be the primary reservoir for Lyme disease bacteria. By feeding on mice, ticks become infected and capable of transmitting the infection to humans, dogs, horses, cattle, and numerous small wild animals.

Drugs That Can Cause This Disorder
Lyme disease is an infection. There are no drugs that can cause Lyme disease, predispose to its development, or cause adverse effects that resemble Lyme disease.

Goals of Treatment

Can This Disorder Be Cured?

If correctly diagnosed in its early stage and adequately treated, this infection can be cured.

Specific Goals

- To initiate appropriate anti-infective drug therapy as early as possible, so as to prevent the development of chronic infection and late stage complications
- To determine the "drug of choice" for each individual, considering:
  - The patient's age (no tetracycline under age of eight years)
  - Pregnancy or breast-feeding (no tetracycline or probenecid)
  - Drug allergies
  - Stage of Lyme infection
- To determine the optimal dosage and duration of drug treatment to maximize the possibility of cure

Health Professionals Who Participate in Managing This Disorder

Family physicians
General internists
Pediatricians
Infectious disease specialists
Rheumatologists
Dermatologists
Cardiologists
Neurologists
Physician assistants
Nurse practitioners

Currently Available Therapies for This Disorder

Anti-Infective Drugs

- doxycycline (the tetracycline of choice)
- tetracycline
- amoxicillin
- erythromycin
- cefuroxime
- ceftriaxone
- cefotaxime
- penicillin G

Anti-Inflammatory Drugs

- aspirin and other salicylates

- nonsteroidal anti-inflammatory drugs (NSAIDs) (see Appendix 8, Nonsteroidal Anti-Inflammatory Drugs: A Guide to Selection for Therapy)

New Drugs in Development for Treating This Disorder

Recent animal studies have shown that two new macrolide antibiotics—azithromycin and roxithromycin—appear to be superior to erythromycin in treating Lyme infection. Clinical trials in humans are currently in progress.

Management of Therapy

Since the discovery of the causative agent (*B. burgdorferi*) in 1982, the most effective drugs for treating Lyme disease have been identified. However, due to the variable nature of this infection—its many manifestations and unpredictable course—definitive treatment programs have not been firmly established for all cases. On occasion, questions still remain as to when treatment should be started, the choice of drug to initiate treatment, the duration of drug courses, etc. The treatment of each patient with known or suspected Lyme disease must be carefully considered and individualized. Close observation and good clinical judgment are essential.

Treatment of Early (Stage 1) Disease

Anti-infective treatment will shorten the course of the rash (EM) and *may* prevent disease progression.

- First choice: doxycycline 100 mg every 12 hours for 21 days (if not contraindicated by allergy, age, pregnancy, or breast-feeding)
- Second choice: amoxicillin 500 mg every 12 hours for 21 days (if not contraindicated by allergy)
- Third choice: erythromycin 250 mg every 6 hours for 21 days (if not contraindicated by allergy); this is less effective than doxycycline or amoxicillin

Treatment of Early (Stage 2) Disease

FOR HEART INVOLVEMENT

- ceftriaxone 2 grams intravenously daily for 14 days, or
- penicillin G 20 million units intravenously for 14 days

FOR NERVOUS SYSTEM INVOLVEMENT

For mild facial paralysis:

- doxycycline 100 mg every 12 hours for 30 days, or
- amoxicillin 500 mg every 12 hours for 30 days (minimum)

For meningitis and other neurologic involvement:

- ceftriaxone 2 grams intravenously daily for 14 to 21 days, or
- penicillin G 20 million units intravenously daily for 14 to 21 days, or
- doxycycline 100 mg by mouth or intravenously twice daily for 30 days

FOR ARTHRITIS

Joint involvement in this stage is often transient and may clear without anti-infective therapy. For arthritis that requires relief or persists, initiate treatment with oral medication: doxycycline 100 mg every 12 hours for 30 days, or amoxicillin and probenecid 500 mg each every 6 hours for 30 days.

Treatment of Late (Stage 3) Disease

FOR NERVOUS SYSTEM INVOLVEMENT

In this stage of infection, symptoms indicating disease of the central or peripheral nervous system are usually more serious and persistent. Treatment should begin with intravenous drug administration using the regimens outlined above for Stage 2.

FOR ARTHRITIS

This is the dominant manifestation of Stage 3 Lyme disease. Joint involvement is usually more intense and chronic, requiring three or more months of drug therapy to obtain improvement. Milder cases may be treated initially with oral medication, but most will require intravenous therapy for significant benefit. Currently recommended regimens are:

- penicillin G 20 million units intravenously in divided doses daily for 14 to 21 days, or
- ceftriaxone 2 grams intravenously daily for 14 to 21 days

Ancillary Drug Treatment (as required)

For persistent arthritis not responsive to anti-infective therapy:

- nonsteroidal anti-inflammatory drugs (see Appendix 8)

For fibromyalgia (chronic):

- tricyclic antidepressants

Note: Drug selection, dosage, and administration schedule must be determined by the physician for each patient individually.

Current Controversies in Management

As with most diseases of this nature, opinions vary regarding drug selection and treatment schedule. However, the most controversial issue at this time is the justification for starting *preventive* drug treatment immediately after a tick bite, before the development of any symptoms indicative of actual Lyme infection. Arguments against this practice are based upon the potential for unwarranted adverse drug effects and that such treatment is not cost-effective. Arguments for prompt drug use cite the significant number of infections (up to 30%) that occur without any indication of stage 1 disease, the frequent delay in properly diagnosing Stage 2 and Stage 3 Lyme infection, the considerable risks involved in untreated late stage infection, and the uncertainty of "cure" when treatment is delayed. The decision to advise preventive drug treatment immediately following tick bite is a matter of clinical judgment that is based upon these considerations:

- identity of the tick (if this can be determined)

- length of time the tick was attached
- technique used to remove the tick
- percentage of infected ticks locally (often unknown)
- prevalence of Lyme disease in the community
- state of health of the individual

Important Points to Consider

- There may be a one- to four-week delay (incubation period) between a tick bite and the development of rash (erythema migrans) indicative of Lyme infection.
- The manifestations of Stage 2 and Stage 3 Lyme disease are frequently unrecognized as being due to Lyme infection (erroneous initial diagnosis).
- When suspected, the diagnosis of Lyme infection may be difficult to establish. Some currently used diagnostic blood tests are not uniformly reliable; the rates of false-negative and false-positive test results are unacceptably high. Request that blood samples be tested by a reputable laboratory.
- The earlier that Lyme infection is treated by appropriate anti-infective drugs, the greater the likelihood of cure. However, treatment failures have occurred with all drug regimens in current use; retreatment is often necessary.
- Early Lyme infection that is successfully treated (cured) does not confer immunity. Reinfection can occur.
- Many cases of Lyme infection include a latent period during which there are no significant symptoms. This state of dormant infection may last for months or years, creating diagnostic dilemmas when symptoms occur at a later time.
- The use of intravenous ceftriaxone in treating some manifestations of Stage 2 and Stage 3 Lyme infection may cause gallbladder disease (inflammation and/or gallstone formation) within 90 days after administration. The risk of this drug-induced complication is approximately 2%, with most cases occurring in females 3 to 40 years of age.

Possible Drug Interactions of Significance

Because of the number of drugs that may be used to manage this disorder, adequate consideration of the volume and complexity of potential drug interactions is beyond the scope of this book. Consult *The Essential Guide to Prescription Drugs*, or a similar drug reference book for possible interactions of significance (see Appendix 17, Drug Information Sources).

Special Considerations for Women

Pregnancy

It has been reported that Lyme disease can cause premature birth, stillbirth, brain infection, and heart birth defects in the fetus, but a cause-

and-effect relationship has not been established. Pending the results of further studies, most authorities recommend that *active* Lyme infection during pregnancy be treated as follows:
- For early localized (Stage 1) infection: amoxicillin 500 mg every eight hours for 21 days
- For early disseminated (Stage 2) or late (Stage 3) infection: penicillin G 20 million units intravenously daily for 14 to 21 days

Breast-Feeding

This consideration depends upon the drugs selected for use. Ask your physician for guidance.

The Role of Prevention in This Disorder

Primary Prevention

When going into wooded or grassy areas, take the following precautions:
- Wear clothing with tight bands around the ankles and wrists.
- Apply a tick repellent (such as DEET) to exposed areas of skin.
- Apply a tick repellent containing permethrin to your clothing.
- On returning home, carefully inspect your hairline and the tops of collars and shoes for ticks.
- When next changing clothes or bathing, inspect your body for ticks.
- If ticks are found, remove them promptly with tweezers. Place the tweezers as close as possible to the skin and pull gently without twisting or crushing the tick. Disinfect the bite with alcohol or Betadine.
- Notify your physician that you have been bitten by a tick and ask for guidance.

Secondary Prevention

If you have been treated for Lyme disease in the past and you develop new symptoms that may possibly be related to your earlier infection, consult your physician promptly for evaluation. The persistence of Lyme disease, in spite of appropriate treatment, is well recognized.

Resources

Recommended Reading

Lyme Disease: The Cause, the Cure, the Controversy, Alan G. Barbour, M.D. Baltimore: Johns Hopkins University Press, 1996.

Coping with Lyme Disease: A Practical Guide to Dealing with Diagnosis and Treatment, Denise Lang and Derrick DeSilva, M.D. New York: Henry Holt, 1993.

Additional Information and Services

Centers for Disease Control and Prevention
1600 Clifton Road

Atlanta, GA 30333
CDC Voice Information System: Phone: (404) 332-4555
CDC FAX Information Service: Phone: (404) 332-4565; follow the prompts
and request documents by number:
   351701 General information and pregnancy
   351702 Symptoms
   351703 Treatment and prevention

Centers for Disease Control and Prevention
National Center for Infectious Diseases
Phone: (303) 221-6453

National Institutes of Health
National Institute of Allergy and Infectious Diseases
Office of Communications
Bethesda, MD
Phone: (301) 496-5717

Lyme Disease Foundation
P.O. Box 462
Tolland, CT 06084
Phone: (203) 871-2900, 1-800-886-LYME; Fax: (203) 870-9789
   Local groups: 130. Provides treatment protocols; offers referral service;
provides videotape and slide programs; maintains registry of infected
pregnant women and congenital cases. Quarterly publication, *Lymelight.*

MANIC-DEPRESSIVE DISORDER

Other Names
Manic depression, bipolar mood disorder, bipolar I disorder, bipolar II
disorder, mania, mood disorder: manic phase of manic-depressive disorder, cyclothymic disorder
   Note: The information in this Profile pertains primarily to the manic
phase of manic-depressive (bipolar) disorder. For information pertaining
to the depressive phase, see the Profile of depression in this section.

Prevalence/Incidence in U.S. The current estimate of prevalence is
1% of the population.

Age Group Onset from 15 to over 50 years of age; mean age of onset is
30 years.

Male-to-Female Ratio Equal incidence in men and women

Principal Features and Natural History

This is the disease suffered by Lord Byron, Robert Schumann, and Vincent van Gogh. It is a fascinating and devastating disorder of the mind, and a living hell for the patient and family. Unlike schizophrenia, the person who lives with manic depression is, for the most part, fully in touch with reality. Between the recurring episodes of emotional highs and lows, he is painfully aware of the anguish imposed by depression and the disruptions that derive from mania. And he is totally dismayed by his inability to avoid or control either phase.

The designation *bipolar* refers to mood disorders having alternating periods of mania (elation, excitement) and depression; the term *unipolar* refers to depression-only mood disorder. Bipolar mood disorder often begins with depression and subsequently switches to mania at least once during the course of the illness. *Bipolar I* disorder is characterized by alternating episodes of full-blown psychotic mania and major depression. In *bipolar II* disorder, depressive episodes alternate with periods of hypomania (mild, nonpsychotic excitement). *Cyclothymic* disorder consists of intermittent periods of alternating mania and depression of mild degree and a few days duration.

Approximately one in five patients with major depressive disorder develops mania or hypomania within 10 years after the onset of depression. This usually occurs in the teens, twenties, or thirties. Episodes of alternating mania and depression occur in cycles of three to six months. The manifestations of the manic phase span a very wide spectrum from mildly exaggerated elation or irritability to truly psychotic delusions and hallucinations. Fortunately, 60–70% of bipolar patients respond well to lithium therapy. Those who respond best display a classic manic syndrome, experience manic episodes less than twice a year, and have a personal or family history of good lithium response on prior use.

Diagnostic Symptoms and Signs

The following manifestations are characteristic of the manic phase in bipolar mood disorder:

Mood Symptoms
elation
euphoria
irritability
hostility

Psychological Symptoms
exaggerated self-esteem and boasting
racing thoughts, distractibility, erratic flight of ideas
unnatural interest in new activities
excessive involvement in religious activities

uninvited and intrusive involvement in social discourse
aggressive behavior
reckless driving
illogical buying sprees
ill-advised business ventures
sexual indiscretions
alcohol and substance abuse

Physical Signs
accelerated physical activities, pacing, unable to remain seated
forced and rapid speech pattern
weight loss
decreased need for sleep
increased sex drive

Psychotic Symptoms
grandiose delusions of intelligence and talent
delusions of exceptional physical strength and agility
delusions of wealth, heritage, and social position
paranoia, delusions of persecution
visual and auditory hallucinations

Diagnostic Tests and Procedures
There are no specific tests that establish the diagnosis of the manic phase
associated with bipolar mood disorder. Your physician will utilize the following procedures to make the diagnosis:

Evaluate your symptoms and signs (as outlined above)

Review your family history regarding medical and mental disorders

Review your personal history of medical and mental disorders

Perform a general physical examination to detect conditions that could
be related to your manic state

Request pertinent laboratory tests to detect conditions that could be
related to your manic state

Elicit information regarding all medications you are taking, your alcohol consumption, and substance abuse

Similar Conditions That May Confuse Diagnosis
Borderline personality disorders
Brain tumors
Head trauma
Huntington's chorea
Hyperthyroidism
Influenza
Multiple sclerosis
Rheumatic chorea

Schizo-affective disorder
Schizophrenia
St. Louis encephalitis
Stroke (cerebral infarction)
Syphilitic infection of the brain
Systemic lupus erythematosus
Temporal lobe epilepsy

Causes

Established Causes
The primary cause of bipolar mood disorder is unknown.

Theoretical Causes
The symptoms of bipolar disorder reflect cyclic disruptions of neuro-transmitter regulation within the brain. The mechanisms responsible for neurotransmitter dysfunction are not understood.

Research indicates that there is a genetic predisposition to the development of bipolar disorder.

Known Risk Factors for Developing This Disorder
A prior history of unipolar depressive disorder
A family history of bipolar disorder

Drugs That Can Cause This Disorder
Most antidepressant drugs, when given in sufficient dosage, can trigger a switch from depression to mania in persons predisposed to bipolar mood disorder.

The following drugs may cause elevated moods (elation, excitement) that resemble bipolar mania:
    amphetamines
    bromocriptine
    cocaine
    cortisonelike drugs (corticosteroids)
    levodopa
    methylphenidate
See Appendix 16, Drug Classes, for specific generic drugs within respective drug classes.

Goals of Treatment

Can This Disorder Be Cured?
Because the primary definitive cause of bipolar disorder is not known, there is no permanently curative therapy.

Can This Disorder Be Treated Effectively?
Currently available drug therapies can provide excellent results in 60–70% of bipolar disorder patients with manic episodes.

Supplemental therapies (psychotherapies, electroconvulsive therapy) can provide additional benefits as needed.

Specific Goals
- Early recognition and treatment of bipolar mood disorder
- Careful monitoring of antidepressant drug therapy to prevent conversion of depressive state to manic state
- Early detection of emerging manic state
- Prompt treatment of manic state
- Establishment of a manic-free and depression-free state
- Provision of a long-term maintenance program with periodic assessment of mood status, lithium blood levels, and general well-being

Health Professionals Who Participate in Managing This Disorder
Family physicians
General internists
Pediatricians
Geriatricians
Gynecologists
Obstetricians
Neurologists
Neuropsychiatrists
Psychiatrists
Clinical psychologists
Pharmacists
Physician assistants
Nurse practitioners
Psychiatric nurse specialists
Medical social workers

Currently Available Therapies for This Disorder

Drug Therapy
- haloperidol (for acute phase of mania)
- lithium (the drug of choice for maintenance)
- fluphenazine decanoate (by injection)
- carbamazepine
- valproate

Nondrug Treatment Methods
- Supportive psychotherapy
- Electroconvulsive therapy (ECT) for severe, unresponsive, life-threatening manic states

Management of Therapy

Use of Lithium

- Can be 70% effective in stabilizing mood in bipolar manic-depressive illness; reduces the frequency and severity of attacks of both mania and depression. When lithium proves to be effective in preventing recurrence of mania and depression, it is very important to continue maintenance treatment when feeling well and free of symptoms.
- Must be taken in divided doses to avoid stomach irritation and excessively high (toxic) blood levels. Early toxic effects include nausea, vomiting, dizziness, unsteadiness, weakness, slurred speech, muscle twitching, and confusion. Periodic measurements of blood levels are mandatory to maintain effective concentrations and to prevent toxicity. Blood samples should be taken 12 hours after the last dose. Recommended therapeutic blood level range: 0.3–1.3 mEq/L.
- Mild side effects (not toxicity) include loss of appetite, metallic taste, indigestion, nausea, thirst, fatigue, tremor, fluid retention, acne.
- While taking lithium, maintain a high liquid intake, but avoid excessive coffee, tea, and cola drinks. Do not restrict your salt intake.
- Lithium should be used cautiously if you have heart disease, kidney disease, or a thyroid disorder. Thyroid and kidney functions should be checked before and during lithium therapy. Lithium can induce hypothyroidism and a loss of kidney concentrating power (excessively dilute urine).

Possible Drug Interactions of Significance

Because of the number of drugs that may be used to manage bipolar disorder, adequate consideration of the volume and complexity of potential drug interactions is beyond the scope of this book. Consult *The Essential Guide to Prescription Drugs*, or a similar drug reference book for possible interactions of significance (see Appendix 17, Drug Information Sources).

Special Considerations for Women

Pregnancy

- Lithium is designated Pregnancy Category D (see Appendix 15, FDA Pregnancy Categories).
- For women who wish to consider establishing pregnancy, it is advisable to attain a two-year period of freedom from manic episodes before discontinuing lithium. Contraceptive measures should be continued until lithium is completely withdrawn.
- If serious symptoms of bipolar disorder recur during the first trimester, ECT is a safer alternative to antidepressant or lithium medication. If necessary, drug therapy could be resumed in the second or third trimester.

- Ask your physician for guidance in making all decisions regarding pregnancy and bipolar therapy.

Breast-Feeding

If bipolar drug therapy is required, it is advisable to refrain from nursing.

Special Considerations for the Elderly

- Manic-depressive illness accounts for approximately 10% of all mood disorders experienced by older people. However, the manic features are less likely to be elation or excitement and more likely to be agitation, irritability, and disturbed sleep.
- Older individuals are more sensitive to the toxic effects of lithium. It is advisable to monitor blood lithium levels more frequently and to maintain levels in the lower half of the recommended range.
- Age alone is not a contraindication to the use of ECT. Older persons generally respond well to this therapy for severe manic episodes that are not adequately controlled by medication.

Quality of Life Considerations

The impaired insight, understanding, and judgment that occur during manic episodes result in major complications for the patient and family. Frequent consequences include divorce, loss of job, financial difficulties, and legal encounters. The only acceptable recourse for the patient with bipolar disorder is the realistic acceptance of his illness and total compliance with an effective treatment program.

The Role of Prevention in This Disorder

Primary Prevention

The only means currently available for the primary prevention of bipolar disorder is genetic counseling and family planning. The evidence for genetic transmission of this illness is the strongest of all psychiatric disorders (see Appendix 11, Genetic Disorders and Gene Therapy).

Secondary Prevention

Effective therapies are available to control the frequency and severity of manic-depressive cycles. Those who are forced to live with this demanding disorder are urged to obtain the help they need to accomplish the following:

- Episodes of mania can become seductive and addictive. Accept your therapist's explanation that you may be using the tool of denial to avoid acceptance and treatment of your disorder.
- Learn to recognize the early signs that indicate a shift in your emotional balance and signal the onset of a manic episode. Report this to your therapist promptly.

- Cooperate fully with your therapist to determine an optimal treatment program.
- Comply honestly with all aspects of recommended therapy. Take your medications exactly as prescribed. Keep all appointments for psychotherapy sessions.

Resources

Recommended Reading
An Unquiet Mind: A Memoir of Moods and Madness, Kay Redfield Jamison. New York: Knopf, 1995.

Living Without Depression and Manic-Depression: A Workbook for Maintaining Mood Stability, Mary Ellen Copeland. Oakland, CA: New Harbinger Publications, 1994.

Additional Information and Services
National Depressive and Manic-Depressive Association
730 North Franklin Street, Suite 501
Chicago, IL 60610
Phone: 1-800-82-NDMDA, (312) 642-0049; Fax: (312) 642-7243

Offers information, one-to-one support, referrals by telephone. Local groups: 190. Publications, audio- and videotapes available.

National Mental Health Information Center
1020 Prince Street
Alexandria, VA 23314-2971
Phone: 1-800-969-6642

Disease Management Expertise
Stanley Center for the Innovative Treatment of Bipolar Disorder
3811 O'Hara Street, Suite 279
Pittsburgh, PA 15213
Phone: 1-800-424-7657, (412) 624-2476; Fax: (412) 624-0493

MENOPAUSE

Other Names Menopausal syndrome, estrogen withdrawal syndrome, female climacteric, change of life

Prevalence/Incidence in U.S. 16.5 million women (candidates for menopause)

Age Group 40 to 60 years; the average age of natural menopause is 51.4 years

Principal Features and Natural History

The term "menopause" refers to the permanent cessation of menstruation and the end of reproductive life. This occurs naturally in most women between 45 and 55 years of age. The characteristic indication of the "change"—altered menstrual pattern with eventual cessation of menstrual periods—usually lasts from 6 to 18 months. The majority of women (85%) experience some physical effects of progressive estrogen withdrawal. These include recurring hot flashes, episodic sweating, shrinkage of breast tissue, and reduction of vaginal secretions. In addition, a variety of nervous and emotional symptoms may occur, such as emotional instability, anxiety, depression, insomnia, headaches, dizziness, and nausea. For approximately 25%, the symptoms are of sufficient intensity to warrant a trial of estrogen replacement therapy (ERT). Up to 35% of menopausal women experience hot flashes for five or more years.

In 1993, the Gallop Organization conducted a national survey of women between 45 and 60 years of age who were perimenopausal (earliest stage), midmenopausal, or postmenopausal. Their greatest concerns regarding the physical and emotional effects associated with menopause were osteoporosis (33%), emotional well-being (28%), and heart disease (27%). When asked about the subject matter of discussions with their physicians, 66% reported osteoporosis, 61% said hot flashes and night sweats, 52% said emotional symptoms, and 46% mentioned heart disease. The survey was sponsored by the North American Menopause Society. Wulf Utian, M.D., founder and executive director of the society, urges physicians to address the full spectrum of menopause-related considerations with their patients. These include the early manifestations that may be baffling for many women, the implications of changing physiology, medications for relief of symptoms, and opportunities for prevention. If women are to actively participate in decision making about such matters as hormone replacement therapy and related issues, they should have ready access to all pertinent information.

Diagnostic Symptoms and Signs

Significant changes in menstrual patterns
Hot flashes, sweating episodes
Emotional instability: mood swings, anxiety, depression, spells of weeping
Fatigability, insomnia, disturbing dreams
Impaired thinking, concentration, and memory
Vaginal dryness, susceptibility to vaginitis
Urinary frequency, urgency, and incontinence

Diagnostic Tests and Procedures

Measurements of female hormone blood levels: estradiol, follicle-stimulating hormone (FSH), and luteinizing hormone (LH)

Cervical cytology (Pap smear) to evaluate the presence of estrogenic effects

Endometrial (uterine) biopsy

Ultrasound studies of the uterus and ovaries

Similar Conditions That May Confuse Diagnosis

Drug-induced suppression of ovarian function (see below).

ALERT!

Altered menstrual patterns during the early stage of menopause can include excessively heavy bleeding. If this occurs, consult your physician regarding the need to determine the cause (hormonal, uterine polyps or tumor) and to evaluate the consequences (significant anemia).

The absence of menstruation for 12 consecutive months is generally recognized as the termination of ovarian function. Any vaginal bleeding that occurs afterward is considered to be postmenopausal and warrants diagnostic evaluation. Report such bleeding promptly to your physician.

Causes

Natural menopause occurs spontaneously to terminate reproductive capability. Smoking can accelerate the onset of menopause by two years.

Therapeutic menopause follows surgical removal of the uterus and/or ovaries, irradiation of the ovaries, or irradiation or removal of the pituitary gland.

Drugs That Can Cause This Disorder

The following drugs can cause cessation of menstruation for varying periods of time, sometimes permanently: busulfan, chlorambucil, cyclophosphamide, mechlorethamine, oral contraceptives, and vincristine. The antiestrogen drug tamoxifen, used for the treatment of breast cancer, can cause hot flashes, dizziness, and menstrual irregularities typical of the menopausal syndrome.

Goals of Treatment

- Reduction in the frequency and severity of hot flashes and night sweats with attendant insomnia
- Relief of nervous and emotional symptoms
- Prevention or relief of atrophic changes of the vulva, vagina, and urethra
- Prevention of thinning of the skin
- Prevention of osteoporosis
- Prevention of coronary artery disease and stroke
- Possible reduction of the risk for developing Alzheimer's disease

Health Professionals Who Participate in Managing This Disorder

Family physicians
General internists
Gynecologists
Clinical endocrinologists
Pharmacists
Physician assistants
Nurse practitioners

Currently Available Therapies for This Disorder

Nondrug Treatment Methods

* Dietary modifications: salt restriction, low-fat and low-cholesterol diet as recommended by your physician
* Nutritional supplements: calcium citrate, up to 1000 mg daily
* Exercise recommendations: 20 to 30 minutes of aerobic, weight-bearing exercise three times a week can reduce hot flashes and help prevent osteoporosis
* Stress reduction techniques
* Smoking cessation

Drug Therapy

Oral contraceptives may be tried to relieve symptoms during the perimenopausal stage (earliest manifestations).

Hormone replacement therapy (HRT):

"Natural-type" estrogens are preferred during the midmenopausal and postmenopausal stages.

* conjugated estrogens (Genisis, Premarin)
* esterified estrogens (Evex, Menest)
* estradiol cypionate (Depo-Estradiol, injection)
* estradiol valerate (Delestrogen, injection)
* estriol (Hormonin, a mixture of estriol, estradiol, and estrone)
* piperazine estrone sulfate (Ogen)
* micronized 17-B estradiol (Estrace)
* transdermal estradiol skin patch (Estraderm-50 and 100)

Nonhormonal therapy for hot flashes:

* clonidine (Catapres): effective in 25% of cases

Management of Therapy

It is now generally held that for the well-informed menopausal woman who has obvious symptoms of estrogen deficiency and does not have any contraindications to its use, the benefits of estrogen replacement therapy outweigh the possible risks. The use of estrogen is considered to be effective and safe when prescribed appropriately and monitored properly.

As each women reaches the menopausal years (late 30s to middle 40s) she should assess her own status and perceived needs. Next she should familiarize herself with the benefits and possible risks of estrogen replacement therapy. If she thinks she needs medical guidance and/or treatment, she should discuss all aspects of her situation with her physician and share in the decision regarding the use of hormones.

A clear indication for the use of estrogen should exist. It should not be given routinely to the menopausal woman, but should be reserved to treat those with symptoms of estrogen deficiency. Estrogen does not retard the natural progression of normal aging. It should not be used for the sole purpose of "preserving femininity."

Before estrogen therapy is started, appropriate examinations should be performed and due consideration given to the following possible contraindications to the use of estrogen:

- pregnancy
- history of deep venous thrombosis or pulmonary embolism
- present or previous cancer of the breast
- cancer of the ovary or uterus
- strong family history of breast, ovarian, or uterine cancer
- current liver disease or previous drug-induced jaundice
- chronic gallbladder disease, with or without stones
- abnormal elevation of blood lipids (total cholesterol, LDL cholesterol, triglycerides)
- history of porphyria
- large uterine fibroid tumors
- any estrogen-dependent tumor
- combination of obesity, varicose veins, and cigarette smoking
- diabetes mellitus
- severe hypertension

In the young woman experiencing premature menopause (destruction or removal of both ovaries), the *long-term* use of estrogen replacement is justified, provided appropriate precautions are observed (see "Guidelines" below).

In the menopausal woman experiencing hot flashes and/or atrophic vaginitis, the *short-term* use of estrogen therapy is generally felt to be acceptable with appropriate supervision and guidance. Estrogen replacement therapy provides symptomatic relief; it is not a permanent cure for hot flashes.

Long-term estrogen therapy for *all* women after the menopause cannot be justified. Treatment must be carefully individualized.

It is generally recommended that estrogens be taken cyclically. The customary schedule is from the 1st through the 25th day of each month, with no estrogen during the remaining days of the month. After 6 to 12 months of continuous use, the estrogen dose should be gradually reduced over a period of 2 to 3 months and then discontinued to assess the individual's need for resumption of use.

The lowest effective daily dose of estrogen should be determined and maintained for the duration of the treatment.

Vaginal cream preparations of estrogen may be considered instead of orally administered estrogen if the only indication is atrophic vaginitis. However, it should be noted that these preparations allow rapid absorption of estrogen into the systemic circulation, and do not permit accurate control of dosage. They should be used intermittently and only as needed to correct the symptoms of atrophic vaginitis. (*Note:* The estrogen in vaginal creams can be absorbed through the skin of the penis and cause tenderness of the breast in men.)

The unnecessary prolongation of estrogen therapy should be avoided. It is advisable to use estrogens in the lowest effective dose and for only as long as necessary to relieve symptoms.

Guidelines for the Use of Estrogens in Specific Deficiency States

I.The young woman (usually under 45 years of age) with both ovaries or ovaries and uterus removed:

- Choice of estrogen: a conjugated "natural" estrogen (see list of estrogen preparations)

  The lowest effective dose should be used. The lowest effective dose is determined by keeping a daily "flash count" to ascertain the lowest daily dose that will reduce the frequency and severity of flashes to an acceptable level.
- Dosage schedule: once daily from the 1st through the 25th day of each month

  Note: If the uterus is present, it is advisable to add a progestin (medroxyprogesterone), 4 to 10 mg daily during the last 7 to 10 days of the estrogen course. The use of a supplemental progestin during the last 7 to 10 days of estrogen administration is still controversial. A possible benefit is the reduced potential for uterine cancer; a possible risk is the increased potential for coronary artery disease; a possible inconvenience is withdrawal bleeding (induced menstruation). The risks of this form of long-term progestin therapy are not known.
- Duration of use: if well tolerated, until 50 years of age, when assessment of continued need is made individually
- Periodic examinations:
  - Baseline mammogram (low-radiation-dose xeroradiography); mammogram should be repeated only as necessary to evaluate possible breast tumor (American Cancer Society guideline)

- Self-examination of breasts monthly
- Physician examination of breasts (and uterus if present) every 6 to 12 months
- Measurement of blood pressure

II. The woman experiencing the "menopausal syndrome" of hot flashes and sweating (usually 45 to 55 years of age):

UTERUS NOT REMOVED:

- Choice of hormones and recommended dosage range:
  - Estrogen: conjugated equine estrogens—0.3 to 0.625 mg daily (see list of alternative estrogen preparations)
  - Progestin: medroxyprogesterone—5 to 10 mg daily
  The lowest effective dose of estrogen should be used. The lowest effective dose is determined by keeping a daily "flash count" to ascertain the lowest daily dose that will reduce the frequency and severity of flashes to an acceptable level.
- Dosage schedule:
  - Estrogen: once daily from the 1st through the 25th day of each month
  - Progestin: once daily during the last 7 to 10 days of the estrogen course. The use of a supplemental progestin during the last 7 to 10 days of estrogen administration is still controversial. A possible benefit is the reduced potential for uterine cancer; a possible risk is the increased potential for coronary artery disease; a possible inconvenience is withdrawal bleeding (induced menstruation). The risks of this form of long-term progestin therapy are not known.
- Duration of use: 6 to 12 months, followed by gradual reduction of dose over a period of 2 to 3 months, and then discontinuation to assess the need for continued use. Treatment should be resumed only if symptoms require it. An attempt should be made to discontinue all hormones after two to three years of continual use, unless a clear need for continuation is apparent.
- Periodic examinations:
  - Baseline mammogram (low-radiation-dose xeroradiography)
  - Low-dose mammogram annually (over 50 years of age) during continuous use of estrogen (American Cancer Society guideline)
  - Self-examination of breasts monthly
  - Physician examination of breasts every 6 to 12 months
  - Cervical cytology and endometrial biopsy (aspiration curettage) annually
  - Blood pressure measurement every three to six months
  - Two-hour blood sugar assay annually

UTERUS REMOVED:

- Choice of estrogen and dose: conjugated equine estrogens—0.3 to 0.625 mg daily

The lowest effective dose should be used. The lowest effective dose is determined by keeping a daily "flash count" to ascertain the lowest daily dose that will reduce the frequency and severity of flashes to an acceptable level.

- Dosage schedule: once daily from the 1st through the 25th day of each month
- Duration of use: 6 to 12 months, followed by gradual reduction of dose over a period of 2 to 3 months, and then discontinuation to assess the need for continued use. Treatment should be resumed only if symptoms require it. An attempt should be made to discontinue all hormones after two to three years of continual use.
- Periodic examinations:
  - Baseline mammogram (low-radiation-dose xeroradiography)
  - Low-dose mammogram annually (over 50 years of age) during continuous use of estrogen (American Cancer Society guideline)
  - Self-examination of breasts monthly
  - Physician examination of breasts every 6 to 12 months
  - Blood pressure measurement every three to six months
  - Two-hour blood sugar assay annually

III. The woman in the "post-menopausal" period (usually over 55 years of age): treatment should be individualized as follows:

- If there are no specific symptoms of estrogen deficiency (hot flashes or atrophic vaginitis), estrogen should not be given.
- If specific symptoms of estrogen deficiency persist to a degree requiring subjective relief, the recommendations in category II apply. However, in addition to limiting courses of estrogen to 6 to 12 months followed by gradual withdrawal, dosage might be limited to three times weekly on a trial basis. Estrogen should be discontinued altogether as soon as possible. If only flashes persist beyond 60 years of age, all estrogen should be discontinued. Nonhormonal drugs such as clonidine and certain sedatives may be substituted for the relief of hot flashes.
- Although we do not yet have accurate and reliable predictive indicators, an attempt should be made to identify the woman who may be at high risk for the development of osteoporosis. The following features suggest the possibility of increased risk:
  - slender build, light-boned, white or Asian race
  - a sedentary lifestyle or restricted physical activity
  - a family history (mother or sister) of osteoporosis (reported by some investigators)
  - a low-sodium diet (also likely to be a low-calcium diet)
  - heavy smoking
  - excessive use of antacids that contain aluminum
  - long-term use of cortisonelike drugs

- habitual use of carbonated beverages (reported by some investigators)
- excessive consumption of alcohol
- increased urinary excretion of calcium
- For the woman thought to be at increased risk for the development of osteoporosis, estrogen treatment should be started within three years after menstruation ceases. The following schedule of estrogen therapy may be recommended for prevention: conjugated equine estrogens— 0.625 mg daily or three times weekly, for the first three weeks of each month. Periodic examinations as outlined in category II above should be performed. Estrogen replacement therapy may continue indefinitely, always with appropriate supervision.
- In addition to the prudent use of estrogen, regular exercise and a daily intake of 1500 mg of calcium and 400 units of vitamin D are generally thought to be beneficial in slowing the development of osteoporosis.
- Periodic examinations:
  - Baseline mammogram (low-radiation-dose xeroradiography)
  - Low-dose mammogram annually during continuous use of estrogen (American Cancer Society guideline)
  - Self-examination of breasts monthly
  - Physician examination of breasts every 6 to 12 months
  - Blood pressure measurement every three to six months
  - Two-hour blood sugar assay annually

Ancillary Drug Treatment (as required)
For anxiety and/or depression:
- alprazolam (Xanax), for intermittent, short-term use
For insomnia:
- doxylamine (Unisom), available over-the-counter (OTC)
- diphenhydramine (Benadryl), available OTC
For headache:
- aspirin
- acetaminophen (Tylenol, Panadol, etc.)
- ibuprofen (Advil, Nuprin, etc.)
For atrophic vaginitis and painful intercourse:
- estrogen creams (Dienestrol, Estrace, Premarin)

   Note: Drug selection, dosage, and administration schedule must be determined by the physician for each patient individually.

Possible Drug Interactions of Significance
Estrogens *taken concurrently* with
- antidiabetic drugs may cause unpredictable fluctuations of blood sugar; close monitoring of blood sugar levels is advised.
- thyroid hormones may require an increase in thyroid dose.

- tricyclic antidepressants may enhance their adverse effects and reduce their antidepressant effectiveness.
- warfarin may cause unpredictable alterations of prothrombin activity; close monitoring advised to achieve satisfactory anticoagulant effect.

The following drugs may *decrease* the effects of estrogens

- carbamazepine (Tegretol)
- phenobarbital (Luminal)
- phenytoin (Dilantin)
- primidone (Mysoline)
- rifampin (Rifadin, Rimactane)

Quality of Life Considerations

If postmenopausal women with their uterus intact elect to use hormone replacement therapy, they will be advised to take progesterone to prevent the possible development of estrogen-induced cancer of the uterus. If estrogen and progesterone are taken in a cyclic regimen, the result is resumption of regular menstruation. While enjoying the "tonic" effects and possible preventive benefits of estrogen, the patient must accept any nuisance and limitations menstruation may cause them. If estrogen and progesterone are taken together continuously (both daily), irregular bleeding may occur for several months and require increased doses of progesterone to eventually abolish menstruation. Progesterone side effects include fluid retention, tender breasts, and reversal of the mental tonic effect of estrogen. Ask your physician for guidance to help you make the decision that is best for you individually.

Resources

Recommended Reading

Managing Your Menopause, W.H. Utian, M.D. Englewood Cliffs, NJ: Simon & Schuster Fireside Press, 1990.

The Menopause Book: A Guide to Health and Well-Being for Women After Forty, S.H. Cherry, M.D. New York: Macmillan, 1993.

The Silent Passage, Gail Sheehy. New York: Random House, 1991.

The Pause: Positive Approaches to Menopause, Lonnie Barbach. New York: Penguin, 1995.

Making Sense of Menopause, Faye Kitchener Cone. New York: Simon & Schuster, 1993.

Without Estrogen: Natural Remedies for Menopause and Beyond, Dee Ito. New York: Carol Southern Books, 1994.

Additional Information and Services

National Institute on Aging Information Center
P.O. Box 8057

Gaithersburg, MD 20898-8057
Phone: 1-800-222-2225

A Friend Indeed Publications, Inc.
P.O. Box 515
Place du Parc Station
Montreal, Canada H2W 2P1
   Monthly newsletter, *A Friend Indeed.*

Disease Management Expertise
North American Menopause Society
University Hospitals of Cleveland
2074 Avington Road
Cleveland, OH 44106
Phone: (216) 844-3334; Fax: (216) 844-3348
   Offers a listing of Menopause Care Providers.

MIGRAINE HEADACHE

Other Names Classic migraine, common migraine

Prevalence/Incidence in U.S. Approximately 23 million; 17.6% of
adult females, 5.7% of adult males

Age Group
Under 18 years—0.8% of population; 18 to 44 years—4.7% of population;
45 to 64 years—5% of population; over 65 years—1.9% of population

Male-to-Female Ratio
With onset at puberty, boys and girls are affected equally.
Over 18 years of age: 1 male to 3 females

Principal Features and Natural History
Migraine headaches may first appear in childhood but usually begin in
the late teens or early twenties; they often cease after menopause. The
migraine attack occurs in one of two patterns:
1. Classic migraine (15% of the total) begins with an "aura" of symptoms that may precede the onset of headache by 15 to 20 minutes.
   These usually consist of visual manifestations described as blind
   spots, zigzag effects, or shimmering lights. The attack may begin at
   any time of the day or night. Approximately 70% of migraine
   headaches are confined to one side of the head; 30% may spread to
   involve both sides before terminating. The pain is usually pulsating

(throbbing) in nature and varies in intensity from mild to severe. The classic migraine episode commonly (90%) includes nausea, vomiting, and increased sensitivity to light and noise. Other associated features are scalp tenderness, dizziness, dry mouth, tremors, sweating, and chilliness.

2. Common migraine (85% of the total) begins as a headache without a warning "aura." Otherwise, the pattern is essentially the same as that with classic migraine. Attacks may occur rarely (one or two a year) or every few days; the average frequency is two to four per month. Individual episodes usually last from 12 to 48 hours.

Diagnostic Symptoms and Signs

Visual "aura:" blind spots, shimmering lights
Deep, throbbing head pain on one or both sides
Photophobia: aversion to light
Phonophobia: aversion to noise
Nausea and vomiting

Diagnostic Tests and Procedures

There are no diagnostic tests that are specific for migraine.

Brain-imaging studies (computed tomography or magnetic resonance imaging) may be used to exclude organic brain disorders.

Similar Conditions That May Confuse Diagnosis

Cerebral hemorrhage (hemorrhagic stroke)
Cerebral infarction (thrombotic stroke)
Cerebral aneurysm (a saccular defect in the wall of an artery, enlarging or leaking blood)
Encephalitis (brain infection)
Meningitis (infection of the brain covering)
Brain tumors
Ménière's disease

ALERT!

The following features suggest the possibility of serious disorders *other than* migraine:

frequent headaches beginning after 30 years of age
frequent headaches localized to one area
headaches associated with altered mental status, seizures, extremity weakness, or paralysis
headaches that are *caused by* bending over, coughing, sneezing, or strenuous physical exertion
headaches that are not relieved by medications used for migraine

Causes

Established Causes

The primary definitive cause that initiates the migraine syndrome is not known.

Theoretical Causes

Migraine is thought to be due to biochemical imbalances in the brain that involve the nerve transmitter serotonin. The resulting disturbance in the autonomic nervous system (serotonin metabolism) causes instability in the control of cerebral arteries. Excessive constriction of arteries initially reduces blood flow, thus producing the characteristic visual "aura." This is followed by excessive dilation of arteries that results in throbbing head pain.

Known Risk Factors for Developing This Disorder

Genetic predisposition: there is a positive family history in 70% of those who experience migraine headaches.

Factors that may "trigger" migraine attacks: emotional stress, excessive fatigue, hunger, erratic patterns of eating and sleeping, bright sunlight, weather changes, loud noises, and the use of alcohol.

The following foods are thought to be responsible for migraine attacks in sensitive individuals: aged cheese, bananas, caffeine-containing beverages, chicken livers, chocolate, citrus fruits, monosodium glutamate, onions, pickled herring, pork, red wine, excessive salt, shellfish, sodium nitrite, vinegar, yogurt. Among the notable offenders are nitrites, tyramine, and monosodium glutamate (see Appendix 9, Tyramine-Free Diet, and Appendix 14, Monosodium Glutamate Syndrome).

Drugs That Can Cause This Disorder

The following drugs may induce migrainelike headaches or aggravate existing migraine syndromes:

aminophylline
analgesics (chronic use of acetaminophen or aspirin)
antihypertensive drugs that cause vasodilation
caffeine (chronic use may cause vascular headache)
estrogens (can worsen migraine in 50% of women)
hydralazine
indomethacin
nifedipine
nitrates
oral contraceptives
prazosin
ranitidine
reserpine

Goals of Treatment

Can This Disorder Be Cured?

There is no therapy known that will permanently eliminate the potential for migraine headaches.

Can This Disorder Be Treated Effectively?

Effective medications are available for (1) preventing migraine attacks; (2) aborting attacks in the early stage of development; (3) relieving the pain of a fully developed headache.

Specific Goals

- Reduction in the frequency and severity of recurrent migraine attacks
- Prompt abortion and relief of the acute migraine attack

Health Professionals Who Participate in Managing This Disorder

Family physicians
General internists
Pediatricians
Gynecologists
Neurologists
Neuropsychiatrists
Clinical psychologists
Pharmacists
Physician assistants
Nurse practitioners
Dietitians

Currently Available Therapies for This Disorder

Nondrug Treatment Methods

- Lifestyle modifications to eliminate factors that predispose to migraine attacks
- Avoidance of specific migraine "triggers" (known foods, beverages, etc.)
- Aerobic exercise programs
- Relaxation techniques: meditation, yoga
- Biofeedback training to abort incipient attacks
- Hypnotherapy

Drug Therapy

FOR PREVENTION OF MIGRAINE ATTACKS
Beta-adrenergic blocking drugs (beta-blockers):
- atenolol (Tenormin)
- metoprolol (Lopressor)

- nadolol (Corgard)
- propranolol (Inderal)
- timolol (Blocadren)

Calcium channel-blocking drugs (calcium blockers):

- diltiazem (Cardizem)
- nifedipine (Procardia)
- verapamil (Calan, Isoptin)

Nonsteroidal anti-inflammatory drugs (NSAIDs):

- aspirin
- fenoprofen (Nalfon)
- ibuprofen (Motrin, Rufen, Advil, etc.)
- ketoprofen (Orudis)
- mefenamic acid (Ponstel)
- naproxen (Naprosyn)

Antidepressants:

- amitriptyline (Elavil, Endep)
- doxepin (Sinequan, Adapin)
- fluoxetine (Prozac)
- nortriptyline (Aventyl, Pamelor)
- sertraline (Zoloft)

Others:

- lithium (Lithane, Lithobid, etc.)
- methysergide (Sansert)
- prednisone for occasional intractable migraine
- valproic acid (Depakene)

FOR ABORTION AND RELIEF OF MIGRAINE ATTACKS

Vasoconstrictor drugs:

- ergotamine: oral (Cafergot, Wigraine); rectal (Cafergot, Wigraine suppositories); sublingual (Ergostat, Ergomar, Wigrettes); inhalant (Medihaler ergotamine)
- dihydroergotamine (DHE-45) for intramuscular injection
- isometheptene (Midrin)
- sumatriptan (Imitrex)

Nonsteroidal anti-inflammatory drugs (NSAIDs):

- aspirin
- diclofenac (Voltaren)
- diflunisal (Dolobid)
- flurbiprofen (Ansaid)
- ibuprofen (Motrin, Rufen, Advil, etc.)
- ketoprofen (Orudis)
- ketorolac (Toradol)
- meclofenamate (Meclomen)
- naproxen (Naprosyn)

Opioid analgesics:
- butorphanol (Stadol-NS), a nasal spray
- codeine
- meperidine (Demerol)

Management of Therapy
Important Note: Not every drug is effective for treating every patient who is subject to migraine attacks. Trial and experimentation may be necessary to determine the most effective treatment for each individual.
- For fewer than three attacks per month of mild to moderate migraine, abortive medications may be used at the onset of symptoms. Ergotamine and anti-inflammatory drugs are the medications of choice.
- For three or more attacks per month and for severe, prolonged migraine, preventive medications may be tried on a continual basis. Beta-blockers are the drugs of choice to reduce the frequency and severity of recurrent migraine attacks.
- Always try to take your medication as soon as possible after the first indications of a developing migraine attack.
- Isometheptene (Midrin) is a mild, well-tolerated and safer drug than ergotamine; it may be used first to determine its effectiveness. Stronger drugs should be used only as needed.
- Metoclopramide (Reglan) is an effective addition to the treatment of migraine attacks; it often controls nausea and vomiting, and it enhances the effectiveness of other oral migraine drugs.
- Antidepressants may be used concurrently with other preventive drugs. They may be very effective *even in the absence of depression.*
- For best results, it is advisable to start the preventive treatment of menstrual migraine three days before the onset of menstruation and to continue it until all spotting has ceased.

Use of Beta-Blockers
- These are the drugs of choice for long-term prevention of migraine attacks. Propranolol (Inderal) is the most widely used; nadolol (Corgard) is a good second choice.
- The preventive dose varies greatly and must be determined by individual trial. Effective dosage ranges from 80 mg to 320 mg daily.
- After a period of 6 to 12 months of good headache control, the dose may be reduced gradually and the drug eventually discontinued.

Use of Calcium Blockers
- The preventive use of this class of drugs has been highly effective in Europe.
- Verapamil (Calan, Isoptin) is the most effective of this class currently available in the United States. Nifedipine (Procardia) has been found

to intensify migraine attacks in some individuals. Its use is not recommended.

- A trial of six to eight weeks is usually required to determine the preventive effectiveness of these drugs.
- Observe for the development of fluid retention and constipation.

Use of Anti-Inflammatory Drugs

- These drugs are useful in both preventing and relieving migraine attacks. They are usually well tolerated and are not habit-forming.
- Meclofenamate (Meclomen) is the fastest acting of the class and is very effective in aborting acute migraine.
- Naproxen (Naprosyn) and fenoprofen (Nalfon) are also effective and widely used for intermittent prevention (as in menstrual migraine).
- The prolonged-action forms of these drugs should be used cautiously, especially in the elderly, because of their potential for reducing kidney blood flow.

Use of Antidepressants

- The long-term use of amitriptyline (Elavil, Endep, etc.) is effective in preventing all types of chronic headaches: tension headaches, migraine attacks, and mixed forms.
- Effectiveness is not dependent upon the drug's antidepressant action; the dose required for headache control is less than the antidepressant dose.
- For migraine patients with sleep problems, the antidepressants of choice are amitriptyline, doxepin, and trazodone because of their sedative effects. The total daily requirement is best given as a single dose at bedtime.
- Desipramine (Norpramin, Pertofrane) is usually considered to have the fewest side effects.

Use of Methysergide

- Although very effective as a migraine preventive, this drug is inherently dangerous. It can cause serious and life-threatening adverse effects with long-term use: formation of scar tissue (fibrosis) involving the heart, lungs, blood vessels, and kidneys. It is usually reserved to treat severe migraine that has not responded to safer drugs. Its use should be limited to courses of no more than four to six months, followed by drug-free intervals of four to six weeks. The smallest effective dose should be determined; the total daily dosage should not exceed 8 mg.
- This drug should not be used in the presence of valvular heart disease or serious blood vessel disorders.

Use of Ergotamine

- This is the most effective abortive drug if taken early in the migraine attack; it can relieve the headache in one to two hours. It tends to be less effective if taken later. Dosage should be limited to no more than

6 mg/24 hours or 10 mg/week to prevent serious adverse effects. It may be taken orally or sublingually in tablet form, rectally in the form of suppositories, by inhalation, or by injection.

- Concurrent use with dopamine, erythromycins, troleandomycin, and beta-blockers should be avoided.
- Frequent and regular use should be avoided. Long-term use on a daily basis can *cause* chronic migrainelike headaches.
- Ergotamine "rebound" (return and intensification of headache) can be prevented by allowing 48 hours between courses of treatment.

Use of Sumatriptan

- This is the most effective drug for relief of acute, manifest headache pain—migraine with or without aura; relief begins within 10 minutes following injection.
- It provides relief at any time during the migraine attack.
- Administration is by self-injection, using a simple push-button autoinjector that injects a single dose (6 mg) beneath the skin from a prefilled syringe.
- It relieves all migraine symptoms: headache, nausea, vomiting, sensitivity to light and noise. It does not cause drowsiness or impair mental function.
- Maximal daily dose: two injections of 6 mg each, given at least one hour apart. Do not use this drug within 24 hours following any ergotamine drug.
- This drug must not be taken concurrently with a monoamine oxidase (MAO) inhibitor drug or within two weeks after discontinuing a MAO inhibitor drug (see Appendix 16, Drug Classes).

Caution: The following are contraindications to the use of this drug: (1) basilar or hemiplegic migraine; (2) uncontrolled hypertension (high blood pressure); (3) any form of angina or indications of coronary artery disease; (4) pregnancy. Before using this drug, consult your personal physician regarding the appropriate use of this drug for you.

Ancillary Drug Treatment (as required)

For nausea and vomiting:
- metoclopramide (Reglan)

For preheadache visual disturbances:
- nitroglycerin, sublingual
- isoproterenol (Isuprel), inhalation

Note: Drug selection, dosage, and administration schedule must be determined by the physician for each patient individually.

Possible Drug Interactions of Significance

Because of the number of drugs that may be used to manage this disorder, adequate consideration of the volume and complexity of potential drug interactions is beyond the scope of this book. Consult *The Essential Guide to Prescription Drugs*, or a similar drug reference book for possible interactions of significance (see Appendix 17, Drug Information Sources).

Special Considerations for Women

Some women notice an increased frequency of migraine headaches associated with the use of oral contraceptives or estrogen therapy. Approximately 60% of women report that migraines often coincide with menstrual periods. Women who are subject to episodes of migraine are advised to keep a log of when their headaches occur in relation to their menstrual cycles. Such information could contribute to therapeutic strategy designed to prevent significant fluctuations in estrogen blood levels.

Pregnancy

As a rule, pregnancy lessens migraine, especially after the first trimester. However, pregnancy may aggravate or precipitate migraine in about 30% of cases.

If you are pregnant, planning pregnancy, or not using contraception, discuss the use of sumatriptan with your physician before using it to treat your migraine.

The following drugs are designated Pregnancy Category D. Consult your physician before using them during pregnancy (see Appendix 15, FDA Pregnancy Categories).

amitriptyline
ergotamine
ibuprofen
naproxen
nortriptyline
sulindac
tolmetin

Breast-Feeding

Consult your physician regarding the compatibility of nursing and any drugs you are taking.

Quality of Life Considerations

According to a survey conducted by the Gallop Organization, more than a third of migraine sufferers said that the pain is so excruciating during an attack that they wished they were dead. Half of those surveyed felt that their families and friends do not fully understand how serious and debilitating an attack can be. A significant number of migraine patients feel that their career and earning potential have been seriously compromised.

Those who find that migraine headaches seriously degrade their quality of life might try the following strategies:

- Closely examine your lifestyle and try to identify those factors that appear to influence the frequency and severity of *your* headaches. Modify your lifestyle accordingly.
- Learn to recognize specific "triggers" that induce *your* migraines. Keeping a food diary can help to identify foods and beverages that you may not have suspected.
- Work with your physician to determine the most effective drugs for aborting *your* migraines. Use these immediately if you detect a warning that a migraine is in the making.

The Role of Prevention in This Disorder

Primary Prevention
There is no method known for preventing the primary predisposition to develop migraine headaches.

Secondary Prevention
Work closely with your physician to utilize the measures and medications outlined above that are designed primarily to prevent the initiation of migraine attacks.

Resources

Recommended Reading
Migraine: Beating the Odds, R.B. Lipton, M.D., L.C. Newman, M.D., and H. MacLean. Reading, MA: Addison-Wesley, 1992.

Headache Relief, A.M. Rapoport, M.D., and F.D. Sheftell, M.D. New York: Simon & Schuster, 1990.

Additional Information and Services
National Headache Foundation
5252 North Western Avenue
Chicago, IL 60625
Phone: 1-800-843-2256 (outside Illinois); (312) 878-7715
Telecommunications services: Fax: (312) 878-2782
Publications available.

MYASTHENIA GRAVIS

Other Names MG, autoimmune myasthenia gravis, childhood myasthenia gravis, myasthenia gravis pseudoparalytica

Prevalence/Incidence in U.S.
Estimated to be 14 in 100,000 people. Approximately 36,000 documented cases. Because many mild forms of this disorder are not recog-

nized or reported, it is estimated that the prevalence may approach 100,000.

Age Group
The autoimmune form of myasthenia gravis (over 90% of all forms of MG) can have its onset at any age from birth to 90 years. Approximately 30% of all cases begin in women between puberty and 40 years of age, with the highest incidence in the twenties. Another 30% of all cases begin in men after the age of 40, with the highest incidence in the fifties.

Male-to-Female Ratio
Age of onset under 40 years: 1 to 3
Age of onset 30–50 years: 1 to 1
Age of onset over 40 years: 3 to 1

Principal Features and Natural History
Myasthenia gravis is a chronic autoimmune disorder of neuromuscular function attributed to the presence of antibodies in the blood that impair the transmission of nerve impulses across the junction of nerve and muscle tissue. The characteristic symptoms are periods of fluctuating fatigue and early exhaustion of affected muscles. Involvement may be restricted to a single muscle group or may gradually expand to affect major muscle groups throughout the body. The first muscles to show abnormal fatigability in 50% of all cases are those of the eye, resulting in drooping eyelids and blurred or double vision. Approximately 25% of cases first become aware of weakness while speaking, chewing, or swallowing. Another 20% first notice unusual weakness and fatigue in the arms or legs.

The course of the disorder varies greatly from one person to another, but the point of maximal involvement is usually reached within three years. Stage 1, the "active" stage, is characterized by increasing disability and fluctuation of symptoms; it may last from 5 to 10 years. Stage 2, the "inactive" stage, is marked by less variation and greater stability. Stage 3, the "burned-out" stage, is usually reached 14 to 20 years after the initial onset of symptoms. It generally represents the residual pattern of the disorder that must be managed for the remaining life of the individual. Spontaneous remissions occur in fewer than 10% of cases, and these may last only two to three years.

There are three types of MG that occur in childhood:
1. Transient newborn MG: Affected mothers pass antibodies to 10–20% of their children.
2. Congenital MG: Caused by congenital defects in the neuromuscular

junctions (the points where nerve fibers join muscle fibers). This is not a form of autoimmune MG.

3. Juvenile MG: This is identical to adult MG, with onset before 12 years of age.

Diagnostic Symptoms and Signs
Drooping eyelids, double vision
Impaired ability to speak clearly, weak voice
Weakness of jaw muscles with chewing
Fluid regurgitation through nose when drinking
Impaired ability to swallow, frequent choking
Muscle weakness that worsens with continued use

Diagnostic Tests and Procedures
Acetylcholine receptor (AChR) antibody assay: increased in 95% of patients with generalized MG
Edrophonium (Tensilon) test: intravenous injection of drug produces a transient improvement in muscle strength in patients with MG
Electromyogram (EMG): repetitive nerve stimulation tests shows a decremental muscle response in patients with MG
X-ray studies of the anterior chest for the presence of a tumor of the thymus gland (thymoma)

Diagnostic "Markers" for This Disorder
Antibodies to acetylcholine receptors (AChR) on muscle endplates; found in 85% to 95% of all MG patients.

Similar Conditions That May Confuse Diagnosis
Eaton-Lambert syndrome
Graves' disease
Muscular dystrophy
Brain tumors
Amyotrophic lateral sclerosis (Lou Gehrig's disease)
Use of penicillamine: causes a drug-induced increase in AChR antibodies

Causes

Established Causes
The primary definitive cause for autoimmunity is not known.

Theoretical Causes
The current belief is that myasthenia gravis is an autoimmune disorder characterized by the formation of antibodies that impair acetylcholine receptors on the nerve-muscle junctions in affected voluntary muscles. Such antibodies are present in 85–95% of all MG patients. Their presence

implies damage or destruction of receptors by autoimmune complexes. The resulting loss of available receptors for nerve impulse transmission is responsible for the muscle weakness and easy fatigability that character- ize this disorder. The mechanisms responsible for the formation of destructive antibodies are not understood. There is no clear pattern of heredity to account for the development of MG (see Appendix 5, The Immune System).

Drugs That Can Cause This Disorder

The drug penicillamine (Cuprimine, Depen), used to treat rheumatoid arthritis and Wilson's disease, can cause true myasthenia gravis in about 1% of users.

The following drugs may impair neuromuscular impulse transmission and should be avoided or used with great caution in patients with myas- thenia gravis:

antihistamines
barbiturates
beta-blocker drugs
calcium channel-blocker drugs
clindamycin
colistimethate
colistin
gentamycin
kanamycin
lidocaine
lithium
magnesium salts
morphine
neomycin
opioid analgesics
phenytoin
polymyxin A and B
procainamide
quinidine
quinine
streptomycin
tetracyclines
thyroid preparations
tobramycin
tranquilizers
trimethadione
tubocurarine

See Appendix 16, Drug Classes, for specific generic drugs within respective drug classes.

Goals of Treatment

Can This Disorder Be Cured?

There is no curative treatment available at this time.

Can This Disorder Be Treated Effectively?

Currently available drugs can significantly improve muscle function and thereby relieve symptoms.

Specific Goals

The primary aim is to minimize disability.

- Prompt determination of the optimal drug regimen for each patient individually
- Smooth control of fluctuating muscle weakness and fatigability; restoration of sustained strength and endurance
- Prevention of both myasthenic crisis and cholinergic crisis
- Achievement of remission of the disease process

Health Professionals Who Participate in Managing This Disorder

Family physicians
General internists
Pediatricians
Geriatricians
Neurologists
Ophthalmologists
Optometrists
Obstetricians
Pharmacists
Physician assistants
Nurse practitioners
Physical therapists
Occupational therapists

Currently Available Therapies for This Disorder

Drug Therapy

CHOLINESTERASE INHIBITORS

- ambenonium (Mytelase)
- neostigmine (Prostigmin)
- pyridostigmine (Mestinon)

CORTISONELIKE DRUG (CORTICOSTEROID)

- prednisone

IMMUNE SUPPRESSIVE DRUGS

- azathioprine (Imuran)
- cyclophosphamide (Cytoxan)
- cyclosporine (Sandimmune)

Nondrug Treatment Methods

- Thymectomy: removal of the thymus gland to blunt autoimmune activities
- Plasmapheresis: used in acute situations to remove immune complexes from the blood

Management of Therapy

- Dosage requirements of drugs may vary from day to day, according to the course of the disorder, the physical demands of daily routines, the emotional state of the patient, etc. Doses should be adjusted according to need, larger doses being taken at times of greatest fatigue, such as just before meals, to facilitate eating.
- Restoration of muscle strength and endurance beyond 80% of normal status (before MG) is usually not possible. Learn by experience the limit of your response to the drugs that work best for you and do not exceed the optimal dose.
- Cholinesterase inhibitors provide only transient symptomatic relief and are of limited usefulness in most cases of moderate to severe MG. They are most useful for nonprogressive eye muscle weakness and mild limb muscle weakness.
- Use caution when taking drugs concurrently that can cause low blood potassium levels (hypokalemia). Many diuretics in wide use can cause potassium loss and thereby increase muscle weakness and fatigue.

Use of Cholinesterase Inhibitors

- These drugs are generally used first to treat the newly diagnosed case of MG. A trial of one to three months is usually sufficient to determine their effectiveness. The drug of choice must be determined for each patient individually by trial and error, as must the optimal dose and administration schedule. These drugs are prone to irregular absorption and consequent variation in therapeutic effect. They are best taken with food to reduce stomach upset.
- Pyridostigmine (Mestinon) is usually preferred by most patients with ocular or mild nonprogressive MG.
- Careful dosage adjustment is mandatory. Underdosage can result in myasthenic crisis. Overdosage can result in cholinergic crisis. Both reactions can cause sudden muscle weakness and be life-threatening if respiration is seriously impaired. Sudden weakness occurring one hour after taking medication usually indicates overdosage (cholinergic crisis).
- After prolonged use, these drugs may lose their effectiveness. Your ability to respond to them can be restored by reducing the dose or withdrawing them for several days. *However, this must be done only under the supervision of your physician.*

- Long-term treatment with high doses of these drugs may itself cause permanent changes in the motor end-plates and adversely affect neuromuscular transmission.

Use of Cortisonelike Drugs (Corticosteroids)

- These drugs have become more widely used within the past five years for treating MG. Some physicians initiate treatment with prednisone if there are no contraindications. The usual course of treatment is two years, to minimize the possibility of relapse.
- Prednisone is given initially in high doses daily until improvement begins, then changed to an alternate-day schedule. With sustained improvement and stabilization of function, the dose is gradually reduced to the smallest effective maintenance level.
- A trial period of 60 days is usually necessary to determine the effectiveness of prednisone therapy for MG. For those who respond favorably, marked improvement occurs within three months and maximal improvement is usually attained within nine months. Favorable results are reported in 80% of patients, with remissions in 25–35%.
- Significant worsening of symptoms can occur in 48% of patients during the early phase of high-dose prednisone treatment. For this reason a trial of prednisone is best initiated in the hospital.
- Approximately 90% of patients remain dependent upon long-term prednisone treatment for sustained improvement. Only 10% can withdraw successfully and remain in remission. Observe carefully for the possible development of adverse effects that often accompany long-term use of cortisonelike drugs.
- Some experts now recommend that thymectomy be done in serious cases *before* corticosteroids are used. A consensus is emerging that long-term corticosteroid therapy should be avoided if possible (see Appendix 6, Long-Term Corticosteroid Therapy).

Use of Azathioprine (Imuran)

- It is now felt that azathioprine is significantly less toxic than long-term steroid therapy. It is useful in reducing steroid requirement, and can produce improvement or remission when used alone.
- It may be used alone or in conjunction with cortisonelike drugs to treat advanced stages of MG with severe disability.
- For those who respond favorably, improvement usually begins within 3 to 12 months; maximal improvement may require continual treatment for 12 to 36 months. Approximately 53% of patients show some improvement using azathioprine alone, with 40% achieving temporary remission. However, continued improvement usually requires high doses. Only 10% of patients show sustained improvement following discontinuation of this drug.
- Observe carefully for the development of serious adverse effects.

Ancillary Drug Treatment (as required)

For apathy, lethargy:

• ephedrine

For hypokalemia:

• potassium supplements

For diarrhea:

• diphenoxylate (Imodium)

Note: Drug selection, dosage, and administration schedule must be determined by the physician for each patient individually.

Possible Drug Interactions of Significance

Because of the number and nature of drugs that may be used to manage this disorder, adequate consideration of the volume and complexity of potential drug interactions is beyond the scope of this book. Consult *The Essential Guide to Prescription Drugs*, or a similar drug reference book for possible interactions of significance (see Appendix 17, Drug Information Sources).

Special Considerations for Women

Pregnancy

The course of MG during pregnancy is unpredictable. It may improve, remain stable, or worsen. MG tends to worsen during the first trimester of first pregnancies. In subsequent pregnancies, it usually worsens during the third trimester and after delivery. However, serious complications are uncommon and therapeutic abortion is rarely needed because of MG.

Azathioprine and cyclophosphamide are designated Pregnancy Category D drugs and should be avoided during pregnancy (see Appendix 15, FDA Pregnancy Categories).

The blood levels of AChR antibodies in the mother with MG and in her newborn child can be about the same. The newborn should be monitored closely for symptoms of neonatal MG.

Breast-Feeding

MG is not a contraindication to breast-feeding. However, you should ask your physician for guidance if you are taking any drugs that are secreted in breast milk.

Special Considerations for the Elderly

One of the most difficult problems to manage in the older person with MG is the impaired ability to chew adequately and swallow without choking. Dietary modifications and assisted eating may be necessary.

Quality of Life Considerations

If the patient has difficulty in communicating verbally, family and friends should understand that overexertion and emotional stress can exacerbate

MG symptoms. Needed assistance with the activities of daily living should be provided, and rest periods should be scheduled appropriately to prevent physical exhaustion.

Resources

Additional Information and Services
Myasthenia Gravis Foundation
222 South Riverside Plaza, Suite 1540
Chicago, IL 60606
Phone: (312) 427-6252, 1-800-541-5454; Fax: (312) 427-8437
Sponsors 54 state groups and low-cost pharmacy service. Publications: physicians' and nurses' manuals, patient handbooks, brochures, pamphlets.

OBSESSIVE-COMPULSIVE DISORDER

Other Names OCD, obsessive-compulsive neurosis, obsessional neurosis

Prevalence/Incidence in U.S. 1–2% of the general population is the current estimate.

Age Group Onset may occur in childhood. 30–50% of adult cases begin before 15 years of age.

Male-to-Female Ratio More common in women

Principal Features and Natural History
Obsessive-compulsive disorder (OCD) is a distinct manifestation of chronic anxiety characterized by the frequent recurrence of persistent thoughts and ideas (obsessions) and repetitive behavior patterns (compulsions). Sufferers experiencing OCD are completely oriented and in touch with reality and recognize that the intrusive thoughts and irresistible urges are irrational and inappropriate, but they feel powerless to resist them. When interrupted or thwarted while performing this ritualistic behavior (compulsively acting out the obsession), the anxiety and agitation increase.

Examples of OCD patterns include repetitive counting, checking, touching while performing the numerous activities of daily living. More serious forms include incessant washing of hands, inspecting the soles of shoes for foreign matter, checking and rechecking stoves, computers, etc., to be certain they have been turned off.

The symptoms of OCD can range from mild annoyance to the individual (and amusement to observers) to severe degrees of agitation and depression that seriously impair social adaptation and effectiveness in the work setting. Dysfunctions of this magnitude require appropriate treatment.

Untreated OCD usually follows a chronic course with unpredictable remissions. Symptomatic periods usually last a year or less. Early treatment usually yields the most favorable results.

Diagnostic Symptoms and Signs

Evidence of recurring episodes of disturbing preoccupation with unreasonable, irrational, bizarre, obsessional thinking, with sense of reality intact

Observation of compulsive, repetitive, ritualistic behavior patterns that reveal an irresistible impulse to perform an irrational act

Demonstration of an ongoing anxiety-tension state; this may intensify if compulsive behavior is thwarted

Diagnostic Tests and Procedures

None required. All routine tests are normal.

Similar Conditions That May Confuse Diagnosis

Compulsive personality disorder: characterized by chronic excessive concern about adherence to standards—overly conscientious. No repetitive, ritualistic, compulsive behavior

Early schizophrenia: thinking is truly delusional; reality awareness is not intact

Causes

Established Causes

None confirmed to date.

Theoretical Causes

Research suggests that impaired function of serotonin receptors in certain brain centers (basal ganglia) may contribute to obsessive-compulsive symptoms.

Known Risk Factors for Developing This Disorder

There is some evidence to suggest that there may be an hereditary predisposition to the development of this disorder.

Drugs That Can Cause This Disorder

None.

Goals of Treatment

Can This Disorder Be Cured?

Although significant improvement can be achieved in responsive patients, permanent cure is unlikely.

Can This Disorder Be Treated Effectively?

Can symptoms be relieved? Approximately 25–30% of patients will achieve marked improvement with available treatments; some of the remainder will show partial improvement; others will show no change.

Specific Goals

- Provide the patient with understanding and insight regarding the nature of OCD
- Teach behavioral techniques designed to achieve control of symptoms
- Determine the drug therapy of choice for each individual

Health Professionals Who Participate in Managing This Disorder

Family physicians
General internists
Clinical psychologists
Psychiatrists
Pharmacists

Currently Available Therapies for This Disorder

Nondrug Treatment Methods

Psychotherapies: insight therapy; supportive therapy; behavioral modification.

Drug Therapy

- clomipramine (Anafranil)
- fluoxetine (Prozac)
- fluvoxamine (Luvox)

Management of Therapy

The three drugs listed above are approved by the FDA for treatment of OCD. Each has a distinct pattern of side/adverse effects. The treating physician will select the most appropriate drug for each patient individually, depending upon the patient's overall status and degree of OCD.

Current expert opinion considers fluvoxamine to be the drug of choice for most cases: it is better tolerated than clomipramine or fluoxetine; it is effective with once-a-day dosing; it can be used safely in combination with antianxiety drugs (benzodiazepines, buspirone).

If taking fluvoxamine, observe the following:

- the total daily dosage should not exceed 300 mg.
- avoid alcoholic beverages.
- use cautiously if you have a seizure disorder.
- avoid concurrent use with monoamine oxidase inhibitor (MAOI) drugs.

Therapeutic Drug Monitoring (Blood Levels)

If fluvoxamine is used concurrently with clomipramine, the blood levels of both drugs may increase; monitoring of blood levels of both drugs is advisable.

Ancillary Drug Treatment (as required)

For anxiety:
- buspirone (Buspar)
- benzodiazepines (diazepam, lorazepam, etc.)

Note: Drug selection, dosage, and administration schedule must be determined by the physician for each patient individually.

Possible Drug Interactions of Significance

Fluvoxamine may *increase* the effects of
- carbamazepine, and cause carbamazepine toxicity.
- warfarin, and increase prothrombin time (risk of bleeding).

Quality of Life Considerations

Mild forms of OCD may consist of nothing more than a minor nuisance without significant impact on daily living. However, more severe forms may actually become disabling. Anyone who exhibits a compulsive personality should be monitored for progression to OCD. If a clear pattern of obsessive and compulsive behavior emerges, early intervention with combined psychotherapy and drug therapy is mandatory to preserve an acceptable quality of life.

The Role of Prevention in This Disorder

Primary Prevention

No preventive measures known.

Secondary Prevention

Recognition and early treatment of compulsive personality disorders, with or without mental depression.

Resources

Recommended Reading

Stop Obsessing! How to Overcome Your Obsessions and Compulsions, Edna Foa, Ph.D., and Reid Wilson, Ph.D. Washington, DC: American Psychiatric Press, 1991.

Additional Information and Services
National Mental Health Association (NMHA)
1021 Prince Street
Alexandria, VA 23314-2971
Phone: 1-800-969-6642

OSTEOARTHRITIS

Other Names Osteoarthrosis, degenerative arthritis, degenerative joint disease, hypertrophic arthritis

Prevalence/Incidence in U.S. Approximately 16 million—8.7% of the adult population; 10% of the elderly population

Age Group 55 years and over

Male-to-Female Ratio Same incidence in men and women

Principal Features and Natural History
Osteoarthritis is the most common joint disease and the major cause of disability in our older population. It is an insidious, slowly progressive deterioration of the surface cartilage on the ends of bones where they come together to form joints. During the early phases of change, there are no symptoms. With progressive destruction of protective cartilage, bone surface becomes exposed and irritated. This results in pain, stiffness, and muscle spasm. As the central area of cartilage is destroyed, new bone and cartilage begin to form on the edges of the joint (spur formation). These degenerative changes can start as early as the fourth decade of life. They usually begin to cause symptoms in sixth and seventh decades. By age 75, all individuals have some degree of osteoarthritis in one or more joints. The most commonly involved joints are: fingers, thumb, shoulders, hips, knees, base of the first toe, neck, and lower (lumbar) spine. Progressive changes in the weight-bearing joints, principally the lower spine, hips, and knees, eventually give rise to pain, deep ache, and muscle spasm. Discomfort grows worse after prolonged activity that involves diseased joints.

Diagnostic Symptoms and Signs
Dull, aching joint pain
Pain worsened by activity, relieved by rest
Transient morning stiffness in affected joints
Loss of range of motion in affected joints

Diagnostic Tests and Procedures

All conventional laboratory tests are normal

X-ray studies of affected joints reveal specific diagnostic changes

Diagnostic "Markers" for This Disorder

The presence of Heberden's nodes (bony prominence) on the distal joints of fingers

The presence of Bouchard's nodes (bony prominence) on the proximal joints of fingers

Bunion formation at the base of the big toe

Similar Conditions That May Confuse Diagnosis

Osteonecrosis

Osteochondritis

Sarcoidosis

Rheumatoid arthritis

Psoriatic arthritis

Systemic lupus erythematosus

Chronic gout

Causes

Established Causes

The initiating cause of primary osteoarthritis is unknown.

Theoretical Causes

The disorder does have a familial pattern, and it is thought that genetic biochemical defects in cartilage structure predispose some individuals to excessive "wear and tear" deterioration of vulnerable joints.

Known Risk Factors for Developing This Disorder

Secondary osteoarthritis is due to congenital joint malformations, joint injuries and infections, and other infrequent causes of bone and cartilage deterioration.

Drugs That Can Cause This Disorder

Although some drugs are capable of causing joint aches and pains (e.g., barbiturates, "sulfa" drugs, oral contraceptives, isoniazid, pyrazinamide), no drugs cause the bone and cartilage destruction characteristic of osteoarthritis. Rarely the systemic (internal) use of cortisonelike steroid drugs can cause aseptic necrosis of bone (destruction without infection); this can initiate a secondary form of osteoarthritis.

Goals of Treatment

Can This Disorder Be Cured?

There is no curative therapy available at this time.

Can This Disorder Be Treated Effectively?
- Currently available medications can relieve pain and stiffness.
- Physical therapy can preserve range of motion and function in some affected joints.
- Surgical procedures in selected cases can remove bone deformities, improve joint function, and remove diseased joints that are unresponsive to medicinal therapy.

Specific Goals
- Relief of pain and stiffness sufficiently to permit continued activity, therapeutic exercise, and physiotherapy
- Relief of associated anxiety and/or depression

Health Professionals Who Participate in Managing This Disorder
Family physicians
General internists
Geriatricians
Rheumatologists
Physiatrists
Orthopedic surgeons
Podiatrists
Pharmacists
Physical therapists
Occupational therapists
Physician assistants
Nurse practitioners
Dietitians
Medical social workers

Currently Available Therapies for This Disorder

Nondrug Treatment Methods
- Weight reduction as appropriate; maintenance of ideal body weight
- Physical therapy to preserve joint function
- Aerobic exercise programs to preserve muscle strength

Drug Therapy
There are no drugs that can prevent, halt the progression of, or reverse the degenerative changes of osteoarthritis. The following drugs are used to relieve pain, stiffness, and muscle spasm.

Initial drug of choice: acetaminophen (Tylenol, etc.)

NONSTEROIDAL ANTI-INFLAMMATORY DRUGS (NSAIDs)
Salicylates:
- aspirin (Bufferin, Ascriptin, Cama, etc.)
- aspirin, enteric-coated (Easprin, Ecotrin, etc.)

- aspirin, zero-order-release (Zorpin)
- magnesium salicylate (Magan, Mobidin)
- choline magnesium salicylate (Trisilate)
- salsalate (Disalcid)
- diflunisal (Dolobid)
- sodium salicylate

Acetic acid derivatives:
- diclofenac (Cataflam, Voltaren)
- etodolac (Lodine)
- indomethacin (Indochron E-R, Indocin SR)
- ketorolac (Toradol)
- nabumetone (Relafen)
- sulindac (Clinoril)
- tolmetin (Tolectin, Tolectin DS)

Propionic acid derivatives:
- fenoprofen (Nalfon)
- flurbiprofen (Ansaid)
- ibuprofen (Motrin, Rufen, Advil, etc.)
- ketoprofen (Orudis, Oruvail)
- naproxen (Aleve, Anaprox, Anaprox DS, Naprosyn)
- oxaprozin (Daypro)
- suprofen (Suprol)

Fenamic acid derivatives:
- meclofenamate (Meclomen)
- mefenamic acid (Ponstel)

Oxicam derivative:
- piroxicam (Feldene)

SIMPLE ANALGESICS
- acetaminophen (Tylenol, Panadol, etc.)
- propoxyphene (Darvon, etc.)
- codeine (Tylenol with codeine, etc.)
- hydrocodone (Vicodin, etc.)
- oxycodone (Percodan, Percocet, Tylox)

MUSCLE RELAXANTS
- carisoprodol (Soma)
- cyclobenzaprine (Flexeril)
- diazepam (Valium)
- methocarbamol (Robaxin)
- orphenadrine (Norflex)

TOPICAL DRUGS
- capsaicin (Zostrix cream)

Management of Therapy

- Osteoarthritis is a chronic and slowly progressive disorder. Although there is no curative treatment available, the symptoms are generally mild for long periods of time and can usually be relieved satisfactorily with available drugs.

- Acetaminophen (Tylenol, etc.) is now the primary drug of choice for pain relief in managing osteoarthritis. Studies have shown that it is just as effective as nonsteroidal anti-inflammatory drugs (NSAIDs) in relieving arthritic pain. Of greater importance is the consideration of safety. Acetaminophen does not cause the pattern of significant adverse effects commonly associated with NSAIDs: stomach ulceration and bleeding, kidney damage, skin rashes, and blood cell disorders.
- Nonsteroidal anti-inflammatory drugs are now considered to be second line therapy for managing advanced osteoarthritis. If acetaminophen does not provide adequate pain relief, NSAIDs may be used cautiously and with close monitoring for adverse effects (see Appendix 8, Nonsteroidal Anti-Inflammatory Drugs: A Guide to Selection for Therapy).
- Other analgesics, such as propoxyphene, codeine, oxycodone, etc., suppress pain perception in the brain. They may be used for pain relief in moderately severe osteoarthritis and to supplement the analgesic effects of acetaminophen or NSAIDs when used for advanced, severe osteoarthritis.
- Cortisonelike steroids by mouth should not be used in the management of osteoarthritis. They may be helpful when injected directly into osteoarthritic joints, sometimes providing prompt and lasting relief of pain and swelling. If effective, steroid injections may be repeated at intervals of three to six months for a limited number of times.
- Symptomatic drug treatment will be more effective if it is supplemented by appropriate physiotherapy and the use of physical aids, such as canes, crutches, walkers, railings, etc.
- Avoid prolonged and repeated overuse of diseased joints to (1) slow the progression of joint destruction and (2) minimize requirements for analgesic drugs.
- Excessive body weight (obesity) can accelerate deterioration of weight-bearing joints. Prudent weight reduction programs are a most important part of treatment for osteoarthritis of the lower spine, hips, and knees.

Use of Nonsteroidal Anti-Inflammatory Drugs (NSAIDs)

- These drugs are not thought to be able to favorably influence the natural course of osteoarthritis, but they can relieve pain and inflammation and thereby improve joint function and mobility.
- Treatment is usually initiated with aspirin (lowest cost). Unfortunately, large doses (two to four tablets of 325 mg each, three to four times daily) are often necessary to achieve satisfactory relief. The high blood levels required can cause ringing in the ears (tinnitus) and loss of

hearing, especially in the elderly. Measurements of salicylate blood levels can be most helpful in establishing correct dosage.

- Soluble aspirin preparations (regular aspirin, Bufferin, Ascriptin, etc.) often cause stomach ulceration and bleeding; they should be taken with food to minimize this effect.

- The preferred forms of aspirin for continual use in large doses include (1) enteric-coated preparations and (2) zero-order-release tablets (see list above).

- Salicylates other than aspirin can also be used (see list above). These cause significantly less stomach irritation; some are effective with twice daily dosage.

- All NSAID aspirin substitutes are better tolerated than aspirin. However, they may share a cross-sensitivity in individuals who are allergic to aspirin and may induce asthmatic reactions.

- An NSAID should be used on a regular schedule for a trial period of three to four weeks. If it is not effective, another one from a different chemical group may be tried. An attempt should be made to find the NSAID that provides the best pain relief with the smallest dose and the fewest adverse effects.

- Authorities do not recommend the use of NSAIDs in combination with each other. A small dose of aspirin taken along with an NSAID may provide additional relief of pain.

- NSAIDs have a potential for injuring the kidney and impairing kidney function. They should be used with caution by individuals over 50 years old; those with hypertension, diabetes, or congestive heart failure; and especially those taking diuretics.

- NSAIDs can increase the effects of oral antidiabetic drugs (sulfonylureas) and anticoagulants. Dosage adjustments may be necessary.

Use of Narcoticlike Analgesics
- In advanced cases of osteoarthritis, mild analgesics such as acetaminophen or NSAIDs may not provide adequate pain relief. Codeine, hydrocodone, or oxycodone may be tried cautiously on an intermittent schedule to avoid *tolerance* and *dependence* (see these terms in the Glossary).

- The use of stronger narcotic (opioid) analgesics (morphine, meperidine, etc.) should be avoided completely. Their potential for causing *addiction* (see Glossary) precludes repetitious, long-term use in chronically painful disorders like osteoarthritis.

Use of Muscle Relaxants
- Muscle spasm prevents exercise and use of affected joints. The cautious use of muscle relaxants in conjunction with physiotherapy may be beneficial in preserving joint mobility and muscle strength.

- Muscle relaxants are most useful in managing osteoarthritis of the lower spine with associated lumbosacral muscle spasm.

Use of Topical Drugs

- The recently introduced capsaicin cream (Zostrix) is a natural chemical derived from plants. It is thought that the local application of this medication to painful skin and joints relieves pain by depleting substance P, the principal transmitter of pain impulses to the brain.
- This product is for external use only. Avoid contact with the eyes. Do not bandage the area tightly. Apply to the affected area no more than three to four times daily. Wash hands immediately after application.

Ancillary Drug Treatment (as required)

For anxiety and/or mild depression:
- alprazolam (Xanax), for intermittent, short-term use

For moderate or severe depression:
- fluoxetine (Prozac)
- trazodone (Desyrel) (see Profile of depression in this section)

For drug-induced constipation:
- docusate with casanthranol (Peri-Colace)

Note: Drug selection, dosage, and administration schedule must be determined by the physician for each patient individually.

Possible Drug Interactions of Significance

Because of the number of drugs that may be used to manage this disorder, adequate consideration of the volume and complexity of potential drug interactions is beyond the scope of this book. Consult *The Essential Guide to Prescription Drugs*, or a similar drug reference book for possible interactions of significance (see Appendix 17, Drug Information Sources).

Resources

Recommended Reading

Reappraisal of the Management of Patients With Osteoarthritis, J.R. Baker, M.D., and K.D. Brandt, M.D. Springfield, NJ: Scientific Therapeutics Information, 1993.

Arthritis Information: Arthritis Answers, The Arthritis Foundation, P.O. Box 7669, Atlanta, GA 30357-0669. For a copy call 1-800-283-7800.

Additional Information and Services

Arthritis Foundation
1314 Spring Street, NW
Atlanta, GA 30309
Phone: (404) 872-7100, 1-800-283-7800
Publications available.

Disease Management Expertise
National Institute of Arthritis and Musculoskeletal and Skin Diseases
Specialized Center of Research in Osteoarthritis
Rush Presbyterian-St. Luke's Medical Center
1653 West Congress Parkway
Chicago, IL 60612-3864
Phone: (312) 942-2711; Fax: (312) 942-3053
   See Appendix 7, Pain Management Centers.

OSTEOPOROSIS

Other Names Osteopenia, type I postmenopausal or spinal osteoporosis (95% of all cases), type II senile osteoporosis

Prevalence/Incidence in U.S.
25 million—approximately 25% of white women over 60 years of age have osteoporosis; 1.3 million fractures due to osteoporosis occur annually.

Age Group
Type I osteoporosis: 50 to 65 years
Type II osteoporosis: 65 years and over

Male-to-Female Ratio Much higher incidence in women: 8 to 1

Principal Features and Natural History
Osteoporosis is a major chronic disorder of bone in the elderly, occurring most often in postmenopausal women. As ovarian function declines and estrogen is withdrawn, the natural loss of bone mass is accelerated. This eventually weakens bone structure and predisposes to fractures that can result from minimal trauma. Osteoporosis can be localized in a single bone (a leg immobilized in a cast), but it is usually more widely distributed, with most fractures occurring in the spine, wrist, and hip. The basic defect is a relative increase in the rate of bone destruction without a compensating increase in the reformation of new bone. There are usually no symptoms prior to the occurrence of a spontaneous or traumatic fracture. A sudden compression fracture of a vertebra in the middle or lower section of the spine can result from such minor strains as bending, lifting, or sneezing. It causes immediate pain and disability lasting several weeks. Gradual compression of the vertebrae (usually painless) causes loss of height and the development of a stooped, rounded back ("dowager's hump"). A spontaneous fracture of a hip (femur) can occur on arising from a chair or while walking. Untreated osteoporosis can cause a loss of 30–60% of bone mass.

Diagnostic Symptoms and Signs

Osteoporosis causes no symptoms to indicate its presence until a bone fracture occurs—either spontaneously or as a result of trauma.

Diagnostic symptoms and signs are directly related to fractures:

acute pain at fracture site: common locations are the spine (vertebra), shoulder (humerus), wrist (radius), and hip (femur);

slow, progressive compression fractures of multiple vertebras in the midsection of the spine can cause constant dull aching and eventual curvature ("dowager's hump");

fractures may occur spontaneously (as a hip fracture while walking) or as a result of very minor trauma (as a vertebral fracture with sneezing or coughing).

Diagnostic Tests and Procedures

All routine laboratory tests (blood cell counts, chemistries, etc.) are usually normal.

Conventional X-ray studies may suggest osteoporosis but are not usually diagnostic.

Bone density measurements (densitometry) are necessary to detect and evaluate osteoporosis. Currently available techniques include:

- single-photon absorptiometry (SPA)
- dual-photon absorptiometry (DPA)
- quantitative computed tomography (QCT)
- dual energy X-ray absorptiometry (DEXA). This technique is the most accurate and precise in measuring bone density at any site.

Similar Conditions That May Confuse Diagnosis

Osteomalacia

Paget's disease

Hyperparathyroidism

Malignant (cancerous) bone disease

Causes

Primary osteoporosis appears to be a normal consequence of aging in predisposed individuals. A woman loses approximately 50% of bone mass, and a man approximately 25% during a normal life span. Type I primary osteoporosis refers to the estrogen withdrawal syndrome following menopause. Type II primary osteoporosis occurs later as a feature of normal aging.

Secondary osteoporosis refers to the bone loss that is associated with other diseases and disorders: hyperthyroidism, hyperparathyroidism, adrenal cortical hormone excess (Cushing's syndrome or drug-induced), multiple myeloma, diabetes, and alcoholism.

Drugs That Can Cause This Disorder

Cortisonelike steroids, especially in immobilized women over 50 years of
  age receiving large doses
Heparin, when used in long-term therapy
Methotrexate, when used in prepubertal children for long-term therapy

Goals of Treatment

Can This Disorder Be Cured?

Currently available treatments can achieve modest improvement in low
bone density, but cannot restore it to normal.

Specific Goals

- Primary prevention: early initiation of estrogen therapy—during or
  immediately after menopause—to prevent acceleration of natural bone
  loss
- Secondary prevention: initiation of estrogen therapy three or more
  years following menopause (after some degree of osteoporosis is present) to arrest or retard progressive bone loss
- Prevention of osteoporosis-related fractures
- Relief of pain and muscle spasm associated with fracture of osteo-
  porotic bone
- Appropriate care to promote satisfactory healing of fractured bone

Health Professionals Who Participate in Managing This Disorder

Family physicians
General internists
Geriatricians
Gynecologists
Endocrinologists
Radiologists
Orthopedic surgeons
Physiatrists
Pharmacists
Physician assistants
Nurse practitioners
Physical therapists
Occupational therapists
Medical social workers

Currently Available Therapies for This Disorder

Nondrug Treatment Methods

- Dietary supplements: calcium and vitamin D

- Regular weight-bearing, aerobic exercise to tolerance
- Avoidance of smoking and alcohol abuse

Drug Therapy

Estrogens ("natural-type" estrogens are preferred):
- conjugated estrogens (Genisis, Premarin)
- esterified estrogens (Evex, Menest)
- estradiol cypionate (Depo-Estradiol, injection)
- estradiol valerate (Delestrogen, injection)
- estriol (Hormonin, a mixture of estriol, estradiol, and estrone)
- piperazine estrone sulfate (Ogen)
- micronized 17-B estadiol (Estrace)
- transdermal estradiol skin patch (Estraderm-50 and 100)

Calcium preparations:
- calcium carbonate (40% calcium) (generic tablets, Alka-2, Biocal, Cal-trate, OsCal-500, Tums)
- calcium citrate (21% calcium) (Citracal)
- calcium gluconate (9% calcium) (generic tablets)
- calcium lactate (13% calcium) (generic tablets)
- dibasic calcium phosphate (31% calcium) (generic tablets)

Vitamin D analogs:
- calcifediol (Calderol)
- calcitriol (Rocaltrol)

Other drugs:
- alendronate (Fosamax)
- calcitonin (Calcimar, Miacalcin)
- fluorides (Slow Fluoride)

New Drugs in Development for Treating This Disorder

A new formulation of slow-release sodium fluoride and calcium citrate has been shown to be clinically effective in producing new growth of stronger bone in aged patients with osteoporosis. The drug is currently under review by the Food and Drug Administration.

Management of Therapy

It is now firmly established that excessive bone loss (osteoporosis) following menopause can be prevented or significantly reduced by the timely administration of low-dose estrogen.

Accurate assessment of bone mass for the detection of osteoporosis can be made by quantitative CT scan of vertebras and by photon absorptiometry of wrist bones. However, these procedures are expensive and not widely available.

Currently it is not feasible to screen all postmenopausal women for osteoporosis. To identify those who may benefit from estrogen used preventively, the following risk factors characterize candidates for post-menopausal osteoporosis:

- slender build, light-boned, white or Oriental race
- a sedentary lifestyle or restricted physical activity
- a family history of osteoporosis (grandmother, mother, aunt, or sister)
- a high-protein diet
- a low-sodium diet (also likely to be a low-calcium diet)
- lifelong avoidance of dairy products
- heavy smoking
- excessive use of antacids that contain aluminum
- long-term use of cortisonelike steroid drugs
- habitual use of carbonated beverages
- excessive consumption of alcohol
- increased urinary excretion of calcium

Thyroid replacement therapy (in appropriate dosage) may increase bone loss and predispose to the development of osteoporosis in the vertebras of the lower spine. If you are taking a thyroid preparation to correct hypothyroidism, consult your physician regarding a possible need for calcium, vitamin D supplements, and estrogen to prevent potential bone loss.

Use of Estrogens

- Estrogen increases the absorption of dietary calcium and reduces the rate of calcium loss from bone. Recent studies have shown that estrogen can reduce the risk of hip fractures by as much as 66%. Estrogen does not substantially increase bone mass; it does not enhance restoration of bone following loss.
- To be effective in preventing significant osteoporosis, estrogen therapy must begin within three years after menopause. Available evidence seems to indicate that continued protection against the development of osteoporosis requires ongoing use of estrogen—probably for life by those at risk.
- Fifty percent of women are protected by 0.3 mg of conjugated estrogens daily. Close to 100% are protected by 0.625 mg daily. Your physician can advise the dose most appropriate for you. For detailed information regarding the use of estrogen, see the Profile of menopause in this section.

Use of Calcium Preparations

- Calcium supplementation of the diet is appropriate for preventing and treating osteoporosis because the calcium content of the diet is usually less than the ongoing requirement for the maintenance of normal bone density. The average dietary intake of calcium by women is 500 to 600 mg daily. The daily requirement for the postmenopausal woman is 1500 to 2000 mg (all sources).

- There is some evidence that calcium supplements (taken alone) may reduce the rate of bone loss and the incidence of fracture, but further proof is needed. Calcium is most effective when taken in conjunction with vitamin D and estrogen.
- Supplemental calcium must not be taken in excessive doses. The recommended daily intake of calcium is approximately 1000 mg if taking estrogen and 1500 mg if not taking estrogen. Excessive intake of supplemental calcium (more than 2000 mg daily) can cause abnormal increases in the blood and urine levels of calcium and predispose to kidney stone formation. The most appropriate calcium preparations to use for supplementation are listed above. Calcium supplements made from bone meal or mineral clay (dolomite, montmorillomite) may contain lead or other toxic metals and should be avoided.
- Calcium supplements may be more effective if taken as a single late-evening dose to suppress the normal nocturnal rise in parathyroid hormone that increases bone loss.
- Calcium may decrease the effects of aspirin (and other salicylates), calcium channel-blocking drugs, iron, and tetracyclines. Do not take calcium preparations within two hours of taking other drugs.

Use of Vitamin D Analogs
- Elderly individuals with osteoporosis who have a normal lifestyle are not likely to a have a vitamin D deficiency. They usually have an adequate supply from their diet and exposure to sunlight.
- Shut-ins (those confined to home, nursing home, or hospital) probably need a supplement of vitamin D. Currently recommended sources include Calderol and Rocaltrol.
- When vitamin D is used, limit calcium intake to 600 to 700 mg daily to prevent excessive absorption and abnormally high calcium levels in blood and urine.

Use of Alendronate
This newly approved drug represents a significant advance in the therapy of osteoporosis. It shifts the balance between bone formation and bone resorption toward the formation of new bone. A 10 mg dose of this drug once daily produced an average increase in lumbar spine bone density of 5% after one year. After three years of treatment, bone density increased 6–8% in the femur. The occurrence of vertebral fractures was reduced by 50% with the use of alendronate. To date, no serious adverse effects have been reported when the drug is taken properly. Follow instructions carefully. Take it with a full glass of water and remain upright for 30 minutes. Do not take it while lying down.

Use of Calcitonin (a Thyroid Hormone That Reduces Bone Loss)
- Studies to date show that calcitonin in doses of 100 units daily can produce an increase in total body calcium (99% in bone) after two

years of treatment. A favorable response was achieved in 70% of users. Calcitonin is given by injection and is used in conjunction with calcium and vitamin D.

- Calcitonin nasal spray became available in 1995, the first dosage form of this drug that does not require injection. Studies confirm its ability to increase bone density in the lumbar spine by 3%. It does not cause nausea, as the injectable dosage form does in some patients.

Use of Fluoride .

- The use of fluoride in the prevention and treatment of osteoporosis is still investigational. Directions for its optimal use have not been established.
- A dose of 40 to 65 mg/day is required to stimulate bone formation. Adverse effects occur in over 30% of users; these include nausea, stomach pain, gastrointestinal bleeding, bone and joint pain, and severe foot discomfort, often intense enough to preclude compliance with treatment.
- If fluoride is used to treat osteoporosis, calcium must always be used concurrently to avoid the development of osteomalacia (abnormal mineral composition of bone).
- A new slow-release form of fluoride and calcium citrate is waiting approval for marketing. Studies have demonstrated that this form of fluoride increases spinal bone density by 4–6% each year for four years. Unlike plain fluoride preparations that can cause serious gastrointestinal adverse effects, the slow-release form is well tolerated.

Ancillary Drug Treatment (as required)

For calcium-induced constipation:
- docusate (Colace, etc.)
- docusate with casanthranol (Peri-Colace, etc.)

For fracture pain:
- acetaminophen with codeine (Tylenol with codeine)
- acetaminophen with propoxyphene (Darvocet-N 100)

Avoid opiate analgesics stronger than codeine.

For muscle spasm:
- diazepam (Valium)

For mild depression:
- alprazolam (Xanax), for intermittent, short-term use

For marked depression:
- fluoxetine (Prozac)
- trazodone (Desyrel)

Note: Drug selection, dosage, and administration schedule must be determined by the physician for each patient individually.

Possible Drug Interactions of Significance

Because of the number of drugs that may be used to manage this disorder, adequate consideration of the volume and complexity of potential drug interactions is beyond the scope of this book. Consult *The Essential Guide to Prescription Drugs*, or a similar drug reference book for possible interactions of significance (see Appendix 17, Drug Information Sources).

Special Considerations for Women

Postmenopausal women who have taken thyroid hormone preparations (Synthroid, etc.) on a long-term basis should be aware that thyroxine dosage of 200 mcg or more daily is associated with significantly lower bone density in the radius (wrist), femur (hip), and lumbar spine. However, women taking thyroxine and estrogen (hormone replacement therapy) concurrently are shown to have significantly higher bone density at all sites than women taking thyroxine only. Estrogen appears to prevent bone loss associated with long-term use of high-dose thyroid hormone.

If you consider yourself to be at increased risk for developing osteoporosis, consult your physician regarding the advisability of using any of the therapies outlined above.

Quality of Life Considerations

Every precaution should be observed to reduce the risk of hip fracture. This is the most serious fracture associated with osteoporosis, causing high morbidity and mortality: 30% of victims are significantly disabled and need assistance to walk; 30% require nursing home placement; 20% die within six months of the event.

Resources

Recommended Reading

Osteoporosis: A Guide to Diagnosis, Prevention and Treatment, Robert Lindsay, M.D. National Osteoporosis Foundation, Washington, DC. For a copy call 1-800-464-6700.

Additional Information and Services

National Institute of Arthritis and Musculoskeletal and Skin Diseases
Information Office: Building 31, Room 4C32B
9000 Rockville Pike
Bethesda, MD 20892
Phone: Information Specialist, (301) 496-8188

Handles inquiries on arthritis, bone diseases (including osteoporosis), and skin diseases.

National Osteoporosis Foundation
1150 17th Street, NW, Suite 500

Washington, DC 20036
Phone: 1-800-464-6700, (202) 223-2226; Fax: (202) 223-2237
  Numerous publications, charts, slides available.

Disease Management Expertise
SPECIALIZED CENTERS OF RESEARCH IN OSTEOPOROSIS
Robert Lindsay, M.D., Ph.D., Director
Helen Hayes Hospital
Route 9W
West Haverstraw, NY 10993
Phone: (914) 947-3000, Ext. 3494; Fax: (914) 947-2485

Robert R. Recker, M.D., Director
Creighton University
601 North 30th Street
Omaha, NE 68131
Phone: (402) 280-4471; Fax: (402) 280-5173

PARKINSON'S DISEASE

Other Names PD, paralysis agitans, parkinsonism, parkinsonian syndrome

Prevalence/Incidence in U.S.
Current estimate: approximately 1.5 million; 1% of the population over 50
  years old
Estimated new cases annually: 50,000

Age Group
10% of cases under 40 years old; 20% of cases 40 to 50 years old; 70% of
cases 50 years old and over. The mean age at onset is 58 to 62 years.

Male-to-Female Ratio More common in men, 3 to 2

Principal Features and Natural History
Parkinson's disease is a slowly progressive, debilitating disorder of certain
brain centers that contribute to the control and regulation of body movement. The earliest symptoms begin very insidiously. One arm or one leg
(or the arm and leg on one side) will gradually develop a sense of weakness, retarded movement, and stiffness. A fine tremor in a hand or foot
will appear in 70% of cases. This occurs at rest and disappears with
intentional use of the affected limb and also while asleep. Symptoms may
remain mild for years or they may progress steadily. Eventually the principal features of the disorder become generalized: the tremor spreads,

most of the body musculature becomes rigid, the posture is stooped, movement is slow and jerky, the gait is shuffling and unsteady. Facial expression is lost. The voice grows weak and speech is indistinct. Withdrawal and depression may occur as disability advances. Loss of mental acuity occurs in 30% of cases within 7 to 10 years. Currently available drug therapy can slow the progress of the disorder significantly for many, and life expectancy has been extended to equal the norms.

Diagnostic Symptoms and Signs
Slowness of movement
Stiffness and rigidity of arms and legs; feel "wooden"
Tremor of head and extremities—worse with anxiety; absent during sleep
Stooped posture; sluggish, short-stepped, unstable gait
Slurred, low volume, monotonous speech
Masklike, expressionless face
Muscle aches and cramps

Diagnostic Tests and Procedures
There are no definitive laboratory or other tests for PD.
Electroencephalogram (EEG), computed tomography (CT scan), and magnetic resonance imaging (MRI) are all normal.

Similar Conditions That May Confuse Diagnosis
Familial essential tremor
Major psychological depression
Secondary parkinsonism due to:
• Head trauma (such as from professional boxing)
• Hypoparathyroidism
• Viral encephalitis (brain infection)
• Exposure to industrial toxins: carbon disulfide, carbon monoxide, carbon tetrachloride, cyanide, manganese, methanol
Drug-induced parkinsonism, the most common type of secondary parkinsonism (see list below)

ALERT!
If you or your family are told that you are developing Parkinson's disease, *ascertain that your symptoms are not due to a drug you are taking.*

Causes

Established Causes
The definitive cause that initiates degeneration of critical brain cells in primary PD is not known.

Theoretical Causes

Primary Parkinson's disease is due to degeneration of the nerve cells in the brain that produce dopamine, one of the major nerve impulse transmitters. Infrequently a virus infection of the brain (encephalitis) may initiate the degenerative process.

Known Risk Factors for Developing This Disorder

Secondary parkinsonism may be caused by hardening of brain arteries, strokes, brain tumors, trauma, and a few rare degenerative disorders of brain tissue.

Drugs That Can Cause This Disorder

The following drugs can block the action of dopamine and cause a form of secondary parkinsonism with features that are indistinguishable from primary Parkinson's disease:

chlorprothixene
droperidol
haloperidol
lithium
methyldopa
metoclopramide
phenothiazines
prochlorperazine
reserpine
thiothixene

See Appendix 16, Drug Classes, for specific generic names within the class of phenothiazines.

Goals of Treatment

Can This Disorder Be Cured?

There is no curative treatment for primary PD known at this time.

Can This Disorder Be Treated Effectively?

Currently available drugs can relieve or moderate some of the symptoms of PD. Smooth continuous control may be difficult. Close monitoring and appropriate adjustments of medications and dosage schedules must be individualized.

Specific Goals
• Improvement of overall function and mobility
• Reduction of muscular rigidity and tremor
• Reversal of slowed movement
• Improvement of posture, balance, gait, speech, and writing

Health Professionals Who Participate in Managing This Disorder
Family physicians
General internists
Gerontologists
Neurologists
Neuropsychiatrists
Physiatrists
Pharmacists
Physician assistants
Neurological nurse practitioners
Physical therapists
Medical social workers

Currently Available Therapies for This Disorder

Drug Therapy
- levodopa (Dopar, Larodopa)
- levodopa + carbidopa (Sinemet, Sinemet CR)
- levodopa + bensarazide (Prolopa in Canada)
- amantadine (Symmetrel)
- anticholinergics (atropinelike drugs): benztropine (Cogentin), diphen-hydraminc (Benadryl), trihexyphenidyl (Artane)
- bromocriptine (Parlodel)
- pergolide (Permax)
- selegiline (Eldepryl)

Nondrug Treatment Methods
- Regular exercise programs to maintain range of motion and muscle strength
- Surgical procedures: thalamotomy to reduce tremors; pallidotomy to reduce tremors, rigidity, and impaired movement
- Transplantation of human fetal brain cells to enhance dopamine production (experimental at this time)

New Drugs in Development for Treating This Disorder
- The Food and Drug Administration is currently reviewing a new drug application (NDA) for pramipexole. Clinical trials have shown this drug to be superior to those currently used to stimulate dopamine receptors in the brain and thus relieve the full spectrum of PD symptoms. It is anticipated to be beneficial in all stages of the disorder and to delay the onset of complications associated with levodopa in advanced stages.
- Apomorphine, an old drug that is widely used to induce vomiting in the treatment of poisoning, has shown promising results during inves-

tigational studies for treating Parkinson's disease with severe motor fluctuations. These studies have utilized subcutaneous injection of the drug. The results of additional studies, using sublingual (under the tongue) administration, indicate that apomorphine may well prove to be safe and effective for treating some aspects of Parkinson's disease.

Management of Therapy

The symptoms of Parkinson's disease are due to a relative increase in the effects of acetylcholine in the brain centers that regulate body movement. The exaggerated acetylcholine effects are the result of a reduced supply of dopamine (primary Parkinson's disease) or to a blocking of dopamine action (drug-induced parkinsonism).

Drugs used to manage parkinsonism utilize three distinct mechanisms of action: (1) anticholinergic drugs reduce the excessive effects of acetylcholine; (2) levodopa is converted to dopamine in the brain, increasing its supply to restore a balance closer to normal; (3) bromocriptine serves as a substitute for dopamine by stimulating its receptor cells directly. Amantadine is thought to have both anticholinergic and direct-stimulating effects.

Appropriate drugs, properly used, can improve function and mobility for significant periods of time; up to 50% of those treated have no major disabilities after 10 years of disease.

The optimal drug program—either one drug used alone or two or more used in combination—is that which provides satisfactory relief of symptoms or the most acceptable compromise between symptom relief and drug side effects. Complete relief of symptoms may not be possible.

Drug selection and dosage schedules *must be carefully individualized*. Adjustments will be necessary throughout the course of this disorder. Daily fluctuations in symptoms and drug responses occur in almost every individual and vary greatly from person to person. A trial-and-error process is unavoidable in determining the best drug(s) and the best dosage schedule. For the best treatment results, keep your physician informed regarding all aspects of your response to the drugs prescribed.

Combinations of several drugs taken in small doses are often more beneficial than a single drug taken in large doses.

Use of Levodopa

• Only 25% of levodopa taken alone by mouth enters the brain. The large doses required to be effective often cause unacceptable side effects. To prevent this, levodopa is combined with carbidopa; the combination (marketed as Sinemet) permits a 75% dosage reduction of levodopa. Levodopa is the most effective drug available in the United States and has been the drug of choice for managing primary parkinsonism for the past 20 years. Approximately 80% of users achieve 80% improvement in muscular rigidity and retarded movement.

- Levodopa may be tried at any time during the course of this disorder. It is most effective during the first two to five years of use. However, authorities differ in their opinions as to the best time to use levodopa. Some advise early use—within the first year of symptoms—to obtain the fullest benefit possible. Others advise later use to delay the onset of side effects and adverse effects that develop with long-term use of levodopa.

- Levodopa is more completely absorbed when taken on an empty stomach. However, it may be necessary to take it following food to prevent nausea. If so, avoid meat when possible; proteins can interfere with absorption of levodopa.

- After a year or more of continual use of levodopa, 80% of users will develop abnormal involuntary movements (dyskinesias) of various muscle groups—jerks and twitches of the head and face or purpose-like movement of the extremities. In 30% of the users these may be severe enough to interfere with normal functioning. They last for a few minutes to several hours and seem to coincide with the times of both high and low blood levels of levodopa.

- Another 20% of users will experience "on–off" episodes—changes from relatively good function and mobility (drug effects "on") to marked loss of function and mobility (drug effects "off"). To minimize these periods of fluctuating effectiveness, levodopa may be taken in small doses every one to three hours throughout the day to maintain a more constant blood level.

- Levodopa can cause a variety of mental disturbances: euphoria, hypo-mania, depression, confusion, nightmares, vivid hallucinations.

- Levodopa should not be used concurrently with those antipsychotic drugs that block the action of dopamine or with monoamine oxidase (MAO) inhibitors that increase the risk of a hypertensive crisis.

- Some authorities advocate the use of "drug holidays" to reduce the toxic manifestations of levodopa. The very gradual withdrawal and reintroduction of the drug are essential to success.

Use of Amantadine

- This drug probably releases dopamine from nerve cells and increases its availability. It may also serve as a dopamine substitute and stimulate receptor cells directly. It has anticholinergic effects that contribute to its effectiveness.

- Amantadine may be tried first in all patients. It can produce a 15–25% improvement in 60% of users. A trial period of one week is usually adequate. If not beneficial or if mentality is adversely affected, discontinue use.

- Amantadine may also be used in conjunction with anticholinergics and levodopa. It is usually well tolerated by the elderly.

- This drug has a low incidence of side effects. Ankle swelling and a reddish-blue mottling of the arms or legs may occur after one month to one year of use. These are not serious and are reversible. Doses over 200 mg can cause excitement, increased tremor, jerkiness, insomnia, and nightmares in sensitive individuals. Amantadine may lose some of its effectiveness after 6 to 12 weeks of continual use.
- In very rare cases the long-term use of this drug is associated with the unexpected development of congestive heart failure. If shortness of breath appears during exertion or while lying down or rouses you from sleep, report this promptly.
- Recent reports indicate that this drug should not be stopped abruptly in the elderly patient (over 70 years of age). Sudden withdrawal can result in the prompt return of parkinsonian features and rapid deterioration.

Use of Anticholinergic Drugs

- These atropinelike drugs are often used to initiate treatment when symptoms are mild. They can produce a 20–30% improvement by suppressing effects due to overactivity of acetylcholine: tremor, excessive salivation, rigidity, and slow movement.
- They may be used alone as long as symptoms remain mild. They may be combined with any of the other drugs used and at any stage of the disorder.
- These drugs are not well tolerated by individuals over 70 years old. They can provoke latent glaucoma and can aggravate urinary retention in men with prostatism (see Glossary).
- Unavoidable side effects include blurring of near vision, dry mouth, constipation, and urinary hesitancy. High doses may cause drowsiness, confusion, impaired memory, hallucinations, and nightmares.
- Following long-term use, these drugs must be discontinued very gradually to avoid a dangerous withdrawal syndrome.

Use of Bromocriptine

- This drug may be used alone but is usually added to the treatment program at a later stage. It is the drug of choice for alleviating the abnormal involuntary movements associated with long-term levodopa use. It can also have a stabilizing effect when the "on–off" effects of levodopa therapy become apparent.
- Bromocriptine is initiated with very small doses, and the dose is increased very slowly. Some individuals develop extreme hypotension (low blood pressure) with the first doses. It is advisable to try a test dose at bedtime for several days to determine individual blood pressure response.
- This drug may not be effective in severe Parkinson's disease or in those with a poor response to levodopa.

- High doses can cause acute personality changes, mood swings, and other intolerable adverse effects. About 40% of users discontinue this drug because of undesirable reactions.
- This drug is an ergot derivative; it should be used with caution in the presence of coronary artery disease, hypertension, or peripheral vascular disease.

Use of Pergolide

- This drug is used adjunctively with levodopa/carbidopa to provide a more uniform control of parkinsonian symptoms and to reduce the adverse effects of long-term levodopa therapy. It permits a 5–30% reduction in the dose of levodopa.
- This drug is an ergot derivative; it should be used with caution in the presence of coronary artery disease, hypertension, or peripheral vascular disease.

Use of Selegiline

- This drug may be used alone to initiate treatment of very early Parkinson's disease, thus delaying the use of levodopa/carbidopa.
- It may also be used later as an adjunct to levodopa/carbidopa therapy when levodopa has lost its effectiveness or is causing serious adverse effects. It permits a 25–30% reduction in the dose of levodopa.

Ancillary Drug Treatment (as required)

For levodopa-induced drowsiness:
- methylphenidate (Ritalin)

For levodopa-induced nausea:
- diphenidol (Vontrol)

For action tremor:
- propranolol (Inderal)

For muscle spasm and rigidity:
- diazepam (Valium)

For constipation:
- docusate (Colace)
- docusate with casanthranol (Peri-Colace)

For insomnia:
- chloral hydrate

For ankle swelling:
- hydrochlorothiazide (generic)

For depression:
- fluoxetine (Prozac)
- amitriptyline (Elavil)
- desipramine (Norpramin)
- imipramine (Tofranil)
- trazodone (Desyrel)

For action tremor (that accompanies resting tremor):

• propranolol (Inderal)

Note: Drug selection, dosage, and administration schedule must be determined by the physician for each patient individually.

Current Controversies in Management

The difference of opinion among authorities regarding the best time to begin treatment with levodopa (Sinemet) has not been resolved to date. Those advocating early use—when symptoms are causing only mild disability—argue that the individual's quality of life is significantly improved and that his or her period of productive functioning is prolonged. Those advocating late introduction of levodopa—when symptoms are causing moderate to severe disability—argue that the early use of levodopa hastens the onset of adverse levodopa effects (abnormal involuntary movements, "wearing-off" effects, "on–off" effects). They propose the use of selegiline, amantadine, and/or anticholinergic drugs to manage the early period of mild disability, and the later use of levodopa only if and when progression of symptoms requires greater relief. Recent studies have shown that selegiline, given as the initial drug at the onset of Parkinson's disease, significantly delayed the time when levodopa treatment had to be started.

One recently published study, however, does show that levodopa treatment started early (one to three years after the onset of symptoms) significantly reduces mortality rates, especially those related to the disease itself.

Comment

The decision as to when levodopa therapy is to be started must be made jointly by the patient and the physician on an individual, case-by-case basis. The patient should be informed of the issues involved in making the decision and should share the responsibility for making the best decision for all concerned.

Possible Drug Interactions of Significance

Because of the number and nature of drugs that may be used to manage this disorder, adequate consideration of the volume and complexity of potential drug interactions is beyond the scope of this book. Consult *The Essential Guide to Prescription Drugs*, or a similar drug reference book for possible interactions of significance (see Appendix 17, Drug Information Sources).

The Role of Prevention in This Disorder

Primary Prevention

There is no method currently known to prevent the development of primary PD.

Some types of secondary PD may be preventable. Monitor your exposure to the industrial toxins cited above. Monitor your response to any of the drugs cited above that can induce parkinsonian adverse effects.

Resources

Additional Information and Services
American Parkinson Disease Association
60 Bay Street, Suite 401
Staten Island, NY 10301
Phone: 1-800-223-APDA, (718) 981-8001; Fax: (718) 981-4399
Available 8:30 A.M.–5:00 P.M. EST, Monday–Friday.

Sponsors 35 information and referral centers. Provides publications, referrals, references, and answers to inquiries regarding research and treatment.

Parkinson's Disease Foundation
Columbia Presbyterian Medical Center
650 West 168th Street
New York, NY 10032
Phone: (212) 923-4700, 1-800-457-6676; Fax: (212) 923-4778

Local groups: 400. Serves as a source of information to patients and physicians on all aspects of Parkinson's disease.

United Parkinson Foundation
360 West Superior Street
Chicago, IL 60610
Phone: (312) 664-2344

Serves 38,000 members (patients, family members, medical personnel); publishes reliable information on all aspects of Parkinson's disease.

National Parkinson Foundation
1501 NW Ninth Avenue
Miami, FL 33136
Phone: (305) 547-6666; 1-800-327-4545; 1-800-544-4882 (in California); 1-800-433-7022 (in Florida); Fax: (305) 548-4403

Publishes *The Parkinson Handbook: How to Start and Run a Support Group.*

PEPTIC ULCER

Other Names Peptic ulcer disease, PUD, duodenal ulcer, gastric ulcer

Prevalence/Incidence in U.S.
Approximately 20 million; 10% of the general population will have a symptomatic peptic ulcer sometime during life; 25% of men and 16% of women have scars of peptic ulcer disease on autopsy examination.

Age Group

Duodenal ulcer occurs most commonly between 25 and 40 years. Gastric ulcer occurs most commonly between 40 and 55 years. Of all ulcers, 1.9% occur under 18 years; 43% occur between 18 and 44 years; 36% occur between 45 and 64 years; 12.8% occur between 65 and 74 years; 6.3% occur at 75 years and over.

Male-to-Female Ratio Duodenal ulcer: higher incidence in men—2 to 1. Gastric ulcer: same incidence in men and women.

Principal Features and Natural History

Peptic ulcer disease refers to an intermittent disorder of the stomach and first portion of the small intestine (duodenum) that is characterized by the formation of ulcers in the lining of these organs. The tissues subject to ulceration are constantly bathed in digestive juices produced in the stomach. The principal components of these juices include hydrochloric acid and the digestive enzyme pepsin (hence "peptic" ulcer). Most individuals with peptic ulcer disease produce excessive amounts of acid and pepsin, which overwhelm the normal protection of the lining tissues and cause erosion (ulceration). The singular feature of an active duodenal ulcer is a gnawing or burning pain in the upper mid-abdomen that usually occurs between meals and in the early morning hours when acid secretion is high. The pain is characteristically relieved by food or antacids. The pattern of pain–food–relief typifies active duodenal ulcer. Episodes of ulcer activation occur unpredictably, but are often more frequent and troublesome in the spring and fall of the year. By nature, peptic ulcer disease is a chronically recurrent disorder. The recurrence rate of duodenal ulcer is approximately 70% within one year and 90% within two years. Frequent recurrence predisposes to serious complications in 30% of ulcer patients: 10–15% will experience bleeding, 5–10% will suffer perforation of the duodenal wall, and 5% will develop obstruction at the stomach outlet (pylorus) due to the extensive scarring that follows ulcer healing.

Within the past 10 years it has been confirmed that infection of the stomach and duodenum by the organism *Helicobacter pylori* is a major cause of peptic ulcer disease. This discovery has revolutionized the management of this disorder and has significantly reduced morbidity and mortality. *H. pylori* is present in 92% of persons with duodenal ulcer and in 73% of those with gastric ulcer. Recent studies show that eradication of *H. pylori* infection reduces the ulcer recurrence rate from 84% to 21%. Currently available medications can eradicate *H. pylori* infections in most cases safely and effectively.

Diagnostic Symptoms and Signs

Gnawing or burning pain in the upper abdomen

Pain occurs one to three hours after eating and during the night

Pain is relieved by food or antacids

Acid indigestion, heartburn, sour stomach

Nausea and vomiting; "coffee grounds" vomitus indicative of stomach bleeding

"Tarry" stools indicative of stomach bleeding

Diagnostic Tests and Procedures

Routine laboratory tests are not diagnostic. Low red blood cell counts and hemoglobin levels may indicate silent stomach bleeding.

Blood test for *H. pylori* antibodies

Upper gastrointestinal endoscopic examination to visualize ulceration and obtain biopsy specimens for detection of *H. pylori* organisms

Upper gastrointestinal X-ray studies

Measurement of blood gastrin levels in recurrent or refractory PUD to evaluate the possibility of Zollinger-Ellison syndrome (see Profile of Zollinger-Ellison syndrome in this section)

Measurement of stomach acid secretion if Zollinger-Ellison syndrome is suspected

Diagnostic "Markers" for This Disorder

Visualization of stomach and/or duodenal ulceration on endoscopic examination

Positive identification of *H. pylori* organisms in biopsy specimens from stomach

Similar Conditions That May Confuse Diagnosis

Gastroesophageal reflux disorder

Gastroduodenitis (without ulcer)

Drug-induced gastritis: caffeine, digitalis, theophylline

Gallbladder disease

Pancreatitis

Crohn's disease

Cancer of the stomach, duodenum, or pancreas

Sarcoidosis

Other infections of the stomach: giardiasis, Mycobacterium avium-intra cellulare, tuberculosis

Causes

Established Causes

Infectious PUD due to *H. pylori* infection of the stomach and duodenum

Drug-induced PUD due to use of nonsteroidal anti-inflammatory drugs (NSAIDs) (see Appendix 8, Nonsteroidal Anti-Inflammatory Drugs: A Guide to Selection for Therapy)

Theoretical Causes

It is now well established that multiple factors contribute to the formation of peptic ulcers. A predisposition to develop peptic ulcer disease appears to be hereditary. Those individuals who produce excessive amounts of stomach acid and pepsin are often prone to the development of duodenal ulcer. Others with normal amounts of acid and pepsin develop ulceration because the protective mechanisms in the lining tissues are defective and inadequate. Certain states of physical stress (burns, trauma, surgery) can increase the incidence of peptic ulcer.

Known Risk Factors for Developing This Disorder

Genetic predisposition: family history of PUD
Blood type O: increased frequency of PUD
Tobacco smoking
Excessive alcohol consumption

Drugs That Can Cause This Disorder

The following drugs can initiate ulceration of the stomach or duodenum in susceptible individuals or aggravate existing ulcers:

aminophylline
aspirin and other nonsteroidal anti-inflammatory drugs (NSAIDs)
nicotine
phenylbutazone
reserpine

Goals of Treatment

Can This Disorder Be Cured?

- PUD due to *H. pylori* infection can be cured with appropriate anti-infective medications.
- PUD due to certain drugs can be cured by drug withdrawal and appropriate use of stomach protective medications.

Can This Disorder Be Treated Effectively?

Currently available medications can relieve symptoms, promote ulcer healing, and prevent complications.

Specific Goals

- Total eradication of *H. pylori* infection
- Short-term control of stomach acidity sufficient to relieve pain and promote ulcer healing
- Long-term control of stomach acidity to prevent ulcer recurrence
- Prevention of complications

Health Professionals Who Participate in Managing This Disorder
Family physicians
General internists
Gastroenterologists
Abdominal surgeons
Pharmacists
Physician assistants
Nurse practitioners

Currently Available Therapies for This Disorder

Drug Therapy
- amoxicillin (Amoxcil, etc.)
- antacids (Delcid, Maalox TC, Mylanta II, etc.)
- anticholinergic drugs (Darbid, Pro-Banthine, Robinul) for adjunctive use
- bismuth preparations
- cimetidine (Tagamet)
- clarithromycin (Biaxin)
- famotidine (Pepcid)
- metronidazole (Flagyl)
- misoprostol (Cytotec); used for prevention and treatment
- nizatidine (Axid)
- omeprazole (Prilosec
- ranitidine (Zantac)
- sucralfate (Carafate)
- tetracycline

Nondrug Treatment Methods
- Smoking cessation programs
- Restriction of alcoholic beverages
- Stress-reduction counseling as appropriate
- Surgical management of complications

Management of Therapy
- Most cases of peptic ulcer disease can be managed successfully by appropriate drug therapy. A treatment program of four to six weeks will heal approximately 90% of peptic ulcers. Surgery is needed only for the management of ulcer complications: uncontrolled bleeding, perforation, obstruction, persistent pain.
- Anti-infective therapy for PUD due to *H. pylori* infection consists of either a two-drug regimen of two weeks duration or a three-drug regimen of one week duration. The two-drug regimen uses amoxicillin and omeprazole and has an eradication rate of 50–84% with fewer

drug side effects. The three-drug regimen uses various combinations of amoxicillin, bismuth, clarithromycin, metronidazole, omeprazole, or tetracycline. It has an eradication rate of 85–90%, but with more drug side effects.

- The four principal histamine-blocking drugs used to promote healing of duodenal ulcer are all equally effective when taken in adequate dosage for four to six weeks. However, some individuals may respond more favorably to two (or more) drugs used concurrently. In the treatment of gastric ulcer, antacids are less effective than cimetidine, ranitidine, or sucralfate.
- Anticholinergic (atropinelike) drugs are used adjunctively only when ulcer symptoms are not adequately controlled by antacids and/or histamine-blocking drugs.
- Tranquilizers and sedatives should not be used routinely but only as necessary to relieve significant anxiety and nervous tension that could possibly contribute to hyperacidity.
- The chronic use of aspirin and other nonsteroidal anti-inflammatory drugs (NSAIDs) increases the chance of developing active peptic ulcer. The concurrent use of cortisonelike (corticosteroid) drugs increases the risk of ulcer recurrence.
- Cigarette smoking doubles the chance of developing peptic ulcer disease; it also delays healing significantly.
- Caffeine-containing beverages (coffee, tea, cola) can stimulate stomach acid production and aggravate an existing ulcer.
- Alcohol (in excess) can aggravate gastric ulcer and increase the risk of bleeding.

Use of Antacids

- These drugs are used to neutralize stomach acids and thereby (1) relieve pain, heartburn, and acid indigestion; and (2) correct hyperacidity and promote ulcer healing.
- The antacids of choice are composed of magnesium and aluminum hydroxide (Delcid, Maalox, Mylanta, etc.). The optimal treatment schedule is 1 ounce taken one hour and three hours after meals and at bedtime until free of pain for two weeks; then one hour after meals and at bedtime for an additional four weeks.
- The long-term (months to years) use of aluminum hydroxide and magnesium trisilicate preparations should be avoided. They may cause depletion of phosphate and increase the risk of osteomalacia (softening of bones).
- Calcium-containing antacids (Alka-2, Titralac, Tums) should be used in moderation. These stimulate secretion of gastrin, a stomach hormone that in turn stimulates production of hydrochloric acid and pepsin, creating a condition referred to as rebound hyperacidity.

- When practical to use, antacid liquids (suspensions) are more effective than tablets.
- Antacids can interfere with the absorption of cimetidine (but not ranitidine), digoxin, iron, isoniazid, and tetracyclines.

Use of Histamine-Blocking Drugs

- These drugs reduce the production of hydrochloric acid by blocking the stomach's response to stimulation by histamine. They promote healing of peptic ulcer in 70–80% of cases when taken for four to six weeks. Treatment with one of these drugs alone is a reasonable alternative to high-dose antacid therapy.
- Cimetidine may cause confusion and unsteadiness in the elderly, especially those with impaired kidney function. Infrequently it can cause breast enlargement and impotence in men. It increases the effects of warfarin when taken concurrently.
- Ranitidine taken in a single dose at bedtime is as effective as other multidose drug regimens for healing peptic ulcer. It is less likely to cause confusion, unsteadiness, breast changes, or altered sexual functions.
- Famotidine and nizatidine are less likely to be involved in any significant drug–drug interactions.
- In the presence of liver disease or impaired liver function, avoid the concurrent use of ranitidine and acetaminophen to reduce the risk of liver toxicity.
- Drugs of this class taken once daily at bedtime can reduce the recurrence rate (in one year) for duodenal ulcer from 70% to 10%, and for gastric ulcer from 56% to 20%.

Use of Sucralfate

- This drug is used for short-term (eight weeks) treatment of active duodenal ulcer. It promotes ulcer healing by forming a dense coating over the ulcer that protects it from the erosive action of hydrochloric acid. Its effectiveness is comparable to antacids and histamine blockers (cimetidine and ranitidine) when used alone. It should not be used in conjunction with antacids or histamine blockers.
- Food may impair the effectiveness of sucralfate. The recommended schedule for use is as follows:
  - If other drugs are being used concurrently, take these one hour before sucralfate.
  - Take sucralfate on an empty stomach, one hour before meals and at bedtime.
  - Food may be taken one hour after sucralfate.
- This drug is very safe. It has no contraindications and minimal side effects: Constipation was reported as a rare occurrence.
- It can interfere with the absorption of tetracyclines and phenytoin.

Use of Omeprazole

This drug is highly effective in suppressing stomach acid secretion and in promoting ulcer healing. It is more effective than histamine-blocking drugs in treating reflux esophagitis and refractory duodenal ulcers.

Ancillary Drug Treatment (as required)

For persistent nocturnal ulcer pain:
- isopropamide (Combid, Darbid) taken at bedtime

For constipation:
- docusate (Colace, etc.)
- docusate with casanthranol (Peri-Colace, etc.)

For anxiety or nervous tension:
- buspirone (Buspar)
- diazepam (Valium)

For headache, minor aches and pains:
- acetaminophen (Tylenol, etc.)
- propoxyphene (Darvon)

  Avoid aspirin.

Note: Drug selection, dosage, and administration schedule must be determined by the physician for each patient individually.

Current Controversies in Management

1. Should histamine-blocking drugs (see above) be used intermittently or continuously in treating peptic ulcer disease?

   Recently completed studies (219 patients followed for five years) have shown that continuous treatment with cimetidine (Tagamet) is significantly more effective than intermittent treatment in preventing recurrence of ulcer activity. Current recommendations call for continuous treatment (daily bedtime maintenance dosing) of anyone who has two or more relapses within two years.

   Such long-term treatment must be individualized; consult your physician regarding its advisability for you. The optimal duration of such treatment and the long-term effects of chronic histamine-blocking drug use have not been determined.

2. Should anti-infective drugs be used routinely to eradicate *Helicobacter pylori* infection in treating active peptic ulcer disease?

   Evidence is mounting to indicate that initial and recurrent duodenal ulcer is probably associated with *H. pylori* infection, and that gastric ulcer is possibly associated with it. Studies show that without eradication of infection, the ulcer recurrence rate is 84%; with eradication of infection the rate is reduced to 21%. Some authorities offer the following guidelines for considering anti-infective treatment:
- Occurrence of two or more episodes of active ulcer, with conventional treatment
- Failure of ulcer to heal after 12 weeks of conventional treatment

- Recurrence of ulcer despite adequate maintenance therapy with conventional drugs
- As an alternative to elective surgery for ulcer complications

To be effective, treatment of *H. pylori* infection must eradicate and not just suppress the presence of organisms. Eradication requires the use of combination drug therapy (see Management of Therapy above).

Possible Drug Interactions of Significance

Because of the number of drugs that may be used to manage this disorder, adequate consideration of the volume and complexity of potential drug interactions is beyond the scope of this book. Consult *The Essential Guide to Prescription Drugs*, or a similar drug reference book for possible interactions of significance (see Appendix 17, Drug Information Sources).

Special Considerations for Women

Pregnancy

Metronidazole is designated Pregnancy Category B. However, the manufacturer advises against its use during the first three months of pregnancy. Consult your physician regarding its use at any time during pregnancy.

Tetracycline is designated Pregnancy Category D. It is advisable to avoid this drug during entire pregnancy.

See Appendix 15, FDA Pregnancy Categories.

Breast-Feeding

Consult your physician regarding the compatibility of nursing and the drugs you are taking.

Special Considerations for the Elderly

Active PUD in older persons may cause few or no significant symptoms, making them vulnerable to serious complications before the disease is detected. If you have a history of PUD earlier in life, monitor your digestion and stools for subtle indications of possible ulcer recurrence.

Resources

Recommended Reading

Helicobacter pylori in Peptic Ulcer Disease, NIH Consensus Statement, Volume 12, Number 1, February 7–9, 1994. National Institutes of Health, Federal Building, Room 618, Bethesda, MD 20892.

Additional Information and Services

American Digestive Disease Society
60 East 42nd Street, Room 411
New York, NY 10165

Telecommunications services: Gutline, available to the public every Tuesday evening from 7:30 to 9:00 P.M. EST. Publications available.

National Ulcer Foundation
675 Main Street
Melrose, MA 02176
Phone: (617) 665-6210
Publication: newsletter concerning peptic ulcer disease.

PROSTATE CANCER

Other Names Adenocarcinoma of the prostate, carcinoma of the prostate

Prevalence/Incidence in U.S.
Current estimate: 240,000
Estimated new cases annually: 165,000
Estimated deaths annually: 40,000

Prostate cancer is the most common cancer currently found in American men. It is estimated that 30–40% of men in the United States over 50 years of age may have prostate cancer. Approximately 60–70% of men over the age of 75 are thought to have some stage of prostate cancer. The lifetime probability of developing prostate cancer is 9.6% in black men and 5.2% in white men in the United States.

Age Group
Prostate cancer is very rare under the age of 50. A small number of cases are first detected in the sixth decade of life. The incidence increases significantly with each subsequent decade. Approximately 95% of prostate cancers are diagnosed in men between 45 and 89 years of age; the median age at diagnosis is 72 years. Studies show that over 40% of men dying in the ninth decade of life have prostate cancer. Age-specific incidence rates (cases per 100,000) are as follows:

Age at Diagnosis	White Males	Black Males
30–34	0.0	0.2
35–39	0.1	0.5
40–44	1.5	3.0
45–49	7.0	9.6
50–54	31.6	61.4
55–59	104.2	167.1
60–64	255.8	412.2
65–69	517.7	819.2
70–74	803.2	1053.4
75–79	1018.9	1357.8

| 80–84 | 1178.9 | 1506.1 |
| 85+ | 1172.8 | 1465.7 |

Principal Features and Natural History

Basic Anatomy and Function

The prostate gland (present only in males) is a walnut-sized organ located at the base of the urinary bladder where the urethra (urine outflow channel) joins the bladder neck. The urethra passes through the body of the prostate; thus the prostate is a "collar" around the first portion of the urethra where it drains urine from the bladder. The primary function of the prostate is to produce an essential portion of the seminal fluid.

Prostate Cancer

Now the most common malignant disease found in American men, cancer of the prostate gland is usually deceptively quiet and slow-growing for long periods of time. When it develops at a relatively early age (fifth and sixth decades of life), it often tends to grow faster and exhibit a higher grade of malignancy. The majority of cases are first recognized in the seventh and later decades and are characteristically slow-growing and less aggressive (lower degree of malignancy). This form can exist for years without producing symptoms.

As with all forms of malignant disease, prostate cancer presents a spectrum of progressive change throughout its course. The degree and rate of change are determined by the interaction of several factors: (1) the basic nature (differentiation) of the cancer cells; (2) the inherent degree ("grade") of malignancy (low to high); (3) the defense systems of the patient. The net effect of these interactions controls the size and extent of the cancer, which in turn determine the "stage" of the cancer at the time of discovery. Appropriate tests can identify the apparent stage of the process and so form a basis for prognosis and treatment.

Stage A

This designation refers to the initiation and early establishment of cancerous tissue within the gland, when the tumor size is too small to be detected by digital rectal examination and there are no symptoms to indicate its presence. It is found (by the pathologist, not the surgeon) in the pieces of prostate tissue removed during transurethral resection of the prostate (TURP) to relieve obstruction of the urethra caused by noncancerous enlargement of the prostate—benign prostatic hyperplasia (BPH). Up to 10% of patients having TURP for BPH will be found to have stage A prostate cancer. Unfortunately, the prostate-specific antigen (PSA) test is not sufficiently sensitive or specific to detect cancer accurately at this early stage. PSA levels above the "normal" range are not always indicative of cancer; prostate infection (prostatitis) and benign prostatic hyperplasia (BPH) can cause elevation of PSA values in the absence of cancer. Also, PSA levels well within the normal range can be found in the presence of verified cancer of the prostate.

Stage B

This is the earliest stage of prostate cancer that can be detected by digital rectal examination. When the cancerous tissue (a nodule or abnormally firm area) is less than 2 centimeters in size and is confined to one side of the gland, it is designated stage B_1. If the area is more than 2 centimeters in size or cancerous areas are found on both sides of the gland, the designation is stage B_2. At this stage it is generally assumed that the cancer is still localized within the prostate and has not spread beyond the outer capsule of the gland. Diagnostic examinations (blood tests, X-ray studies, bone scans, etc.) are used to evaluate this assumption. It has been reported that up to 35% of stage B_2 cancers have already spread to regional lymph glands. Approximately 20–30% of all prostate cancers are first detected in stage B. The PSA test, though not completely reliable, does have greater utility in monitoring the progress of cancer in this stage of disease. Serial measurements of PSA values made periodically may be helpful in judging the stage and severity of the malignant process in stage B and subsequent stages of disease.

Stage C

This designation indicates that digital rectal examination reveals extensive cancerous involvement throughout the prostate, often with extension into adjacent tissues and the seminal vesicles. Up to 85% of patients in this stage can have spread to regional lymph nodes. As with stages A and B disease, confirmatory tests are mandatory for accurate staging. Approximately 30–40% of all prostate cancers are first detected in stage C.

Stage D

When confirmatory studies reveal that the cancer is no longer localized within the gland and has spread beyond the capsule and seminal vesicles, the designation is stage D. If the spread can be shown to be only regional—adjacent tissues and lymph glands—the designation is stage D_1. If there is evidence of spread (metastasis) to distant sites—bones, lungs, liver, etc.—the designation is stage D_2. Nearly 20% of newly diagnosed patients with prostate cancer have stage D_1 disease. PSA levels are usually found to be elevated in the majority of patients with stage D disease.

Note: Once the presence of prostate cancer is confirmed, appropriate studies are performed to determine: (1) the "stage" of the disease—an indication of tumor size and extent; (2) the "grade" of the malignant process—an indication of the tumor's propensity for growth and spread. Examination of cancer cells (obtained by needle biopsy of the prostate) enables the pathologist to determine the grade on a scale of 1 to 4: grades 1 and 2—low potential for growth and spread; grades 3 and 4— high potential for growth and spread. Knowing the "stage" and "grade" permits the development of optimal treatment strategies. Current methods of treatment include surgery, radiation, and drugs, used singly and in combination.

Diagnostic Symptoms and Signs
There are usually no specific symptoms during early stage disease.
With urinary tract obstruction: frequency, urgency, and hesitancy of urination; occasional urination during the night
With local spread of disease: bloody urine, swelling of the legs
With systemic spread of disease: weakness, weight loss, back pain due to spine involvement

Diagnostic Tests and Procedures
Digital rectal examination (DRE)
Needle biopsy of prostate gland
Measurement of prostate-specific antigen (PSA) blood level
Measurement of prostatic acid phosphatase (PAP) blood level
Transrectal sonogram to detect prostatic tumor
Bone scans, liver scans to detect metastatic disease

Diagnostic "Marker" for This Disorder
Detection of prostate cancer cells in biopsy specimen.

Similar Conditions That May Confuse Diagnosis
Chronic prostatitis (low-grade infection)
Benign prostatic hyperplasia (BPH)

ALERT!
Prostatitis and benign prostatic hyperplasia (noncancerous conditions) can cause an abnormally high PSA test result—a false positive.
    A normal PSA test result is found in 40% of cases of prostate cancer.

Causes
The primary cause of prostate cancer is not known. Apparently its development is dependent upon the presence of male sex hormones (androgens), since prostate cancer rarely occurs in eunuchs. Studies have identified a few possible "contributing" factors such as genetic predisposition and high-fat diets, but no significant evidence of specific cause. Benign prostatic hyperplasia (BPH) occurs during the same period of life as prostate cancer, but there appears to be no causative relation-

ship. Two recent studies suggest a possible link between vasectomy and an increased risk for developing prostate cancer up to 20 years later. No rational explanation for this association is yet apparent, and no definitive evidence has been found to establish a cause-and-effect relationship.

Drugs That Can Cause This Disorder

There are no drugs that are known to induce prostate cancer. However, several widely used drugs can produce effects that resemble symptoms associated with bladder neck obstruction such as that caused by an enlarged prostate gland, benign or malignant. Decongestant drugs used to treat head colds, sinus congestion, and allergic rhinitis may increase muscle tone within the prostate and cause contraction of the bladder neck, actions which could impede the flow of urine. These drugs include pseudoephedrine (Sudafed), phenylephrine (Sinex, etc.), and phenyl-propanolamine (Contac, Ornade, etc.); the latter is also used to control appetite (Dexatrim). Drugs with an atropinelike (anticholinergic) action may inhibit contraction of bladder muscle and impair its ability to overcome urethral compression, thus enhancing the pattern of prostatism.

Goals of Treatment

Can This Disorder Be Cured?

Only by surgical resection of all malignant tissue during the early stage of disease.

Can This Disorder Be Treated Effectively?

Currently available medications and therapeutic radiation can control prostate cancer for varying periods of time.

Specific Goals

- To achieve "medical" castration as completely as possible: the total suppression of androgens (male sex hormones) that stimulate the activity and growth of prostate cancer cells
- To determine the "drugs of choice"—those most appropriate for each patient individually
- To determine the optimal time for initiating drug treatment for each patient individually
- To provide the best quality of life consistent with optimal drug therapy

Health Professionals Who Participate in Managing This Disorder

Family physicians
General internists
Geriatricians
Urologists

Medical oncologists
Radiation oncologists
Surgical oncologists
Nurse oncologists
Physician assistants
Nurse practitioners
Medical social workers

Currently Available Therapies for This Disorder

Drug Therapy

Drugs for medical castration:
- estrogens (diethylstilbestrol)
- hormonal drugs:
  - buserelin (Suprefact)
  - goserelin (Zoladex)
  - leupolide (Lupron)
  - nafarelin (Synarel)
- ketoconazole (Nizoral)

Antiandrogens:
- finasteride (Proscar)
- flutamide (Eulexin, Euflex)
- nilutamide

Mixed-mechanism-of-action drugs:
- cyproterone (Androcur, Cyproteron)
- progestins (hydroxyprogesterone, medrogestone, megestrol)

Drugs to suppress adrenal androgens:
- aminoglutethimide (Cytadren)
- glucocorticosteroids
- ketoconazole (Nizoral)

Nondrug Treatment Methods

- Watchful waiting: palliative treatment for symptoms as required
- Radiation therapy
- Radical prostatectomy: surgical removal of entire prostate
- Bilateral orchiectomy: surgical removal of testicles
- Chemotherapy
- Cryotherapy

New Drugs in Development for Treating This Disorder

Several new antiandrogens are under study: Anandron, Casodex, and Win. They are similar to flutamide, inhibiting the growth-stimulating effects of androgens on prostate cancer cells. An unrelated drug, suramin, is currently being evaluated in the management of prostate cancer that does not respond to conventional hormone therapy. Suramin inhibits the growth of prostate cells and suppresses the production of androgens by the adrenal glands.

Management of Therapy

Established procedure in the United States at this time is to recommend "definitive" treatment for localized (stages A and B) prostate cancer— either radical surgery (total prostatectomy) or radiation—in the belief that such treatment can be "curative." Stages C and D disease cannot be cured surgically. Selected cases of stage C may be treated by a combination of radiation and hormonal drug therapy. The current treatment of choice for stage D prostate cancer is the use of drugs to produce "medical" castration—the abolition of androgen influence to the greatest extent possible. In some instances, surgical removal of the testicles (orchiectomy) is recommended in conjunction with selected drug therapy.

"Medical" Castration

- This is accomplished by the combined use of (1) a hormonelike drug that suppresses the production of testosterone by the testicles, and (2) an antiandrogen drug that blocks the biological effects of testosterone on the prostate gland.
- Leuprolide (Lupron) or goserelin (Zoladex) is given by injection once a month. This causes the pituitary gland (in the brain) to produce increased amounts of the hormone that stimulates testosterone production by the testicles. Continued use of leuprolide or goserelin soon creates a supersaturation state in the pituitary which then shuts down production of the hormone that stimulates testosterone production. The initial (and transient) rise in testosterone production can cause a "flare" reaction in cancerous prostate tissue—both locally within the gland and in metastatic cancer sites in bone—resulting in bladder neck obstruction and scattered bone pain. This "flare" response can be minimized by the simultaneous administration of an antiandrogen drug (such as flutamide) when leuprolide or goserelin injections are begun.
- Flutamide (Eulexin) is taken daily by mouth. It suppresses the biological effects of testosterone by blocking its uptake and binding in target tissues—benign or cancerous prostate cells in the gland or elsewhere in the body (metastases). Continual use on a regular schedule for two to three months is necessary to determine its effectiveness. In some individuals this drug may become less effective after several months of continual use.
- For optimal results, flutamide and leuprolide (or goserelin) should be started together and continued together for the duration of treatment. Response to this drug regimen is monitored by periodic measurement of prostate-specific antigen (PSA) blood levels. Prior to drug therapy, PSA levels are usually found to be above the normal range, indicating

prostate cancer activity. Good response to treatment is indicated by a significant decrease in PSA levels. When values stabilize in the normal range, dosage schedules of the above medications may be modified.

- If "total" elimination of androgens is considered appropriate, their production by the adrenal glands (which is considerably less than by the testicles) can be suppressed by the use of aminoglutethimide or keto-conazole.

Alternative Drug Therapy

Conventional hormonal drug therapy (as above) is usually effective in the majority of stage C and D cancers during the initial periods of treatment. However, the drugs in current use can lose their effectiveness in time and many prostate cancers will become "resistant" to hormonal therapy. When this occurs, the following drugs may be tried in selected cases:

- Megestrol (Megase), a progestin that (1) inhibits the secretion of the pituitary hormone that stimulates testosterone production and (2) blocks the androgen receptor sites on prostate cells.
- Diethylstilbestrol (DES), a synthetic estrogen (given intravenously in high doses) that has a direct toxic effect on prostate cancer cells.
- Cyproterone (Androcur), an antiandrogen that (1) competitively blocks testosterone at receptor sites and (2) partially suppresses pituitary hormone secretion. It is used singly and in combination with hormonal drugs and surgical castration. This drug is available in Canada but not in the United States.

Ancillary Drug Treatment (as required)

For mild to moderate pain:
- acetaminophen or nonsteroidal anti-inflammatory drugs (NSAIDs); alone or in combination with opioid drugs; may be especially effective for bone pain

For moderate pain:
- codeine, oxycodone, alone or in combination with nonopioid drugs

For severe pain:
- morphine, hydromorphone, oxycodone, levorphanol, methadone, fentanyl (avoid pentazocine and meperidine)

For chronic neuropathic pain:
- nortriptyline, desipramine, amitriptyline, imipramine, doxepin

Note: Drug selection, dosage, and administration schedule must be determined by the physician for each patient individually (see Appendix 3, Cancer Pain Management, and Appendix 7, Pain Management Centers).

Current Controversies in Management

Approximately 60% of patients with untreated stage C prostate cancer will experience disease progression within five years; with stage D_1 disease about 85% of patients will show progression within five years. Those with stage D_2 disease have a five-year survival rate of 20%. Currently available treatment—"total" removal or suppression of androgen activity—can achieve beneficial responses (but not cure) in 70% of those with stages C and D prostate cancer. The duration of improvement ranges from several months to several years. However, therapists do not agree as to when drug therapy should be started. Early studies were interpreted to show that the outcomes were about the same for early and delayed treatment. Reanalysis of older studies, conclusions from recent studies, and the availability of improved drugs establish clearly that early treatment offers significant advantages over delay. Benefits of early treatment include a marked delay of disease progression in the majority of treated patients, and a significantly better quality of life during the extended symptom-free period. The benefit–risk analyses provided by knowledgeable specialists strongly support early hormonal drug treatment for appropriate cases of advanced prostate cancer.

Note: The decision of when and how to initiate treatment for advanced-stage prostate cancer should be made jointly by the physician and the patient. The periodic use of PSA measurements provide one indicator of disease status and can frequently detect any tendency to progression. The physician should discuss fully his analysis of the individual's disease state and fully inform the patient regarding the known benefits and risks of current drug therapy. The quality of life should be a paramount consideration of any extension of life.

Important Points to Consider

Based upon the assumption that the early discovery of "localized" prostate cancer (stage A or B) provides an opportunity for "cure," it is currently standard practice in many areas of the United States to initiate prompt and aggressive methods of treatment—radical surgery or radiation (X-ray therapy)—at the time of diagnosis. Recently published reviews of the consequences (benefits and risks) challenge the efficacy and wisdom of these procedures for many patients. Most prostate cancers are slow-growing, and the vast majority of those who have prostate cancer never develop symptoms indicative of their disease. Only 8% of patients with stage A disease develop metastases within 10 years and only 2% die from it. Of those with stage B disease, 30% develop metastases within five years and 20% die from it. Radical surgery carries the risk of a 2% mortality rate and a 5–10% complication rate. Radiation therapy imposes a major complication rate of 10%. Given the natural history of most prostate cancers, can these risks be justified in the absence of symptoms or evidence of disease progression? At the time of diagnosis of "localized" prostate cancer, some pathologic features of the disease can be determined. The majority of patients with "well-differentiated" tumors will not die from their disease; early radical treatment is not mandatory. For those with "poorly differentiated" tumors, neither radical surgery nor radical radiation therapy has been shown to be significantly effective. A consensus is emerging that the decision to advise "watchful waiting" (surveillance) rather than radical treatment at the time of diagnosis is in the best interest of elderly men (75 years and older) with slow-growing prostate cancer. Radical therapies may be selectively appropriate for younger men with fast-growing tumors. It is advisable for anyone diagnosed to have "localized" prostate cancer to seek a physician who will provide clear, objective information regarding the benefits, risks, outcomes, and uncertainties of all treatments currently available.

Possible Drug Interactions of Significance

Because of the number and nature of drugs that may be used to manage this disorder, adequate consideration of the volume and complexity of potential drug interactions is beyond the scope of this book. Consult *The Essential Guide to Prescription Drugs*, or a similar drug reference book for possible interactions of significance (see Appendix 17, Drug Information Sources).

Resources

Recommended Reading

The Prostate Book: Sound Advice on Symptoms and Treatment, Stephen J. Rous, M.D. New York: Norton, 1988.

The Prostate Sourcebook: Everything You Need to Know, S. Morganstern, M.D., and A. Abrahams, Ph.D. Los Angeles: Lowell House, 1994.

Additional Information and Services

American Cancer Society
1599 Clifton Road, NE
Atlanta, GA 30329-4251
Phone: 1-800-ACS-2345, (404) 320-3333; Fax (404) 325-0230

American Foundation for Urologic Disease
300 West Pratt Street, Suite 401
Baltimore, MD 21201
Phone: (410) 727-2908, 1-800-242-2383; Fax: (410) 783-1566

Sponsors "US TOO" patient support groups for prostate cancer survivors.

National Cancer Institute
Cancer Information Service
Bethesda, MD
Phone: 1-800-422-6237

National Kidney and Urologic Diseases Information Clearinghouse
P.O. Box NKUDIC
9000 Rockville Pike
Bethesda, MD 20892
Phone: (301) 468-6345
    Established by the National Institutes of Health. Provides direct
responses to written and telephone inquiries.

Disease Management Expertise
    See Appendix 2, Part One: National Cancer Institute Designated Cancer
Centers and Part Two: Clinical Trials.

PROSTATE ENLARGEMENT

Other Names Benign prostatic hyperplasia, benign prostatic hypertro-
phy, BPH

Prevalence/Incidence in U.S.
The most prevalent disease occurring in older men.
    The following statistics represent findings at autopsy:

Age	% with BPH
31–40	8
41–50	22
51–60	42
61–70	72
71–80	82
81–90+	88

Age Group The following statistics represent clinical diagnosis of BPH
and prostatectomy for BPH:

Age	Incidence of BPH per 1,000 person-years	Incidence of BPH Surgery per 1,000 person-years
40–49	9.4	0.2
50–59	31.3	4.1
60–69	51.3	12.1
70–87	59.2	19.4

Principal Features and Natural History

Basic Anatomy and Function
    The prostate gland (present only in males) is a walnut-sized organ
located at the base of the urinary bladder where the urethra (urine out-

flow channel) joins the bladder neck. The urethra passes through the body of the prostate; thus the prostate is like a "collar" around the first portion of the urethra where it drains urine from the bladder. This portion is known as the prostatic urethra. At the outer end of the prostatic urethra where it emerges from the gland, a circular muscle (the external urethral sphincter) is located. Voluntary contraction of this sphincter shuts off the flow of urine. The primary function of the prostate is to produce an essential portion of the seminal fluid.

Benign Prostatic Hyperplasia

The process of enlargement usually begins between 40 and 45 years of age. Like all tubular structures in the body, the prostatic urethra has a lining. New and excessive growth of prostate tissue (referred to as hyperplasia) begins just beneath (outside) this lining. This new tissue is predominantly glandular in nature—responding to the growth-stimulating effects of dihydrotestosterone (a male sex hormone). Once started, the growth process continues slowly (though not uniformly) in all directions. Eventually this results in (1) enlargement of the prostate gland outwardly (which can be detected by digital rectal examination) and (2) narrowing of the prostatic urethra due to inward growth of tissue that compresses (constricts) it. Over a period of years the progressive constriction of the urethra (obstruction to the outflow of urine) gradually affects the function of the bladder, and a characteristic pattern of changes in urination develop. Often the initial symptom is the need to urinate during the night (nocturia); the frequency of night urination increases with time. The next symptom is the development of a sense of urgency when the desire to urinate becomes apparent; it becomes increasingly difficult to delay voiding. As the prostate continues to enlarge and the degree of urethral obstruction increases, there is a delay in the flow of urine when voiding is attempted (hesitancy). In addition, the size and force of the urinary stream are significantly reduced. Once this degree of obstruction is reached, the flow of urine may stop and restart several times before the bladder feels empty (intermittency). At this point it becomes difficult to know when the bladder is truly empty, and small amounts of urine will pass without effort after voiding is thought to be complete (terminal dribbling). If treatment is not sought and the obstruction is not relieved at this point, the bladder loses its ability to empty completely at the time of voiding. This results is urinary retention—a serious and potentially dangerous condition. This late manifestation of BPH causes marked daytime frequency of urination and involuntary leakage of urine (overflow incontinence). It is at this stage of prostate enlargement that an episode of acute urinary retention can occur. Suddenly and without warning a full bladder creates extreme urgency to void, but the individual is unable to start any flow of urine. This emergency situation requires immediate catheterization to empty the bladder. The chronic retention of urine predisposes to bladder and prostate gland infection and, less frequently, to the formation of bladder stones. Continuous bladder filling (without adequate relief) can eventually lead to sufficient back pressure within the kidneys to seriously impair kidney function and threaten the development of kidney failure (uremia).

Note: Once it becomes apparent that prostate enlargement has reached the point of causing symptoms, it is advisable to consult a urologist for evaluation. Ask for a thorough determination of your status and a review of appropriate treatment options. Choices include both medical and surgical therapies. Together with the urologist decide which treatment is in your best interest, considering carefully all aspects of the problem.

Diagnostic Symptoms and Signs
All of the following are directly due to the irritation and obstruction of the urethra caused by the enlarging prostate gland:
   Nighttime urination (nocturia)
   Urinary urgency
   Urinary frequency
   Pain during urination (dysuria)
   Urinary hesitancy (delay in starting urine flow)
   Urinary intermittency (flow starting and stopping)
   Urinary dribbling at end of flow
   Straining to empty bladder
   Overflow incontinence (leakage of urine with full bladder)
   Acute urinary retention (inability to void)

Diagnostic Tests and Procedures
Digital rectal examination (DRE) to determine size and consistency of
   prostate gland
Urine analysis and culture for possible infection
Measurement of prostate-specific antigen (PSA) blood level
Abdominal sonogram to detect incomplete emptying of urinary bladder
Transrectal sonogram to estimate size of prostate gland
Kidney function tests: measurement of blood urea nitrogen (BUN) and
   creatinine

Similar Conditions That May Confuse Diagnosis
Acute or chronic prostatitis
Prostate cancer

Causes
It is known that normal development and growth of the prostate gland is dependent upon the presence of testosterone and its derivative dihy-

drotestosterone, the principal male sex hormones. However, the true cause of enlargement of the prostate with aging is not known. BPH does not occur in eunuchs. We know that gradual enlargement requires the continued presence of male sex hormones (androgens). It appears that inherent changes in aging prostate tissue are somehow responsible for abnormal growth and enlargement. The degree and nature of sexual activity or prior prostate infection are not causally related to BPH.

Drugs That Can Cause This Disorder

There are no drugs known to be capable of initiating the process of benign prostatic hyperplasia. Medicinal forms of testosterone may enhance BPH if given in sufficient dosage for an extended period of time.

Several decongestant drugs commonly used to treat head colds, sinus congestion, and allergic rhinitis may increase muscle tone within the prostate and cause contraction of the bladder neck, actions which could enhance constriction of the urethra due to BPH. These drugs include pseudoephedrine (Sudafed), phenylephrine (Sinex, etc.), and phenyl-propanolamine (Contac, Ornade, etc.); the latter is also used to control appetite (Dexatrim).

Drugs with an atropinelike (anticholinergic) action may inhibit contraction of bladder muscle and impair its ability to overcome urethral compression, thus enhancing the pattern of symptoms due to BPH (see anticholinergic drugs in Appendix 16, Drug Classes, and the term "prostatism" in the Glossary).

Goals of Treatment

Can This Disorder Be Cured?

There is no curative treatment available at this time.

Can This Disorder Be Treated Effectively?

There are drugs currently available that are capable of relieving the urinary obstructive features of BPH sufficiently to defer or avoid surgery.

If drug therapy proves to be inadequate, currently available surgical procedures are safe and very effective.

Specific Goals

- Arrest and reversal of the process causing benign hyperplasia of prostate tissue
- Relief of symptoms due to prostatic urethral compression
- Prevention of complications and consequences of urinary obstruction

Health Professionals Who Participate in Managing This Disorder

Family physicians
General internists

Geriatricians
Urologists
Pharmacists
Physician assistants
Nurse practitioners
Radiologists

Currently Available Therapies for This Disorder

Drug Therapy
Alpha-adrenergic blocking drugs:
- doxazosin (Cardura)
- prazosin (Minipress)
- terazosin (Hytrin)

Antiandrogen drugs:
- finasteride (Proscar)
- flutamide (Eulexin, Euflex)
- nilutamide (Anandron)

Surgical Procedures
- Open prostatectomy: removal of prostate gland via external incision
- Transurethral resection of prostate (TURP): removal of obstructing prostate fragments via the urethra; no external incision
- Transurethral incision of prostate to relieve obstruction
- Transurethral laser resection to relieve obstruction

ALERT!
If you are taking any drugs that could possibly cause or contribute to your prostatism, discontinue them completely for one week and then reevaluate the need for surgery.

New Drugs in Development for Treating This Disorder
The following alpha-adrenergic blocking drugs are under investigation: alfuzosin, indoramin, ketanserin, nicergolin, and thymoxamine.

The following androgen-reducing drugs are under investigation: buserelin, leuprolide, nafarelin, cyproterone (Androcur), hydroxyprogesterone (Delalutin), and megestrol (Megace).

Management of Therapy
At this time, the definitive treatment for BPH that is significantly symptomatic is surgical—transurethral resection of the prostate (TURP). About 29% of those with symptomatic disease will require surgery. The role of drug therapy is limited to treating (1) the early manifestations of BPH (before surgery is necessary); (2) temporizing situations until surgery is possible.

A reasonable criticism of electing drug therapy for early BPH is the lost opportunity to detect early (stage A) cancer—no surgically removed tissue specimens (via TURP) for pathologic examination. Before starting drug treatment, the following procedures are advisable:
- thorough digital rectal examination
- transrectal ultrasound imaging of the prostate gland
- measurement of the prostate-specific antigen (PSA) blood level

It is recommended that these tests be performed periodically during drug therapy to monitor the course of BPH. Any suspicious findings in the prostate should be evaluated by needle biopsy.

Use of Alpha-Adrenergic Blocking Drugs
- These drugs are used to reduce the muscle tone of the prostate gland and bladder neck. By blocking stimulation to the muscle fibers within the gland, they exert a modest "relaxation" effect that partially reduces the constriction of the urethra and improves urine flow. They are suitable for trial in those with moderate BPH.
- It is important to take an initial "test" dose of these drugs at bedtime to detect the possibility of a first-dose drop in blood pressure. Use caution on arising the following morning. Observe for any indication of light-headedness or impending faint due to drop in blood pressure (see orthostatic hypotension in Glossary). Consult your physician if this occurs.

Use of Androgen-Reducing Drugs
- These drugs are used to reduce the size (tissue bulk) of the prostate. By several different actions the drugs of this group decrease the production of androgens and/or block the effects of androgens on prostate cells. The net result is reversal of the hyperplasia process and reduction in prostate size.
- The only drug of this group currently approved in the United States for treatment of BPH is finasteride (Proscar). This drug inhibits the conversion of testosterone to dihydrotestosterone, the principal androgen responsible for prostate growth. Because testosterone levels remain within the normal range, this drug does not cause significant loss of libido or impotence. Because this drug does reduce levels of dihydrotestosterone (by 70%), prostate growth is reversed. About 50% of patients experience an increase in urine flow and lessening of symptoms.
- Drugs of this group can cause a 30–40% decrease in prostate size within three to six months of treatment. However, any improvement depends upon continual use of the drug. Prostatic regrowth occurs quickly after discontinuation of drug therapy.

Ancillary Drug Treatment (as required)
For bladder infections:
- appropriate anti-infective drugs determined by urine culture and bacterial sensitivity testing

Note: Drug selection, dosage, and administration schedule must be determined by the physician for each patient individually.

Current Controversies in Management

Current options for treating BPH include (1) "watchful waiting," (2) drug therapy (surgery deferred), or (3) surgical procedures. For those with advanced BPH experiencing severe and possibly life-threatening symptoms, surgery is certainly the treatment of choice. For those with early BPH and mild symptoms, watchful waiting (observation) is advisable. For the large majority of those with moderate BPH who are experiencing significant symptoms that require relief, a trial of drug therapy is now accepted as an appropriate and reasonable alternative to immediate surgery (TURP). During the trial of medication, periodic evaluation to monitor the course of BPH is mandatory. It will be shown that many individuals may never require surgery.

Transurethral resection of the prostate (TURP) is the most commonly performed surgery for BPH. Approximately 85% of patients having TURP are markedly improved. However, it does carry the risk of possible complications: urinary incontinence, urethral stricture, impotence, infection, and serious bleeding. The overall complication rate is 16.1%. Approximately 10% of patients require reoperation within 10 years. In comparison, 67% of patients treated medically with terazosin are markedly improved. There are no serious complications, drug side effects are minimal and reversible, and the majority of patients are extremely satisfied. Those with moderate symptoms of BPH who *do not have* urinary retention, recurrent urinary tract infection, or impaired kidney function (due to bladder outlet obstruction) are logical candidates for a trial of drug therapy.

Drugs currently in use to treat BPH include the alpha-adrenergic blockers and the antiandrogen finasteride. All are well tolerated and easily managed. Alpha-adrenergic blockers have been in use to treat BPH for more than 15 years. Finasteride, released in 1993, has been shown in premarketing studies to be safe and effective drug therapy for 50% of patients with BPH. Used singly or in combination, a trial of these alternative treatments to surgery is a reasonable and appropriate recommendation for properly selected patients.

When competing methods of treatment are being considered, decisions must be made jointly by the knowledgeable (and altruistic) physician and the informed patient.

Important Points to Consider

• Those with manifestations indicating the development of BPH should be aware that the following can significantly intensify symptoms: exposure to cold, emotional stress, nervous tension, overdistention of the bladder (ignoring the urge to urinate).

- Keep in mind that many drugs in common use can affect bladder function. "Drugs" includes those prescribed by a physician *and* those purchased over-the-counter (OTC). Many products used to treat head colds, cough, and allergies contain antihistamines and decongestants. Some antihistamines can inhibit contraction of the urinary bladder; some decongestants can tighten the bladder neck. The net effect is significant impairment of urination. Obviously such medications can enhance the symptoms of BPH. If your condition requires medical attention, be certain you inform attending physicians regarding *all* medications you have taken recently.
- The prostate-specific antigen (PSA) test, although helpful in some situations, is not totally reliable and must be interpreted with caution. Increased PSA test results are found in 9–21% of men with BPH (no cancer). Approximately 40% of men with early cancer will have normal PSA levels. The PSA test is only one factor to be considered in deciding the "treatment of choice" on an individual basis.

Possible Drug Interactions of Significance

Because of the number and nature of drugs that may be used to manage this disorder, adequate consideration of the volume and complexity of potential drug interactions is beyond the scope of this book. Consult *The Essential Guide to Prescription Drugs*, or a similar drug reference book for possible interactions of significance (see Appendix 17, Drug Information Sources).

Resources

Recommended Reading

The Prostate Book: Sound Advice on Symptoms and Treatment, Stephen N. Rous, M.D. New York: Norton, 1988.

The Prostate Sourcebook: Everything You Need to Know, S. Morganstern, M.D., and A. Abrahams, Ph.D. Los Angeles: Lowell House, 1994.

Treating Your Enlarged Prostate: Patient Guide, Public Health Service, Agency for Health Care Policy and Research, Rockville, MD. AHCRP Publication No. 94-0584, 1994. For a copy call 1-800-358-9295.

Additional Information and Services

American Foundation for Urologic Disease
300 West Pratt Street, Suite 410
Baltimore, MD 21201
Phone: (410) 727-2908, 1-800-242-2383; Fax: (410) 783-1566

National Kidney and Urologic Diseases Information Clearinghouse
P.O. Box NKUDIC
9000 Rockville Pike

Bethesda, MD 20892
Phone: (301) 468-6345
Established by the National Institutes of Health. Provides direct responses to written and telephone inquiries.

PSORIASIS

Other Name Psoriasis vulgaris

Prevalence/Incidence in U.S.
Current estimate: between 3 and 4 million
Estimated new cases annually: 150,000
Approximately 2–4% of the white population; less than 1% of the black population. About 7% of individuals with psoriasis have associated arthritis (psoriatic arthritis).

Age Group The usual onset is between 10 and 40 years of age. However, psoriasis may begin at any age.

Male-to-Female Ratio Slightly more common in men in all age groups

Principal Features and Natural History
Psoriasis is the most common type of chronic, recurrent scaling dermatitis. It begins gradually, often with one or two small patches, and follows a course of irregular and unpredictable remissions and recurrences throughout life. The characteristic skin change consists of a well-demarcated pink to reddish patch (plaque), one to three inches in size, which is covered almost completely by dry, silvery scales. Removal of the scales exposes numerous small, red, bleeding points. Itching, if present at all, is usually mild. The size, number, and distribution of the patches varies greatly. They may remain localized to a few small areas or they may spread to involve the entire body surface. The areas most commonly involved include the scalp, back of the neck, and the outer surfaces of the arms and legs, especially the elbows, knees, and shins. Less commonly, psoriasis may involve the eyebrows, armpits, palms of the hands, soles of the feet, fingernails, umbilicus, and the anal and genital areas. A rare form may involve the back, hips, and thighs. Very rarely patches may occur in the mouth or on the tongue. During remission the patches fade and clear, the skin heals without scarring, and there is no alteration of hair in involved areas. Permanent remission is rare. Currently there is no curative treatment, but most cases can be controlled satisfactorily.

Usually the general health is not affected. Infrequently a more serious and extensive form of psoriasis may develop. An acute, generalized, pustular form with fever, weakness, and systemic debility can occur. Another unusual type causes extensive inflammation and peeling of the skin. Approximately 7% of cases will develop a form of arthritis that resembles rheumatoid arthritis. This varies in severity from relatively mild to permanently disabling.

Diagnostic Symptoms and Signs

Symmetrical distribution of thickened, reddish plaques that are covered
  with silvery scales
Pitting and degeneration of nails
Joint swelling, inflammation, and pain resembling rheumatoid arthritis
  (infrequent)

Diagnostic Tests and Procedures

There are no specific laboratory tests for the diagnosis of psoriasis.
Skin biopsies taken from plaques reveal diagnostic features.

Diagnostic "Markers" for This Disorder

Auspitz sign: the removal of scales from the surface of plaques will cause small areas of bleeding. This is fairly specific for psoriasis.

Similar Conditions That May Confuse Diagnosis

Eczema
Tinea corporis ("ringworm" fungus infection of skin)
Drug-induced skin eruptions
Syphilis
Lichen planus
Mycosis fungoides

Causes

Established Causes

The primary definitive cause for the development of psoriasis is not known.

Theoretical Causes

Psoriasis is thought to be a genetically determined, hereditary defect of the factors that regulate skin growth. The characteristic scaly patch is caused by a tenfold increase in the turnover rate of the surface cells of the skin. Precipitating factors that can "trigger" the development of psoriasis plaques include excessive sunburn, acute respiratory infections (such as "strep" throat), local injury to the skin, surgical incisions, and vaccination.

ALERT!
Human immunodeficiency virus (HIV) infection can cause new-onset psoriasis or flares of preexisting psoriasis.

Drugs That Can Cause This Disorder
Drugs cannot cause or initiate psoriasis in an individual with normal skin (hereditary defect absent). However, a few drugs can exacerbate existing psoriasis. These include beta-blockers, chloroquine, hydroxychloroquine, indomethacin, lithium, quinidine, and the withdrawal of cortisonelike drugs.

Goals of Treatment

Can This Disorder Be Cured?
There is no curative treatment known at this time.

Can This Disorder Be Treated Effectively?
Most patients respond well to the topical use of medicinal creams, lotions, and ointments. More severe forms of psoriasis will benefit from the use of ultraviolet light and relatively potent systemic drug therapy.

Specific Goals
- Acceleration of clearing of active plaques; this can usually be achieved in close to 90% of cases
- Prevention of recurrence of plaques; although remissions of several months can be achieved, permanent remission is not possible with currently available drugs

Health Professionals Who Participate in Managing This Disorder
Family physicians
General internists
Pediatricians
Dermatologists
Pharmacists
Physician assistants
Nurse practitioners

Currently Available Therapies for This Disorder

Drug Therapy
- Lubricants: lotions, creams, ointments; used to reduce water loss from psoriasis plaques. Examples: Lac-Hydrin, Moisturel lotion, Eucerin Creme, Aquaphor Creme, Vaseline Petroleum Jelly
- Keratolytic agents: used to remove scale. Examples: 6% salicylic acid (Keralyt Gel), 10–20% urea in petrolatum

- Coal tar preparations: used with and without ultraviolet light. Examples: Aquatar, Estar, Fototar, psoriGel, P&S Plus, T-gel, others
- Anthralin preparations: used with and without ultraviolet light. Examples: Anthra-Derm, Dithroceme, Lasan
- Cortisonelike preparations: topical creams, gels, and ointments for local use. Examples: Aristocort, Cyclocort, Diprolene, Kenalog, Lidex, Topicort, Valisone, others
- Vitamin D_3 derivative: calcipotriene (Dovonex), slows the turnover of skin cells; used as an alternative to corticosteroids
- Psoralen preparations: used with ultraviolet light. Example: methoxsalen, topical and oral forms
- Fish oil containing eicosapentanoic acid (EPA): for relief of itching and inflammation
- Methotrexate
- Etretinate

New Drugs in Development for Treating This Disorder
- Vitamin A derivatives similar to etretinate and isotretinoin are currently under investigation.
- Cyclosporine, a drug in current use to prevent rejection in organ transplant surgery, appears to be effective for psoriasis when used in small doses. This use is currently under investigation. It can cause dramatic clearing of generalized psoriasis, but its long-term adverse effects preclude its use except in very severe and resistant cases.

Management of Therapy

Topical Use of Drugs
- Coal tar preparations: method of action is not fully known. Available in solutions, bath oils, shampoos, lotions, and ointments. When used in conjunction with ultraviolet light (UVL), they can produce remissions lasting 6 to 12 months. Can cause burning, stinging reactions ("tar smarts") in skin on exposure to sun or large doses of UVL.
- Anthralin preparations: interfere with DNA synthesis and skin cell reproduction. Available in creams, ointments, and paste. Apply only to psoriasis plaques; can irritate normal skin and stain it brown. More effective when used in conjunction with UVL.
- Cortisonelike preparations for local use: reduce inflammation, swelling, and itching of psoriasis plaques. These are the drugs most commonly used in the current management of mild to moderate psoriasis. Available in lotions, creams, and ointments. Lotions are preferred for treating the scalp; creams are preferred for treating the armpits and groin; ointments are preferred for remaining skin areas. The ointment is more effective when used under occlusive dressings.

- These drugs are used primarily when (1) the skin is "sore" and vulnerable to the irritant effects of other drugs; (2) other drugs are unacceptable for cosmetic reasons; (3) results with coal tar or anthralin preparations alone are unsatisfactory.
- Prolonged use without interruption can cause skin atrophy and loss of drug effectiveness.
- Possible side effects: rosacealike skin changes, excessive hair growth (at point of application), lowered resistance to infection, systemic absorption, glaucoma (when applied around eyes).
- Calcipotriene ointment (Dovonex), a vitamin D_3 analog, is used to treat moderate plaque psoriasis. Used twice daily for eight weeks, it has produced complete healing in 10% of patients, and marked improvement in 70%.

Systemic Use of Drugs

- Psoralens: inhibit DNA synthesis and suppress skin cell reproduction. Available as methoxsalen and trioxsalen for both local and systemic use. These are photosensitizing drugs and are used in conjunction with ultraviolet light in the A range; the combined treatment program is referred to as PUVA. The drug is taken orally two hours before UVL exposure; food impairs absorption and should be avoided. Treatments are given two to four times per week until the skin is clear. Maintenance treatment is given every one to three weeks to prevent recurrence. Protective glasses should be worn during treatment and for eight hours following treatment to prevent cataracts.

  Side effects include itching, nausea, and accelerated aging of the skin. When properly used, this form of treatment produces improvement in two to three weeks and clearance of plaques within one to three months in 75–80% of cases.
- Methotrexate: reduces the turnover rate of superficial skin cells. This drug is reserved for use in treating severe, resistant cases of psoriasis, especially the generalized pustular forms and those with chronic extensive plaque formation that have not responded to safer treatment measures. It may also be beneficial in cases of psoriatic arthritis.

  This drug can be highly effective. However, it has very serious potential toxicity. It can depress bone marrow function, damage liver tissue, and impair kidney function. Avoid alcohol, aspirin, and aspirin substitutes while taking this drug.
- Etretinate: This vitamin A derivative may be used alone or in conjunction with other appropriate treatments, especially PUVA. It provides excellent relief in severe pustular psoriasis and when there is involvement of the palms and soles. This drug should be used only to treat severe, resistant forms of psoriasis that have failed to respond to standard treatments. It can cause major birth defects; significant elevations

of blood triglycerides; and toxic effects on bone marrow, liver, and kidney tissue.

Therapeutic Drug Monitoring (Blood Levels)
The recommended blood level range for methotrexate is up to 0.1 mcmol/L.

Ancillary Drug Treatment (as required)
For itching:
- hydroxyzine (Atarax, Vistaril)

Note: Drug selection, dosage, and administration schedule must be determined by the physician for each patient individually.

Current Controversies in Management
Should doses of psoralen and ultraviolet light (PUVA) and the duration of treatment be reduced to lessen the long-term risk of developing skin cancer?

Comments
PUVA treatment is an established, highly effective therapy for severe psoriasis. The best results are obtained when relatively high doses and extended treatment periods are used. Two recently published research reports demonstrate a significantly increased risk of developing two types of skin cancer five years after initial treatment with PUVA. The risk for squamous cell skin cancer was 12 times greater for those who received over 260 PUVA treatments than for those who received 160 or fewer treatments. The risk for basal cell skin cancer was moderately increased and also dose-related. It is recommended that PUVA treatment dosage be reduced by alternating it with other treatment methods, even if this means less than complete clearing of the skin.

Possible Drug Interactions of Significance
Because of the number and nature of drugs that may be used to manage this disorder, adequate consideration of the volume and complexity of potential drug interactions is beyond the scope of this book. Consult *The Essential Guide to Prescription Drugs*, or a similar drug reference book for possible interactions of significance (see Appendix 17, Drug Information Sources).

Special Considerations for Women
Psoriasis is common in the anogenital area. Recommended treatment is the topical use of low-potency corticosteroid (cortisonelike) preparations. Higher potency preparations should be limited to short-term use. Tar or anthralin preparations are too irritating to use for vulvar psoriasis.

Pregnancy

Methotrexate and etretinate are both designated Pregnancy Category X drugs. Avoid use completely during pregnancy (see Appendix 15, FDA Pregnancy Categories).

Breast-Feeding

Consult your physician regarding the compatibility of nursing and any of the drugs you are taking.

Resources

Additional Information and Services

National Institute of Arthritis and Musculoskeletal and Skin Diseases
Information Office: Building 31, Room 4C32B
9000 Rockville Pike
Bethesda, MD 20892
Phone: Information Specialist, (301) 496-8188
Handles inquiries on arthritis, bone diseases, and skin diseases (including psoriasis).

National Psoriasis Foundation
6443 SW Beaverton Hwy, Suite 210
Portland, OR 97221
Phone: (503) 297-1545; Fax: (503) 292-9341
Patient-oriented publications and services.

Psoriasis Research Association
107 Vista del Grande
San Carlos, CA 94070
Phone: (415) 593-1394
Publications available.

Psoriasis Research Institute
600 Town and Country Village
Palo Alto, CA 94301
Phone: (415) 326-1848; Fax: (415) 326-1262
Maintains Psoriasis Medical Center, providing advanced treatment programs. Publications available.

RECTAL CANCER

Other Names Carcinoma of rectum, adenocarcinoma of rectum

Prevalence/Incidence in U.S.

Estimated new cases annually: 45,000
Estimated deaths annually: 7,300

Age Group Median age is 60 years old

Male-to-Female Ratio Slightly higher incidence in men

Principal Features and Natural History

The rectum is composed of the last 6 inches of the lower intestinal tract, with the anus being the terminal 1.5 inches. Unlike the colon, which is very accessible for surgical procedures, the rectum lies deep within the cramped space of the pelvic basin. This imposes critical consequences on the evolution of malignant disease and its management. Direct invasion by cancer of the rectum can involve the urinary bladder, the prostate gland, seminal vesicles, urethra, ureters, uterus, vagina, sacrum, and small intestine. Unlike colon surgery, rectal surgery does not permit the attainment of adequate disease-free tissue margins during tumor resection. Local failure rates within the pelvis following rectal cancer surgery are quite high: 25–40% for stage II and 40–65% for stage III disease. Postoperative complications of pain, bladder dysfunction, and infection are frequent, hence the importance of adjuvant therapy following surgery.

The primary site for the initiation of cancer is usually well localized within the surface tissues (the mucosa) that cover the inner wall of the rectum. The primary tumor usually begins in the lower part of the rectum adjacent to the anus. Like colon cancer, the characteristic growth pattern of rectal cancer is to first invade the layers of tissue that comprise the wall, and then to extend concentrically around the wall and upward along the wall.

In time the invasive nature and increasing size of the tumor begin to cause symptoms. Early indications of its presence include bright red blood on the surface of the stool (and toilet paper), mild to moderate discomfort with stool passage, and eventual tenesmus—painful, ineffective straining during defecation. If discovery and treatment of the tumor are delayed, additional symptoms related to local invasion of adjacent tissues develop: pelvic pain, impaired urination, vaginal discharge, local infection.

At the time of discovery, rectal cancer can be found in any of the following stages:

Stage 0, carcinoma-in-situ: localized within surface cells of the rectal wall; no invasion; no spread to lymph nodes; no distant metastases

Stage I: tumor invades into the muscle layer of the rectal wall and extends around the rectal–anal junction; no spread to lymph nodes; no distant metastases

Stage II: tumor penetrates through all layers of the rectal wall and extends a greater distance upward into the rectal pouch; no spread to lymph nodes; no distant metastases

Stage III: tumor increases in size; spread to regional lymph nodes; no distant metastases

Stage IV: tumor of any size; spread to regional lymph nodes; regional invasion of adjacent tissues; distant metastases to liver, lung, etc.

Diagnostic Symptoms and Signs

Rectal bleeding (65–90%)

A change in the pattern of bowel movements: looseness or constipation (45–80%)

Rectal pain or pressure sensation (10–25%)

Change in stool caliber or shape

Rectal discharge

A feeling that the rectum does not empty completely on defecation

Tenesmus—prolonged, ineffective straining at stool

A mass that can be felt on digital rectal examination (65–80%)

ALERT!

It is not uncommon for rectal bleeding to be attributed to hemorrhoids and the true source of the bleeding (rectal cancer) to go undetected for long periods of time. All episodes of rectal bleeding should be investigated promptly to determine their cause.

Diagnostic Tests and Procedures

Battery of laboratory tests: complete blood cell counts, urine analysis, liver function tests, appropriate blood chemistries, CEA assay (carcinoembryonic antigen)

Digital rectal examination

Anoscopic, proctoscopic, and sigmoidoscopic examinations.

Transrectal sonography

X-ray studies of the colon: barium enemas with air contrast to detect polyps and tumors at higher levels in the bowel

X-ray studies of the lungs for metastases

CT scans of the pelvis for tumor extension and of the liver for metastases

Diagnostic "Markers" for This Disorder

The identification of cancer cells in biopsy specimens obtained during proctoscopic or sigmoidoscopic examination.

Similar Conditions That May Confuse Diagnosis

Diverticulitis of the descending or sigmoid colon with bleeding

Active ulcerative colitis or proctitis

Active Crohn's disease involving the rectum and anus

Causes

Established Causes

The definitive cause of rectal cancer is not known at this time.

Theoretical Causes

Genetic predisposition

High-animal-fat, low-fiber diet: causes increased concentration of bile acids in the colon and rectum, slows passage of food residues, enhances the action of carcinogenic (cancer-causing) agents

Known Risk Factors for Developing This Disorder

Family history of colon or rectal cancer in a parent or sibling

Family history of familial polyposis (very strong risk factor)

Personal history of ulcerative colitis or Crohn's disease of colon (strong risk factor)

Personal history of colon or rectal polyps

For women: personal history of breast, ovarian, or uterine cancer

High intake of salt-cured, salt-pickled, and smoked foods

Excessive alcohol consumption

Goals of Treatment

Can This Disorder Be Cured?

Disease-free periods of five years ("cures") can be achieved in 75–100% (average 85%) in Stage I rectal cancer when:

- the cancer has been detected early.
- the cancer is confined to a relatively small area of the rectum.
- the tumor can be carefully removed with wide clear margins.
- there has been no spread to regional lymph nodes.
- there has been no distant spread to other organs.
- postoperative radiation therapy or chemotherapy was used as warranted.

Can This Disorder Be Treated Effectively?

Appropriate use of surgery, radiation therapy, and adjuvant chemotherapy can significantly reduce morbidity and improve survival in selected patients.

Specific Goals

- Early diagnosis of operable cases
- Accurate staging to determine optimal therapy
- Successful removal of all malignant tissues
- Optimal use of radiation therapy and adjuvant chemotherapy
- Maximal periods of disease-free postoperative life
- Maintenance of an acceptable quality of life

Health Professionals Who Participate in Managing This Disorder

Family physicians
General internists
Gastroenterologists
Radiologists
General surgeons
Proctologists
Colon/Rectal surgeons
Pathologists
Medical oncologists
Surgical oncologists
Radiation oncologists
Nurse oncologists
Enterostomal therapists
Psychiatrists
Dietitians
Medical social workers
Pastoral counselors

Currently Available Therapies for This Disorder

Surgery

- Polypectomies: removal of polyps from the rectum
- Abdominoperineal resection or low anterior resection of the rectum
- Colostomy: surgical creation of an opening (stoma) between the colon and the surface of the abdomen to facilitate defecation
- Resection of selected metastases in liver or lung

Radiation Therapy

- Preoperative X-ray treatment to reduce the size of tumors in preparation for removal
- Postoperative X-ray treatment to destroy cancer cells remaining in the operative area
- Palliative X-ray treatment to relieve pain or control bleeding in patients whose tumors cannot be removed

Chemotherapy

The following drugs are used in various combinations as adjuvant therapy following surgery or as palliative therapy for inoperable cancer.

- 5-fluorouracil
- folinic acid
- leucovorin
- levamisole
- methotrexate
- vincristine

Management of Therapy

The optimal treatment of rectal cancer is determined by the stage of disease at the time of discovery. The following treatment options are those in current use.

For Stage 0, Carcinoma-in-situ

- Local excision (tissue removal) or simple polypectomy (polyp removal) with clear margins

For Stage I

- Abdominoperineal or low anterior resection; removal of lymph nodes
- Radiation therapy for selected cases
- Chemotherapy not recommended

For Stage II

- Abdominoperineal or anterior resection; removal of lymph nodes
- Adjuvant (auxiliary) radiation therapy postoperatively
- Concurrent chemotherapy and radiation therapy

For Stage III

- If tumor is nonresectable, perform colostomy
- Adjuvant radiation therapy preoperatively with surgical reassessment
- If tumor is then resectable, use adjuvant radiation therapy postoperatively
- Concurrent chemotherapy and radiation therapy

For Stage IV

- This stage denotes significant local disease and spread (metastasis) to distant organs
- If tumor is nonresectable, perform colostomy
- Palliative radiation therapy to control pain or bleeding
- Referral to clinical trials investigating new drugs and biological therapies

Ancillary Drug Treatment (as required)

For pain management:

see Appendix 3, Cancer Pain Management

For control of nausea and vomiting:

see Appendix 4, Management of Nausea and Vomiting Associated with Cancer Chemotherapy

Note: Drug selection, dosage, and administration schedule must be determined by the physician for each patient individually.

Treatment Outcomes

For stage I disease: five-year survival averages 85% (range 75–100%)
For stage II disease: five-year survival averages 65% (range 40–80%)

For stage III disease: five-year survival averages 40% (range 15–60%)
For stage IV disease: five-year survival is less than 5%

Special Considerations for Women

A personal history of breast, ovarian, or uterine cancer may increase your
risk for developing colon/rectal cancer. Observe all preventive measures.
Utilize early detection procedures.

Pregnancy

Drugs used for cancer chemotherapy are contraindicated during pregnancy (see Appendix 15, FDA Pregnancy Categories).

Breast-Feeding

Avoid chemotherapeutic drugs or refrain from nursing.

Special Considerations for the Elderly

Age greater than 70 years is not a contraindication for standard treatments
for colon/rectal cancer. Long-term survival is clearly achievable in the
elderly.

Quality of Life Considerations

For some patients who undergo abdominoperineal resections for rectal
cancer, a permanent colostomy may be unavoidable. Enterostomal therapists are available to teach patients how to manage colostomies properly
and how to resume a fully active and acceptable way of life. The United
Ostomy Association is a national support group that provides information
and services for ostomy patients; see "Resources" below.

The Role of Prevention in This Disorder

Primary Prevention
- Eat a low-fat, high-fiber diet: fruits, vegetables, and whole grain
  cereals;
- Avoid salt-cured, salt-pickled, and smoked foods.
- Avoid excessive alcohol consumption.
- Maintain bowel regularity with diet and fiber; avoid constipation.
- Obtain prompt removal of all polyps when found.

Secondary Prevention
- Fecal test for occult (hidden) blood annually beginning at age 40
  years, which may be of limited value because of frequent false-positive
  and false-negative test results
- Digital rectal examination annually beginning at age 40 years
- Sigmoidoscopy every three to five years beginning at age 50 years
- Colonoscopy every three to five years beginning at age 18 years if
  there is a history of familial polyposis or a personal history of adeno-

matous polyps or ulcerative colitis; beginning at 40 years of age if there is a history of two or more first-degree relatives with colon cancer

Resources

Recommended Reading

What You Need to Know About Cancer of the Colon and Rectum, National Cancer Institute, NIH Publication No. 94-1552, April 1994. For a copy call the Cancer Information Service, 1-800-4-CANCER.

The Cancer Patient's Handbook: Everything You Need to Know About Today's Care and Treatment, Mary-Ellen Siegel, M.S.W. New York: Walker and Company, 1986.

Additional Information and Services

The Cancer Information Service
Phone: 1-800-422-6237, 1-800-4-CANCER
Questions answered in English or Spanish.

American Cancer Society (ACS)
1599 Clifton Road, NE
Atlanta, GA 30329
Phone: 1-800-ACS-2345

United Ostomy Association
36 Executive Park, Suite 120
Irvine, CA 92714
Phone: (714) 660-8624

Disease Management Expertise

See Appendix 2, Part One: The National Cancer Institute Designated Cancer Centers and Part Two: Clinical Trials.

RHEUMATOID ARTHRITIS

Other Names RA, atrophic arthritis, chronic inflammatory arthritis, proliferative arthritis

Prevalence/Incidence in U.S. Approximately 2.1 million—1% of the general population

Age Group Affects all ages, infancy to senescence. Usual onset is between 20 and 50 years. Mean age at onset is 30 to 40 years.

Male-to-Female Ratio In 20- to 50-years-old age group, more common in women, 3 to 1. Over 50 years, same incidence in men and women.

Principal Features and Natural History

Rheumatoid arthritis is a highly complex, chronic inflammatory disorder that can affect several systems of the body simultaneously. It is quite variable in its manifestations. It may last a few days or up to 50 years. It may affect a single joint or up to 60 joints. It may involve the skin, eyes, nervous system, lungs, heart, blood vessels, and spleen. It can be mild, moderately severe, or life-threatening in its most virulent forms. It usually begins with fatigue, poor appetite, loss of weight, morning stiffness, and joint pains. Initially the small joints of the hands, wrists, and feet are affected. Larger joints may be affected later. The painful and destructive disease of the joints is the major feature of this disorder. The disease process begins with a severe inflammation of the joint lining (synovial membrane). This is followed by the formation of thick granulation tissue that ultimately destroys joint cartilage, bone, and adjacent ligaments. The affected joints are swollen, warm, tender, stiff, and painful to use. After a sustained period of active disease, joint destruction results in irreversible deformity. All of the joints that are affected will show evidence of disease within the first two years. Ten percent of cases will have a spontaneous complete remission (recovery) within 6 to 24 months after the onset of symptoms.

Diagnostic Symptoms and Signs

Malaise, fatigability, weakness, low-grade fever

Loss of appetite and weight

Morning stiffness in joints

Painful, swollen, inflamed joints in fingers, wrists, and feet of symmetrical distribution

Rheumatoid nodules adjacent to involved joints

Eventual joint deformities

Diagnostic Tests and Procedures

Blood test for presence of rheumatoid factor (RF); positive in 80% of RA patients

Red blood cell sedimentation rate (see Glossary) characteristically elevated; useful in judging severity of disease and monitoring disease activity

Blood assay of antinuclear antibodies (ANA); positive in 30% of RA patients

Synovial (joint) fluid examination: high white blood cell counts indicative of active inflammation

X-ray examination of affected joints: characteristic findings consistent with RA

ALERT!

Rheumatoid factor (RF) is the single most useful test for diagnosing RA. However, it is often negative during the first several months of active disease. It may remain negative in 20% of RA patients; this does not exclude the diagnosis of RA. Rheumatoid factor is also found in numerous other systemic diseases.

Similar Conditions That May Confuse Diagnosis

Osteoarthritis
Ankylosing spondylitis
Psoriatic arthritis
Reiter's syndrome
Systemic lupus erythematosus
Systemic sclerosis (scleroderma)
Lyme disease
Gout
Pseudogout (calcium pyrophosphate deposition disorder)

Causes

Established Causes

A specific definitive cause for rheumatoid arthritis has not been established.

Theoretical Causes

There is evidence to support the theory that the disease process is initiated by a virus that infects the joints of individuals who are genetically susceptible because of a defective immune system. RA is now considered to be an autoimmune disease (see Appendix 5, The Immune System).

Drugs That Can Cause This Disorder

There are no drugs that induce true rheumatoid arthritis. The following drugs may aggravate an active or latent arthritis: BCG vaccine, iron-dextran (Imferon), isoniazid and pyrazinamide (in combination), levamisole.

Goals of Treatment

Can This Disorder Be Cured?

There is no curative treatment available at this time.

Can This Disorder Be Treated Effectively?

Available medications can relieve symptoms effectively and in some cases arrest progression of the disease.

Specific Goals
- Relief of pain, tenderness, and stiffness
- Control of inflammation in joint tissues
- Production of remission; arrest of active disease
- Prevention of joint destruction; preservation of joint function

Health Professionals Who Participate in Managing This Disorder

Family physicians
General internists
Pediatricians
Rheumatologists
Clinical immunologists
Hand surgeons
Orthopedic surgeons
Physiatrists
Pharmacists
Physician assistants
Nurse practitioners
Physical therapists
Occupational therapists
Medical social workers

Currently Available Therapies for This Disorder

Drug Therapy

There are no drugs that can cure rheumatoid arthritis. The drugs currently available for use in managing this form of arthritis fall into two groups: (1) those that relieve symptoms but do not alter the basic disease process (do not produce remission); (2) those that *may* retard or arrest the disease and initiate remission.

DRUGS USED TO RELIEVE SYMPTOMS

Salicylates:
- aspirin (Bufferin, Ascriptin, Cama, etc.)
- aspirin, enteric-coated (Easprin, Ecotrin, etc.)
- aspirin, zero-order-release (Zorprin)
- magnesium salicylate (Magan, Mobidin)
- choline magnesium salicylate (Trisilate)
- salsalate (Disalcid)
- diflunisal (Dolobid)
- sodium salicylate (Pabalate)

Other nonsteroidal anti-inflammatory drugs (NSAIDs):
- Acetic acid derivatives:
  - diclofenac (Cataflam, Voltaren)

- etodolac (Lodine)
- indomethacin (Indochron E-R, Indocin SR)
- ketorolac (Toradol)
- nabumetone (Relafen)
- sulindac (Clinoril)
- tolmetin (Tolectin, Tolectin DS)
- Propionic acid derivatives:
  - fenoprofen (Nalfon)
  - flurbiprofen (Ansaid)
  - ibuprofen (Advil, Motrin, Rufen, etc.)
  - ketoprofen (Orudis, Oruvail)
  - naproxen (Aleve, Anaprox, Anaprox DS, Naprosyn)
  - oxaprozin (Daypro)
  - suprofen (Suprol)
- Fenamic acid derivatives:
  - meclofenamate (Meclomen)
  - mefenamic acid (Ponstel)
- Oxicam derivative:
  - piroxicam (Feldene)

Cortisonelike steroid drugs:
- prednisone
- triamcinolone (Aristocort)
- dexamethasone (Decadron)
- methylprednisolone (Medrol)

Immunosuppressive drugs:
- azathioprine (Imuran)
- chlorambucil (Leukeran)
- cyclophosphamide (Cytoxan)
- cyclosporine (Sandimmune)
- methotrexate (Mexate)

DRUGS USED TO PRODUCE REMISSION
- Gold preparations:
  - auranofin (Ridaura)
  - aurothioglucose (Solganal)
  - gold sodium thiomalate (Myochrysine)
- hydroxychloroquine (Plaquenil)
- penicillamine (Cuprimine, Depen)
- sulfasalazine (Azulfidine)

Nondrug Treatment Methods
- Physical therapy is a most important part of management.
- Surgical procedures to remove diseased tissues and repair damaged joints.

Management of Therapy

Rheumatoid arthritis can be the most difficult of all arthritic disorders to control. In its more severe forms, it is the most damaging to joint tissues. Its course is usually intermittent to chronic. If the diagnosis is made early and if adequate treatment is started promptly, severe crippling can often be prevented or minimized.

Every case of rheumatoid arthritis is a unique, individual problem. Successful management depends upon a treatment program that is carefully individualized. Many drugs are available to treat rheumatoid arthritis. None is curative, and none is effective in all cases. Drugs that control inflammation can provide symptomatic relief but do not modify the underlying disease process; they cannot induce a remission. Disease-altering drugs are used in an attempt to modify the actual disease process and thereby initiate a remission. If successful, maintenance drug treatment may be continued for months or years.

Treatment is usually started with the safest and best tolerated drugs. There is marked individual variation in response to most drugs. This is very apparent with the use of the nonsteroidal anti-inflammatory drugs (aspirin substitutes). Trial-and-error experimentation is necessary to find the most effective and acceptable anti-inflammatory drug for each person.

Drug treatment of rheumatoid arthritis often requires a combination of drugs. The more severe forms of RA respond most favorably when a disease-modifying drug is added to an established program of salicylates or NSAIDs (see drugs listed above).

Use of Salicylates

- Aspirin is often the first drug used to provide adequate anti-inflammatory effects. It must be taken in large doses. A trial of salicylates is indicated in all cases of rheumatoid arthritis unless there is a history of aspirin allergy, peptic ulcer disease, gastritis, or gastrointestinal bleeding.

- Aspirin preparations that are designed for absorption in the small intestine (instead of in the stomach) are preferred: Disalcid, Easprin, Ecotrin, Zorprin. The measurement of salicylate blood levels is advisable to determine the optimal dose of the salicylate used and to avoid serious toxicity. Warning symptoms of early salicylate toxicity are ringing in the ears (tinnitus) and loss of hearing. However, these may not occur in the very young or in the elderly. Approximately 50% of patients cannot tolerate the large doses of aspirin required to achieve adequate anti-inflammatory effects. Other salicylates may be tried or a nonsteroidal anti-inflammatory drug may be substituted.

Use of Other Nonsteroidal Anti-Inflammatory Drugs (NSAIDs)

- These may be used as substitutes for aspirin by those who cannot tolerate (or should not take) salicylates, or they may be used to initiate treatment at the outset. As a group the NSAIDs are not superior to salicy-lates in anti-inflammatory effect, but they are generally better tolerated.

- These drugs produce significant decrease in morning stiffness, improve comfort and function, and may be more effective than aspirin for some. Fenoprofen and naproxen are among the more active NSAIDs. A trial of two weeks will identify those who can respond favorably.
- Response to NSAIDs is highly variable from person to person. If an NSAID from one chemical class proves to be ineffective or unaccept-able, a drug from another class within the NSAID group should be tried. A trial of two weeks is usually adequate to determine effective-ness and tolerance (see Appendix 8, Nonsteroidal Anti-Inflammatory Drugs (NSAIDs): A Guide to Selection for Therapy).

Use of Cortisonelike Steroid Drugs

- Steroids are used infrequently and for short periods of time in both acute and chronic stages of rheumatoid arthritis. They are always added to existing drug programs as needed. Their use is justified, in small doses, to control acute "flares" of inflammation that prevent any degree of mobility in severely diseased joints.
- Steroids provide a powerful anti-inflammatory effect, but they do not alter the underlying disease process or induce remission. They should be used to provide short-term comfort as necessary but not to abolish all symptoms.
- Long-term maintenance use of steroids—even in small doses—must be avoided. Risks of excessive use include cataracts, osteoporosis, muscle wasting, atherosclerosis (see Appendix 6, Long-Term Corticosteroid Therapy).

Use of Immunosuppressive Drugs

- These highly toxic and hazardous drugs are used only when arthritis activity persists in spite of combined treatment with NSAIDs and dis-ease-modifying agents. They are used in an attempt to prevent further joint destruction, deformity, and disability.
- Methotrexate is often the first choice of this group to try in the treat-ment of severe rheumatoid arthritis that has not responded to conven-tional therapy. In low dosage it can be very effective in approximately 50% of patients. Potential risks include severe depression of the bone marrow, liver damage, ulceration of the mouth and intestine, and birth defects. Avoid alcohol and salicylates during methotrexate therapy.
- Cyclophosphamide is the most effective drug of this group. Its use is reserved for patients with disabling systemic complications of rheuma-toid arthritis.

Use of Gold Preparations

- Based upon long experience with its use, gold is the standard disease-modifying drug for treating rheumatoid arthritis. It is often the first choice to add to an established program of NSAID therapy. Gold is used only when arthritis cannot be controlled with safer drugs. A trial of six months or longer is necessary to determine its ability to induce remission. Approximately 50% of patients respond favorably.

- Risks of gold therapy include dermatitis, kidney damage, and blood cell and bone marrow toxicity. Treatment should be stopped immediately if any of the following develop: skin rash, mouth ulcers, fever, sore throat, abnormal bleeding or bruising.

Use of Hydroxychloroquine

- This drug is used to treat mild or moderately severe rheumatoid arthritis. It can be very effective in some cases, relieving symptoms and retarding disease activity. A trial of six months is necessary to determine this drug's ability to induce remission.
- After one year of continual use, this drug can (rarely) damage eye structures and impair vision. Corneal deposits, retinal pigmentation, and optic neuritis have been reported. The estimated incidence is 1 in 1,000 to 1 in 2,000 patients. Other possible adverse drug effects include skin rash, abnormally low white blood cell count, and peripheral neuritis (see Glossary).
- This drug can aggravate existing psoriasis.

Use of Penicillamine

- This drug is an effective substitute for gold therapy when a disease-modifying drug is needed. A trial of 6 to 12 months is necessary to determine its ability to induce remission. For maximal effectiveness, this drug should be taken on an empty stomach.
- This is a potent drug! It can cause the following adverse effects: dermatitis, kidney damage, blood cell and bone marrow toxicity, bronchiolitis (dry cough and shortness of breath), and a pattern of muscular weakness similar to myasthenia gravis.

Therapeutic Drug Monitoring (Blood Levels)

Recommended blood level range for salicylates: 100–250 mcg/ml.

Ancillary Drug Treatment (as required)

For additional analgesia:
- propoxyphene (Darvon)
- hydrocodone (Vicodin) (for short-term, intermittent use only)

For night pain:
- indomethacin (Indocin) (taken with food at bedtime)

For anemia:
- iron preparations
- folic acid (if appropriate for type of anemia)

For anxiety and tension:
- diazepam (Valium)

For depression:
- fluoxetine (Prozac)
- tricyclic antidepressants (see Profile of depression in this section)

For drug-induced peptic ulcer:
- cimetidine (Tagamet)
- famotidine (Pepcid)
- nizatidine (Axid)
- ranitidine (Zantac) (see Profile of peptic ulcer in this section)
- See Profile of peptic ulcer in this section.

Note: Drug selection, dosage, and administration schedule must be determined by the physician for each patient individually.

Possible Drug Interactions of Significance

Because of the number and nature of drugs that may be used to manage this disorder, adequate consideration of the volume and complexity of potential drug interactions is beyond the scope of this book. Consult *The Essential Guide to Prescription Drugs*, or a similar drug reference book for possible interactions of significance (see Appendix 17, Drug Information Sources).

Special Considerations for Women

Pregnancy

Many of the drugs used to treat RA are contraindicated during pregnancy. Ask your physician for guidance if you are pregnant or planning pregnancy.

Breast-Feeding

Consult your physician regarding the compatibility of nursing and any of the drugs you are taking.

Resources

Recommended Reading

Primer on the Rheumatic Diseases, 10th edition, H.R. Schumacher, M.D. Atlanta: The Arthritis Foundation, 1993.

The Duke University Medical Center Book of Arthritis, D.S. Pisetsky, M.D., Ph.D., and S.F. Trien. New York: Fawcett-Columbine, 1992.

Arthritis: A Comprehensive Guide to Understanding Your Arthritis, J.F. Fries, M.D. Reading, MA: Addison-Wesley, 1990.

Additional Information and Services

Arthritis Foundation
1314 Spring Street
Atlanta, GA 30309
Phone: (404) 872-7100, 1-800-283-7800; Fax: (404) 872-0457
Publications available.

National Arthritis and Musculoskeletal and Skin Diseases Information
Clearinghouse
9000 Rockville Pike
P.O. Box AMS
Bethesda, MD 20892-2903
Phone: (301) 495-4484; Fax: (301) 587-4352

Disease Management Expertise
SPECIALIZED CENTERS OF RESEARCH
Duke Medical Center
Box 3258
Durham, NC 17710
Phone: (919) 684-5093; Fax: (919) 684-5230

University of Michigan
4570 Kresge 1
Ann Arbor, MI 48109-0531
Phone: (313) 763-0308; Fax: (313) 763-8974

University of Tennessee
956 Court Avenue, G326
Memphis, TN 38163
Phone: (901) 448-5774; Fax: (901) 448-7265

University of Texas SW Medical Center
5323 Harry Hines Boulevard
Dallas, TX 75235-8884
Phone: (214) 648-8350; Fax: (214) 648-7995

SCHIZOPHRENIA

Other Name Dementia praecox

Prevalence/Incidence in U.S.
Current estimate: approximately 2.4 million—1% of the general population
Estimated new cases annually: 100,000

Age Group Onset most common between 16 and 25 years of age.
Onset uncommon after 30 and rare after 40 years of age.

Male-to-Female Ratio Equal incidence in men and women

Principal Features and Natural History
Schizophrenia refers to a group of disorders of the brain manifested by
severe disturbances of the mind and personality. Cardinal features are

abnormal thinking, behavior, and mood. The schizophrenic pattern is characterized by misinterpretation of reality, withdrawal, delusions, hallucinations (usually auditory), and bizarre or regressive behavior. It usually begins early in life, may be mild and transient in nature, or may develop into a psychosis of major dimension that is intermittent or chronic for life.

The first group—referred to as schizophreniform—experiences one episode of varying severity (often in response to stress), responds well to treatment, and has no relapse after treatment is stopped.

The second group—classical chronic schizophrenia—experiences recurrent episodes of disabling symptoms that require long-term antipsychotic drug therapy for control. Most of this group will relapse if maintenance treatment is stopped.

A variety of subtypes are identified according to their dominant features: delusions of persecution and grandeur (paranoid type); primitive mentality, markedly disorganized thought and behavior (hebephrenic type); withdrawn, negativistic, uncommunicative, apathetic behavior pattern (catatonic); disorganized thinking, delusions, hallucinations accompanied by either mania or depression (schizo-affective); insidious loss of motivation and ambition, avoidance of interpersonal relationships (simple type); mixed or indefinite symptom complex (undifferentiated type).

Though the presentations may vary according to type, the same group of antipsychotic drugs is used to treat all types without distinction.

Diagnostic Symptoms and Signs
Inability to recognize and identify with reality
Vivid hallucinations
Bizarre delusions
Disorganized speech, irrelevance, and incoherence
Markedly disorganized behavior
Impaired ability to function appropriately in all settings: social, occupational, self-care

Diagnostic Tests and Procedures
There are no routine laboratory tests that diagnose schizophrenia.
Detailed psychological examinations are usually diagnostic.
Electroencephalograms (EEG): abnormal but not diagnostic findings in many cases.
Computed tomography of brain (CT scans): evidence of decreased brain mass.
Positron emission tomography (PET scans): decreased metabolism in the frontal lobes of the brain.

Similar Conditions That May Confuse Diagnosis
Substance abuse: intoxication or withdrawal symptoms

Schizo-affective disorder: features of manic-depressive illness
Personality disorders with periods of psychotic symptoms

Causes

Established Causes

The fundamental cause of schizophrenia is unknown. No specific diagnostic anatomical or biochemical abnormality of the brain has been identified.

Theoretical Causes

Studies suggest that a genetic predisposition is necessary for the development of schizophrenia, rendering the subject vulnerable to disturbances of neurochemical transmission of nerve impulses or to alterations of brain circuitry. Effective antipsychotic drugs block dopamine receptors in certain brain cells. This suggests that altered dopamine activity is somehow responsible for the schizophrenic syndrome.

Known Risk Factors for Developing This Disorder

A positive family history of schizophrenia. Identical twin pairs who are genetically predisposed will develop schizophrenia in 47% of cases.

Drugs That Can Cause This Disorder

The following drugs may aggravate existing schizophrenia or produce schizophrenialike symptoms in normal individuals:

albuterol
alcohol (intoxication)
amantadine
amphetamines (abuse)
anticonvulsants
apomorphine
atropinelike drugs
bromides
bromocriptine
cimetidine
cocaine
cortisonelike steroids
digitalis
disopyramide
disulfiram (toxicity)
indomethacin
isoniazid
levodopa
methyldopa
propranolol

tocainide
triazolam

Goals of Treatment

Can This Disorder Be Cured?

There is no curative treatment available at this time.

Can This Disorder Be Treated Effectively?

Available medications and counseling can control symptoms of this disorder in approximately 70% of cases. However, satisfactory control depends upon long-term compliance with recommended therapy: combined psychotherapy and antipsychotic drug therapy.

Specific Goals

- Good control of symptoms with the lowest possible doses of antipsychotic drugs
- Determination of the most effective drug and dosage schedule for each individual: intermittent dosage (as needed) versus continual long-term dosage
- Prevention of relapse (recurrent psychotic episode)
- Improvement of capacity to function in society as normally as possible

Health Professionals Who Participate in Managing This Disorder

Family physicians
General internists
Psychiatrists
Neuropsychiatrists
Neurologists
Pharmacists
Physician assistants
Psychiatric nurse practitioners
Mental health social workers

Currently Available Therapies for This Disorder

Drug Therapy

PHENOTHIAZINES
Aliphatic type:
- chlorpromazine (Thorazine)
Piperazine type:
- perphenazine (Trilafon)
- trifluoperazine (Stelazine)
- fluphenazine (Prolixin, Permitil)

Piperidine type:
- thioridazine (Mellaril)
- mesoridazine (Serentil)

THIOXANTHENES
- thiothixene (Navane)

BUTYROPHENONES
- haloperidol (Haldol)

DIBENZOXAZEPINES
- loxapine (Loxitane)

DIHYDROINDOLONES
- molindone (Moban)

DIBENZODIAZEPINE
- clozapine (Clozaril)

BENZISOXAZOLE
- risperidone (Risperdal)

Nondrug Treatment Methods
- Hospitalization as required for diagnosis, determination of optimal drug therapy, and patient safety (in the event of suicidal ideation)
- Psychotherapy to improve compliance with all aspects of the treatment program
- Electroconvulsive therapy (ECT) in severe cases that are unresponsive to conventional drug therapy.

Management of Therapy
- The primary management of schizophrenia is based upon the rational use of antipsychotic drugs. Psychotherapy and drug therapy are considered to be complementary. Psychotherapy can improve the patient's social adjustment; drug therapy can control disabling symptoms and make the situation somewhat manageable. Neither therapy is curative.
- If appropriate drug treatment is started early, 30–50% of patients will have a satisfactory remission. Another 30% will improve sufficiently to live outside of a hospital. Drug therapy can abolish delusions, hallucinations, hyperactivity, and combative behavior. Approximately 10–20% of patients do not respond to any drugs currently available.
- The initial treatment of an acute psychotic episode consists of a course of carefully selected antipsychotic drugs taken for 6 to 12 months. Many individuals will respond favorably to one drug and not at all to another. History of previous drug use and response can be very helpful in selecting a drug for the management of recurrent episodes.
- Current practice is to attempt withdrawal of antipsychotic drugs from all patients who have had a good response to drug treatment during their first episode of schizophrenia. This allows identification of those who will have a self-limited type of schizophrenia (schizophreniform

disorder) and will do well without maintenance drug therapy. Fifteen to thirty percent of patients will recover spontaneously following the initial episode and drug withdrawal. Antipsychotic drugs should be discontinued gradually over a period of one to two weeks.

- The majority of schizophrenic patients will require continual drug therapy for long periods of time—possibly for life. Many will relapse rapidly and severely after drugs are discontinued. The nature of the drug maintenance program is determined by the type and frequency of continuing psychotic symptoms and the pattern of relapses experienced by each individual. When the patient complies well, maintenance drug therapy is successful in 85% of cases.

- The principal action of antipsychotic drugs is to block dopamine receptors in the brain. By blocking dopamine action in the mesolimbic system, the drugs control the abnormal manifestations of schizophrenia. By blocking dopamine action in the nigrostriatal system, the drugs cause parkinsonism (and related adverse effects). Thus parkinsonism is now recognized as an *unavoidable* side effect of most antipsychotic drugs. It is usually very responsive to the anticholinergic drugs used to treat Parkinson's disease, but not to levodopa (see Profile of Parkinson's disease in this section).

- It is generally recommended that antiparkinsonism drugs *not* be used routinely while taking antipsychotic drugs. Reasons given are: (1) antiparkinsonism drugs can produce toxic brain syndromes; (2) they can interfere with the effectiveness of antipsychotic drugs; (3) they may increase the risk of developing tardive dyskinesia. This condition (see Glossary) is one of the most serious adverse effects of long-term antipsychotic drug use. The reported incidence ranges from 3% after one year of medication to 21% after seven years of medication. It appears to occur more frequently in elderly women.

- "Drug holidays" of four to six weeks without medication are being used by some physicians treating chronic schizophrenia to reduce the risk of developing tardive dyskinesia. Among those who have been on maintenance therapy for one year without relapsing, 66% will not relapse within six months after stopping medication. For this group of patients, a "drug holiday" is feasible and possibly beneficial.

- Antipsychotic drugs usually improve behavior. However, excessively high doses can cause a toxic state that worsens behavior. Drug response and tolerance vary greatly from person to person and must be monitored carefully in each individual.

- Patients with schizo-affective disorders will probably require an antipsychotic drug and an additional drug for the affective component—mania or depression. This could be either lithium or an antidepressant.

- Lithium may aggravate the neurological complications of antipsychotic drug therapy. The concurrent use of these two drugs requires caution and careful monitoring.

Use of Phenothiazines

- Because of its numerous side effects, chlorpromazine (the first phenothiazine) is used less frequently.
- Because of its relatively greater sedative effects, thioridazine is favored for treatment of acute psychotic episodes. It causes parkinsonism (and possibly tardive dyskinesia) less frequently.
- Fluphenazine is less sedating but is thought to have a higher risk for causing parkinsonism and tardive dyskinesia.
- Trifluoperazine is thought to be preferable for the elderly schizophrenic because it has less sedative and atropinelike side effects.

Use of Thiothixene

- This antipsychotic drug is thought to be more effective for the retarded and regressed schizophrenic. It has less sedative and atropinelike side effects, but a higher risk for causing parkinsonism.
- Because of its mild antidepressant effect, this drug is preferred for the schizo-affective patient who has features of depression.

Use of Haloperidol

- This drug is reported to be effective in patients who are not responsive to chlorpromazine, as it can control aggressive behavior without causing significant sedation.
- Although it has a relatively high potential for causing parkinsonism (and related effects), it is useful in the elderly because it is less sedating and has fewer atropinelike side effects.

Use of Loxapine

- This drug is especially useful in treating the paranoid schizophrenic.
- It is less sedating than chlorpromazine and equal to haloperidol in effectiveness.

Use of Molindone

- This is the only antipsychotic drug that appears to contribute to weight loss. Many antipsychotic drugs tend to promote weight gain.
- This drug is as effective as other major antipsychotics and is less sedating than many.

Use of Clozapine

- This drug is very effective in treating patients who have hallucinations, delusions, and thought disturbances that have not responded to conventional drug therapy.
- It also has a significantly lower potential for causing tardive dyskinesia (see Glossary) with long-term use.

- During the first year of use, this drug can induce a serious decrease in certain white blood cells (granulocytes) in 1–2% of patients. For this reason patients taking clozapine are required to have weekly white blood cell counts to detect this adverse effect early.
- Concurrent intake of caffeine-containing beverages may cause marked increase in clozapine blood levels with toxic effects.

Use of Risperidone
- This drug is effective in treating both the "positive" and the "negative" features of schizophrenia. "Positive" features include delusions, hallucinations, and disordered thinking; "negative" features include depression, social withdrawal, and apathy.
- It has a low potential for causing Parkinson-like side effects. Possible adverse effects include fatigue, excessive sleep, nervousness, loss of appetite, and decreased libido.

Therapeutic Drug Monitoring (Blood Levels)
- Recommended blood level range for chlorpromazine: 50–300 ng/ml
- Recommended blood level range for thioridazine: 50–300 ng/ml

Ancillary Drug Treatment (as required)
For anxiety:
- buspirone (Buspar)

For depression:
  see Profile of depression in this section

For insomnia:
- chloral hydrate
- temazepam (Restoril)

For constipation:
- docusate (Colace, etc.)
- docusate with casanthranol (Peri-Colace)

For parkinsonism:
- benztropine (Cogentin)
- trihexyphenidyl (Artane)

For akathisia (marked restlessness):
- propranolol (Inderal)
- diphenhydramine (Benadryl)

Note: Drug selection, dosage, and administration schedule must be determined by the physician for each patient individually.

Current Controversies in Management
Is "low-dose" antipsychotic drug therapy feasible for maintenance following release from the hospital?

The vast majority of schizophrenic individuals will experience a return of symptoms shortly after discontinuing a stabilizing maintenance dose of effective medication. Conventional practice has not favored reduction of dosage that proved effective for long-term maintenance. Recent studies have shown that many responsive and stabilized schizophrenic patients can be maintained satisfactorily at home (following hospital discharge) with one-fifth of the usually prescribed dose of injectable, long-acting fluphenazine: 5 mg every two weeks instead of the standard 25 mg dose. Patients on low-dose maintenance therapy adjusted better to family and work situations, were less apathetic, and experienced fewer adverse drug effects. The lower dosage may also reduce the potential for the development of tardive dyskinesia (see Glossary).

Possible Drug Interactions of Significance

Because of the number and nature of drugs that may be used to manage this disorder, adequate consideration of the volume and complexity of potential drug interactions is beyond the scope of this book. Consult *The Essential Guide to Prescription Drugs,* or a similar drug reference book for possible interactions of significance (see Appendix 17, Drug Information Sources).

Special Considerations for Women

Pregnancy is ill-advised for the woman with schizophrenia. Discuss all aspects of this with your personal physician (see Appendix 11, Genetic Disorders and Gene Therapy, for recommendations regarding genetic counseling).

Quality of Life Considerations

Depending upon the type and severity of schizophrenia that you are experiencing, its impact on the quality of your life will be proportionately negative. To the greatest extent possible, take advantage of the supportive psychotherapy available to you. Gaining insight and understanding of your situation will enhance your compliance with treatment programs. This is the key to achieving the acceptance and stability you need to pursue an acceptable lifestyle.

Resources

Recommended Reading

Surviving Schizophrenia: A Manual for Families, Consumers and Providers, 3rd edition, E.F. Torrey, M.D. New York: HarperCollins, 1995. Very highly recommended.

Caring for the Mind: The Comprehensive Guide to Mental Health, Dianne Hales and Robert E. Hales, M.D. New York: Bantam Books, 1995.

Additional Information and Services

American Schizophrenia Association
900 North Federal Highway, Suite 330
Boca Raton, FL 33432

Phone: (407) 393-6167
    State groups: 35. Publications available.

National Mental Health Association
1021 Prince Street
Alexandria, VA 22314-2971
Phone: (703) 684-7722, 1-800-969-NMHA; Fax: (703) 684-5968
    State groups: 650. Publications: *FOCUS*; also provides pamphlets and films.

Schizophrenics Anonymous
1209 California Road
Eastchester, NY 10709
Phone: (914) 337-2252
    Twenty-five local groups. A self-help organization sponsored by the American Schizophrenia Association. Conduct meetings for discussion of all aspects of managing and coping with schizophrenia.

Disease Management Expertise
Alliance for the Mentally Ill
Phone: 1-800-950-NAMI
    A national referral resource.

SICKLE CELL DISEASE

Other Names
Sickle cell anemia, hemoglobin SS disease, hemoglobin SC disease, sickle beta-thalassemia, S-D Punjab, S-O Arab, S-Lepore, S-E disease

Prevalence/Incidence in U.S.
Current estimate: approximately 60,000; 1,000 new cases annually. One black child in every 375 has sickle cell disease; it is estimated that 8% of the black population carries the sickle cell trait.
    Prevalence per 100,000 population by race/ethnic group:

Race/Ethnic Group	Prevalence
White	2
Black	289
Hispanic, eastern U.S.	90
Hispanic, western U.S.	3
Asian	8
Native American	36

Age Group
The disorder is present at birth; initial disease manifestations occur in infancy and early childhood. Average life expectancy is 20 to 50 years.

Male-to-Female Ratio Both sexes are affected equally.

Principal Features and Natural History

Sickle Cell Disease

The term sickle cell disease is used to designate a group of genetic disorders that are characterized by abnormal forms of hemoglobin, the red pigment in red blood cells. The principal member of the group is sickle cell anemia, so named because red blood cells contain inherited sickle hemoglobin (Hgb S). This abnormal hemoglobin causes red blood cells to change from their usual biconcave disc shape to a crescent or sickle shape when they are passing through portions of the circulation where oxygen content is low. Upon returning to areas where sufficient oxygen is available, the red blood cells initially resume their normal configuration. After repeated cycles of "sickling and unsickling," red blood cells are permanently damaged and ultimately disintegrate. Continuous loss of red cells leads to anemia.

Infants born with sickle cell disease tend to be free of symptoms at birth. The onset of symptoms usually occurs between three months and two years of age. During periods of sickling, hemoglobin S red cells lose their flexibility and cannot readily pass through the small vessels of the microcirculation. Aggregates of sickle cells can actually block the flow of blood and cause serious damage to vital tissues throughout the body. Such manifestations include painful crises involving the chest, back, and extremities; seizures; stroke; impaired vision; engorgement of the spleen; liver and kidney damage; and predisposition to pneumonia. Chronic anemia impairs immunity and increases susceptibility to deadly viral and bacterial infections.

Sickle Cell Trait

In contrast with the individual who has inherited Hgb S from both parents and has sickle cell anemia (Hgb SS disease), the person who inherits normal hemoglobin (Hgb A) from one parent and Hgb S from the other parent is known as a carrier of Hgb S and has sickle cell trait. This is not considered to be a form of sickle cell disease. In those with sickle cell trait, normal hemoglobin (Hgb A) is the dominant type and none of the symptoms of sickle cell disease occur; life expectancy is normal. However, when both parents have sickle cell trait (Hgb AS), there is a 25% chance with each pregnancy that the infant will have sickle cell anemia. One in 12 black Americans has sickle cell trait.

Diagnostic Symptoms and Signs

Fever, malaise, weakness
Loss of appetite, stomach pain, nausea, vomiting
Swelling in hands and feet

Pain crises involving the chest, back, arms, and legs
Abdominal distention, jaundice
Enlargement of the heart, spleen, and liver

Diagnostic Tests and Procedures

Complete blood cell counts; detection of sickled red blood cells
Hemoglobin electrophoresis
Thin-layer isoelectric focusing analysis
High-performance liquid chromatography
Hemoglobin DNA analysis
X-ray studies of bones

Diagnostic "Markers" for This Disorder

Confirmation of hemoglobin S genotype by electrophoresis.
For sickle cell anemia, the mutant gene is on chromosome 11.
For the thalassemias, the mutant genes are on chromosome 16.
    See Appendix 11, Genetic Disorders and Gene Therapy.

Similar Conditions That May Confuse Diagnosis

Rheumatic fever, pericarditis
Infectious hepatitis, meningitis, osteomyelitis
Acute appendicitis, gallbladder disorders
Leukemias

ALERT!

It is mandatory that the correct diagnosis be made as early as possible so
that prophylactic medication can be started promptly. Screening for sickle
cell disease can be done before birth and anytime after birth.

Causes

Established Causes

    Inheritance of mutant genes for hemoglobin S and other abnormal
hemoglobins.

Known Risk Factors for Developing This Disorder

    Parents with sickle cell trait.

Drugs That Can Cause This Disorder

There are no drugs that can cause sickle cell disease.

Goals of Treatment

Can This Disorder Be Cured?

    There is no standard curative treatment at this time. Bone marrow
transplants and stem cell transplants are being evaluated.

Can This Disorder Be Treated Effectively?

With early diagnosis, prophylactic antibiotics and immunizations can be given to prevent infections. Close monitoring for onset of acute pain episodes ensures appropriate pain management.

Specific Goals

- Maintenance of optimal nutrition, growth, and development
- Maintenance of long-term immunity to infectious diseases
- Prevention of infections by long-term antibiotic medication
- Prevention of chronic anemia
- Avoidance of acute pain episodes; prompt and adequate management of pain crises as necessary
- Close monitoring for complications that require immediate evaluation and treatment

Health Professionals Who Participate in Managing This Disorder

Family physicians
Pediatricians
Pediatric surgeons
Pediatric nurses
General internists
Hematologists
Clinical geneticists
Genetic counselors
Medical social workers

Currently Available Therapies for This Disorder

Nondrug Treatment Methods

- Long-term exchange blood transfusions to keep hemoglobin S level below 30%
- Standard immunizations: diphtheria-tetanus-pertussis, hemophilus influenza type B, hepatitis, measles, mumps, polio, rubella, and pneumococcal vaccine

Drug Therapy

- Anti-infectives: oral penicillin
- Analgesics: acetaminophen, nonsteroidal anti-inflammatory drugs, codeine, morphine, oxycodone, propoxyphene
- Corticosteroids: methylprednisolone—short-course, high-dose therapy to treat acute pain crises
- Adjuvant drugs: antihistamines, antiemetics, antidepressants
- Nutritional supplements: iron, folic acid, multiple vitamins (recommended dietary allowances)

- Hydroxyurea: used to increase levels of fetal hemoglobin (Hgb F) that inhibits the sickling effects of Hgb S and reduces the occurrence of acute pain crises by 50%

New Drugs in Development for Treating This Disorder

Combination therapy using hydroxyurea and erythropoietin has shown beneficial effects in raising the level of fetal hemoglobin (Hgb F). Further studies are needed to determine if treatment benefits justify the high cost of medications.

Management of Therapy

- The patient and family should receive genetic counseling regarding the transmission of sickle cell disease. They should also be taught the nature and course of the disease, with emphasis on the recognition of complications that can occur abruptly and be life-threatening.
- It is essential to begin prophylactic oral penicillin twice daily as early as possible, but no later than two months of age. This should be continued on a regular basis until at least five years of age.
- Begin the full schedule of infant immunizations as early as possible; complete the full series of each vaccine. Begin pneumococcal vaccine at 12 months (optional) or 24 months (certain) of age, followed by booster doses every five years for life. Influenzal vaccine should be given at 12 months of age and repeated annually.
- Monitor closely for indications of infection: fever, malaise, headcold, cough, loss of appetite, diarrhea, etc. Consult your physician and request an evaluation.
- Treat acute pain episodes promptly and adequately. Learn by experience which drugs and what dosages are most effective.
- Monitor for the development of priapism (painful erection of the penis) (see Glossary for description and list of drugs to avoid).
- The following developments require urgent medical evaluation and treatment:
  - Fever with progressive rise in temperature
  - Sudden weakness, lethargy, abdominal pain, nausea, vomiting
  - Headache, impaired vision, facial distortion, loss of use of arm or leg, inability to speak, seizures
  - Painful swelling of hands and/or feet
  - Acute chest pain, difficult breathing
  - Enlargement of liver or spleen. Your physician can teach you how to detect this.

Special Considerations for Women

Menstruation may provoke acute pain crises.

Oral contraceptives may be used safely in carefully selected patients.

Pregnancy

Women with sickle cell trait are at increased risk for kidney infection (pyelonephritis) during pregnancy.

Women with sickle cell disease may experience increased frequency of acute pain episodes and infections of the respiratory and urinary tracts.

Spontaneous abortion occurs in 10–20% of pregnancies, even with the best of care.

The Role of Prevention in This Disorder

Primary Prevention

Individuals with sickle cell disease (Hgb SS) or sickle cell trait (Hgb AS) should seek genetic counseling regarding family planning and the potential for transmission of mutant genes to offspring.

Secondary Prevention

Close observation of the treatment principles outlined above.

Helpful Suggestions for Daily Living

Your Environment

Avoid prolonged or unprotected exposure to markedly hot or cold environments.

Your Diet

Eat a balanced, highly nutritious diet, including recommended dietary allowances of vitamins and minerals.

Your Lifestyle

Avoid strenuous exercise and excessive physical activity. Avoid situations that cause emotional or physical stress. Maintain as normal a lifestyle as possible, participating in social and educational activities at a comfortable pace.

Resources

Recommended Reading

Sickle Cell Disease Guideline Panel, *Sickle Cell Disease: Screening, Diagnosis, Management, and Counseling in Newborns and Infants. Clinical Practice Guideline No. 6.* AHCPR Pub. No. 93-0562. Rockville, MD: Agency for Health Care Policy and Research, U.S. Department of Health and Human Services. April 1993.

Additional Information and Services

Sickle Cell Disease Association of America Inc.
200 Corporate Pointe, Suite 495
Culver City, CA 90230-7633
Phone: 1-800-421-8453, 8:30 A.M. to 5:00 P.M. (Pacific time) Monday–Friday

Provides materials, trains counselors, and offers programs to medical professionals and the public. Also supports research, conducts public education campaigns, and provides diagnostic screening.

Disease Management Expertise
Comprehensive Sickle Cell Disease Center
Meharry Medical College
Nashville, Tennessee
Director: Ernest A. Turner, M.D., Associate Professor of Pediatrics, Medicine, and Pathology
Phone: (615) 555-1212

SJÖGREN'S SYNDROME
(SHER grenz SIN drome)

Other Names Sjögren's disease, sicca syndrome, SS

Prevalence/Incidence in U.S.
Primary SS: 1 in 2,500; secondary SS: 20% of rheumatoid arthritis patients and 30% of systemic lupus erythematosus patients have sicca (dryness) syndrome.

Age Group Peak onset during sixth decade of life; less frequent onset in childhood, third and fourth decades

Male-to-Female Ratio Male—10% of cases, female—90% of cases

Principal Features and Natural History
Sjögren's syndrome is a chronic autoimmune disorder that consists primarily of marked dryness of the eyes and mouth—the sicca complex. It occurs in three relatively distinct forms: primary SS, secondary SS, and lymphoproliferative SS (see Appendix 5, The Immune System).

Primary SS
This designation refers to the form of the disorder that is limited primarily to disease of the tear-producing (lacrimal) glands in the eye and the saliva-producing (salivary) glands in the mouth and jaw. As the autoimmune process destroys the functional tissues within these glands, the production of tears and saliva is greatly reduced. The resulting combination of dry eyes and dry mouth is known as the sicca (dry) complex: *keratoconjunctivitis* in the eyes and *xerostomia* in the mouth. Over time, this form of SS may extend to involve other systemic tissues and organs: skin, lungs, digestive tract, liver, pancreas, kidneys, genital tract, and nervous system.

Secondary SS

This form consists of the sicca complex associated with another con-current autoimmune disease, most commonly rheumatoid arthritis (RA), systemic lupus erythematosus (SLE), or progressive systemic sclerosis (PSS). These are multisystem disorders with many diverse symptoms that reflect disease in the numerous organs involved.

Lymphoproliferative SS

This uncommon form of SS consists of the sicca complex and a coex-isting abnormal proliferation of lymphatic cells and tissues. These are usually benign tumors, but a small percentage of them can become can-cerous (malignant lymphomas).

Diagnostic Symptoms and Signs

Primary SS

The most common eye symptoms include severe dryness, gritty feeling, itching, burning, sensitivity to light, thick mucous strings, and blurred vision.

The most common mouth symptoms include varying degrees of dryness, altered taste, difficulty in chewing and swallowing food, burning of the mouth lining, inability to wear dentures, frequent tooth and gum prob-lems, and yeast (*Candida*) infections of the lips, mouth, tongue, and throat.

Other manifestations include swelling of the salivary glands, dryness of the skin and nasal passages, lung infections with cough and difficult breathing, vaginal dryness, and peripheral neuritis (see Glossary) in the legs.

Secondary SS

In addition to the above symptoms and signs, any manifestations of other coexisting autoimmune disorders (rheumatoid arthritis, lupus, etc.) can occur. The clinical features of many connective tissue diseases over-lap. See the respective Disorder Profiles in this section.

Lymphoproliferative SS

The hallmark of this form is the development of tumors in the salivary glands and lymph glands, in conjunction with the features described above. Such tumors may be benign or malignant. SS patients experience a 44-fold increase in the occurrence of lymphoma (lymphatic cancer).

Diagnostic Tests and Procedures

For Keratoconjunctivitis Sicca (Dry Eye)

Slit lamp examination of eyes: magnification without direct illumination to determine the status of the conjunctiva and tear volume

Schirmer test: a filter paper wick is placed in the trough of the lower eyelid to measure the volume of tear production; a positive result is less than 8 mm of wetting per five minutes

Fluorescein or rose bengal stain is placed in the eye to detect corneal abrasion or ulceration

Tear osmolarity test: this measures the salt concentration in tear film; this concentration is abnormally high in the dry eyes of SS

For Xerostomia (Dry Mouth)
Techniques that measure the rate of salivary production
Testing the ability to chew and swallow a dry cracker without water
Determination of salivary response to the presence of candy

Diagnostic "Markers" for This Disorder
Tissue biopsies of the minor salivary glands are taken from inside the lower lip. A positive diagnostic finding is the presence of an average of two aggregates of lymphocytes per 4 square mm area, each containing more than 50 lymphocytes.

Significant results of blood tests:
* Positive rheumatoid factor (RF)—90% of cases
* Positive antinuclear antibodies (ANA)—80% of cases
* Presence of anti-SS A (Ro) or anti-SS B (La) antibodies
* Human leukocyte antigens HLA-B8 and HLA-DR3 are associated with primary SS; HLA-DR4 is associated with secondary SS.

Possible Effects of Drugs on Test Results
The following drugs may reduce the production of saliva (see Appendix 16, Drug Classes, for names of specific drugs in each class):

atropine derivatives and drugs with atropinelike (anticholinergic) side effects
antispasmodics
tricyclic antidepressants
antihistamines
decongestants
over-the-counter cold remedies
some antihypertensives
muscle relaxants
narcotic analgesics
diuretics

Similar Conditions That May Confuse Diagnosis
Sarcoidosis
Tuberculosis
HIV infection/AIDS
Other bacterial and viral infections

ALERT!

Persons who wear contact lenses and use antihistamines, estrogen skin patches, or oral contraceptives may experience the "dry eye syndrome:" scratchy sensation in the eyes, blurred vision, excess watering, and increased eye infections. This is not indicative of Sjögren's syndrome.

Causes

Established Causes

The specific causes that initiate this autoimmune disorder are unknown.

Theoretical Causes

It is thought that multiple factors are involved in the development of this disorder: genetic predisposition, altered immune system functions, hormonal influences, environmental exposures (see Appendix 5, The Immune System).

There is some evidence to indicate that the Epstein-Barr virus (the cause of infectious mononucleosis) may contribute to the initiation of SS in some cases.

Known Risk Factors for Developing This Disorder

Other autoimmune connective tissue disorders are frequently associated with the secondary forms of SS. These include rheumatoid arthritis, systemic lupus erythematosus, progressive systemic sclerosis (scleroderma), polyarteritis nodosa, and polymyositis.

Drugs That Can Cause This Disorder

There are no drugs that cause the fundamental disease states responsible for SS.

The drugs that can cause dry mouth (xerostomia) are listed above (see "Possible Effects of Drugs on Test Results").

Goals of Treatment

Can This Disorder Be Cured?

No curative treatment is available at this time.

Can This Disorder Be Treated Effectively?

- Can symptoms be relieved?
  - Eye dryness can be relieved by artificial tears during the day and by ointments during the night.
  - Mouth dryness can be relieved by frequent sips of water, artificial saliva, sugarless candy, and pilocarpine mouthwash.
  - Vaginal dryness can be relieved by sterile, greaseless, water-soluble lubricants: K-Y Jelly, H-R Jelly, Surgilube, Maxilube.

- Can the mechanism(s) of the disorder be:
  - controlled? Partially, depending upon the degree and duration of disease activity.
  - arrested? Not completely or permanently.
  - reversed? No.

Specific Goals
- Relief of symptoms
- Limitation of damage to diseased organs and tissues
- Control of the underlying autoimmune activity to the greatest extent possible

Health Professionals Who Participate in Managing This Disorder
Family physicians
General internists
Allergists
Clinical immunologists
Ophthalmologists
Optometrists
Opticians
Otolaryngologists
Dentists
Rheumatologists
Pulmonologists
Gastroenterologists
Gynecologists
Dermatologists
Oncologists
Pharmacists

Currently Available Therapies for This Disorder

Nondrug Treatment Methods
- Room humidifiers
- Moisture chamber eyeglasses
- Closure of the tear ducts (punctal occlusion), temporary or permanent; this prevents drainage of tears from the eye via the nasolacrimal canal (nasal passage)

Drug Therapy
Artificial tears:
- Teargard (hydroxyethylcellulose)
- Lacrisert (hydroxypropylcellulose)
- Isopto Tears (hydroxypropyl methylcellulose)

- Liquifilm Tears (polyvinyl alcohol)
- Tears Plus (polyvinyl alcohol)
- Refresh (polyvinyl alcohol and povidone)
- numerous others

Ocular ointments:

- Duratears Naturale (preservative-free petrolatum, lanolin, mineral oil)
- Refresh P.M. (preservative-free petrolatum, lanolin, mineral oil)
- several others

Artificial saliva:

- Mouth Cote
- Salivart

Disease-modifying drugs:

- prednisone (generic)
- hydroxychloroquine (Plaquenil)
- azathioprine (Imuran)
- chlorambucil (Leukeran)
- cyclophosphamide (Cytoxan)

New Drugs in Development for Treating This Disorder

- Bromhexine has been studied in Europe to evaluate its ability to increase tear production in SS patients with mild to moderate kerato-conjunctivitis sicca. Results to date are inconclusive. It has not yet been approved for marketing in the United States.
- Anetholetrithione (Sulfarlem in Europe, Sialor in Canada) is able to increase salivary flow in SS patients with mild, but not severe, xerostomia. It is not available in the United States.

Management of Therapy

As with all autoimmune diseases, there are no drugs that can cure the fundamental causes of Sjögren's syndrome. The drugs currently available for managing SS fall into two groups: (1) those designed primarily to relieve the symptoms of mild to moderate disease and (2) more potent drugs that are somewhat capable of modifying the inflammation and tissue destruction associated with the underlying autoimmune activity.

Every case of SS is a unique, individual mixture of manifestations. Successful management depends upon the accuracy of diagnosis, the assessment of disease activity, and an appropriately individualized treatment program.

There is considerable variation in response to the drugs utilized to manage SS. Optimal treatment often requires a mixture of drugs, usually on a trial-and-error basis.

Use of Artificial Tears

- Currently there are 30 brand formulations of artificial tears available. These vary in composition; some contain preservatives, others are preservative-free. Some individuals find certain preservatives to be irritating; a preservative-free solution should be sought that will provide adequate relief.
- Observe sterile technique: wash hands thoroughly before use; do not allow the tip of the applicator to touch any surface; replace top immediately after use. The usual dose is one or two drops into the eye three or four times daily. With initial use, mild stinging and blurred vision may occur temporarily. If these symptoms persist, discontinue the product and consult your physician or pharmacist for guidance.

Use of Ocular Lubricants

- Currently there are 15 brand formulations of ocular lubricants and emollients available. Generally they share the same ingredients. A few contain preservatives which may be irritants for some users.
- Do not use with contact lenses. These are intended for night use to moisten and protect the eye surface during sleep. Use sterile technique when applying: wash hands thoroughly, do not allow the tip of the applicator to touch any surface, replace cap promptly.

Use of Cortisone Derivatives

- When symptomatic treatment fails to give adequate relief, prednisone may be added to the treatment regimen to reduce inflammation in actively diseased tissues.
- Prednisone is usually effective in conditions of mild to moderate severity. Once a favorable response is obtained, the lowest effective dose should be determined. Courses of prednisone should be as short as possible. Avoid prolonged, uninterrupted use (see Appendix 6, Long-Term Corticosteroid Therapy).

Use of Immunosuppressant Drugs

- Hydroxychloroquine (Plaquenil) has been shown to be effective in relieving the mild to moderate symptoms of systemic SS; blood tests such as the sedimentation rate (see Glossary) and the level of immunoglobulin G (IgG) confirm that this drug can provide significant anti-inflammatory action in autoimmune-diseased tissues.
- If prednisone fails to control disease activity satisfactorily or excessive dosage is required, a trial of other immunosuppressant drug therapy is considered. Azathioprine (Imuran) and chlorambucil (Leukeran) are potent immunosuppressant drugs that are usually reserved to treat more serious manifestations of autoimmune disease: vasculitis, hemolytic anemia, and pleuropericarditis.

- Because of its potential for causing cancer, cyclophosphamide (Cytoxan) is reserved for treating life-threatening vasculitis. It is advisable to avoid daily dosage; the preferred method is single intravenous dosage at intervals of one to three months.

Ancillary Drug Treatment (as required)
For mouth angle infection (cheilitis):
- Lotrimin or Mycelog ointment

For oral yeast (*Candida*) infections:
- clotrimazole (Gyne-Lotrimin) vaginal tablets
- nystatin vaginal tablets, dissolved in mouth

For vaginal yeast (*Candida*) infections:
- clotrimazole (Gyne-Lotrimin) cream or suppositories

For muscle and joint pains:

see Nonsteroidal Anti-Inflammatory Drugs (NSAIDs) in the rheumatoid arthritis Profile in this section and Appendix 8.

Note: Drug selection, dosage, and administration schedule must be determined by the physician for each patient individually.

Current Controversies in Management
Probably the most significant area of difficulty is establishing the initial diagnosis of SS—obtaining a consensus among consultants regarding the interpretation of tests and an appropriate treatment program. The manifestations of this disorder are so variable among patients and so prone to fluctuations over time that frequent, careful monitoring is essential. If possible, anyone thought to have primary SS should seek evaluation and guidance at a Sjögren's Syndrome Clinic similar to those listed at the end of this profile. Once the correct status of the disorder is established, an appropriate treatment program can be carried out under the supervision of the patient's primary physician.

Important Points to Consider
- The following factors can aggravate keratoconjunctivitis sicca (dry eyes):
  - low humidity
  - air-conditioning
  - air currents
  - dust, smoke, fumes
  - excessive eye makeup
  - prolonged reading
  - concentrated and prolonged use of computer terminals
- The xerostomia (dry mouth) of SS predisposes to serious deterioration of teeth and gums. Regular dental checkups every four months are essential. Consult your dentist regarding the use of fluoride applications to teeth, fluoride-containing toothpastes, and other measures to prevent cavities.

- Marked reduction of salivary flow and mucous production in the esophagus (food tube) can cause significant difficulty in swallowing tablets and capsules. This creates a risk for lodging of the medication in the esophagus before it reaches the stomach. If this should occur, some drugs are capable of initiating erosion and ulceration at the point of contact. The following suggestions are advisable:
  - Swallow some water to moisten the mouth and throat immediately before taking the medication.
  - Stand or sit upright as you take the medication.
  - Use 4 to 6 ounces of water to swallow the medication. After three to five minutes, drink another 4 ounces of water.
  - Remain upright for another three to five minutes.
  - If you have discomfort in the chest that suggests the medication may be lodged in the esophagus, eat some soft food (bread, cottage cheese, gelatin, etc.) and drink water with it. Repeat as needed until the discomfort is relieved.
  - Rinse the mouth thoroughly after taking liquid medications.
- Significant hypothyroidism develops in 10–20% of patients with SS. Appropriate thyroid function studies are warranted if symptoms of thyroid deficiency appear: fatigue, increased sleep requirement, weight gain, intolerance to cold, dry skin, elevated blood cholesterol level, etc.

Possible Drug Interactions of Significance

Chlorambucil *taken concurrently* with
- aspirin may increase the risk of bruising or bleeding; the platelet-reducing effects of chlorambucil and the antiplatelet action of aspirin are additive; avoid aspirin while taking chlorambucil.
- antidepressant or antipsychotic drugs requires careful monitoring; these drugs can lower the threshold for the occurrence of seizures and increase the risk of chlorambucil-induced seizures.

The following drugs may *decrease* the effects of prednisone:
- antacids—may reduce its absorption
- barbiturates
- phenytoin (Dilantin, etc.)

Special Considerations for Women

Sjögren's syndrome is predominantly a woman's disorder. Primary concerns include the potential for (1) vaginal dryness with attendant painful intercourse (dyspareunia); (2) vaginal yeast infections (candidiasis); (3) vaginal atrophy at the time of menopause and the question of estrogen replacement therapy; (4) increased risk for SS-induced congenital heart block in the fetus during disease activity.

Pregnancy

The autoantibodies associated with the mother's Sjögren's disease—anti-SS-A/Ro and anti-SS-B/La—are present in 50–70% of women with SS. They can attack the heart tissues of the developing fetus and damage the conduction system that regulates the rate and rhythm of the functioning heart. The result is a permanent, complete heart block which is potentially life-threatening. The risk of this occurring is estimated to be 1 in 60 pregnancies. Women with SS, of childbearing age, and planning pregnancy should be tested for the presence of autoantibodies against Ro and La. Test results should be reviewed by appropriate consultants and guidance sought regarding the advisability of establishing pregnancy.

Breast-Feeding

If any of the disease-modifying drugs listed above are being taken, breast-feeding should not be attempted.

Special Considerations for the Elderly

Normal aging causes a reduction in both tear and saliva formation. This should not arouse concern regarding the possible development of SS. The elderly also tend to be more susceptible to the drying effects of the drugs listed above.

Xerostomia (dry mouth) can cause considerable difficulty for the elderly who wear dentures. A satisfactory saliva substitute should be sought and used regularly.

The Role of Prevention in This Disorder

Primary Prevention

Since the primary causes of autoimmune disease are unknown, there are no primary preventive measures available at this time.

Secondary Prevention

The principal aspect of SS that provides opportunity for secondary prevention is the practice of good oral hygiene and routine dental prophylactic care every four months.

Resources

Recommended Reading

The Sjögren's Syndrome Handbook: An Authoritative Guide for Patients, Elaine K. Harris, ed. Sjögren's Syndrome Foundation, Inc., 333 North Broadway, Jericho, NY 11753.

Additional Information and Services

Sjögren's Syndrome Foundation, Inc.
The Moisture Seekers

333 North Broadway
Jericho, NY 11753
Phone: (516) 933-6365

National Sjögren's Syndrome Association
3201 West Evans Dr.
Phoenix, AZ 85023
Phone: 1-800-395-6772, (602) 993-7227

Sjögren's Syndrome Clinical Trials
Philip C. Fox, D.D.S., Director
National Institute for Dental Research
National Institutes of Health
9000 Rockville Pike
Building 10, Room 1N-113
Bethesda, MD 20892
Phone: (301) 496-4278

Disease Management Expertise
Sjögren's Syndrome Clinic
Paula Rackoff, M.D., Director
Hospital for Joint Diseases
301 East 17th Street
New York, NY 10003
Phone: (212) 598-6516

Sjögren's Syndrome and Dry Mouth Center
Frederick Vivino, M.D., Director
Presbyterian Medical Center
MAB Building 107
Philadelphia, PA 19104
Phone: (215) 662-9292

The Duke Sjögren's Syndrome Clinic
E. William St. Clair, M.D., Director
Box 3874
Durham, NC 27710
Phone: (919) 684-4499

Sjögren's Syndrome Treatment Center
Norman Talal, M.D., Director
University of Texas Health Sciences Center
7703 Floyd Curl Drive
San Antonio, TX 78284
Phone: (210) 567-4656

Sjögren's Syndrome Clinic
Troy Daniels, D.D.S., M.S., Director

University of California
San Francisco, CA 94143
Phone: (415) 476-5756

Sjögren's Syndrome Treatment Center
Robert I. Fox, M.D., Director
Scripps Clinic & Research Foundation
10666 North Torrey Pines Road
La Jolla, CA
Phone: (619) 554-8639

Sjögren's Syndrome Treatment Center
Alan Slomovic, M.D., Director
Toronto Western Hospital
399 Bathurst Street
Toronto, Ontario, Canada, M5T 2S8
Phone: (416) 639-5892

SPINAL STENOSIS
(SPY nal ste NO sis)

Other Names
Cervical spinal stenosis, lumbar canal stenosis, lumbar spinal stenosis, lumbosacral spinal stenosis, tandem spinal stenosis, thoracic spinal stenosis

Age Group
Symptomatic congenital stenosis: 20 to 40 years of age
Degenerative spinal stenosis: 50 to 80 years of age

Male-to-Female Ratio More common in males

Principal Features and Natural History
The term spinal stenosis is used to designate a localized narrowing or constriction of the spinal canal (within the vertebral column) that houses the spinal cord as it emerges from the brain at the base of the skull and extends downward to the end of the spine. If the narrowing is confined to the central area of the canal, it is called central stenosis; if the narrowing involves the perimeter of the canal at points where the spinal nerve roots leave the spinal cord and exit between the bones of the spine (vertebras), it is called lateral stenosis. Central stenosis may cause compression of the spinal cord; lateral stenosis (also known as the "lateral recess" syndrome) may cause compression of the nerve roots. Central and lateral stenosis can occur separately or together at any level of the spinal canal. However, the most common sites of significant stenosis occur in the neck

(cervical stenosis) and lower spine (lumbar stenosis). Stenosis of the mid-spine (thoracic stenosis) due to noncancerous disease is relatively rare.

The pattern of symptoms due to spinal stenosis is determined by the site and degree of constriction (cervical, thoracic, or lumbar spine) and whether the stenosis is central (spinal cord compression) or lateral (nerve root compression) or both. Stenosis can occur at two or more levels of the spine concurrently, causing serious diagnostic confusion. When symptomatic stenosis is present in the cervical and lumbar spine at the same time, the condition is referred to as tandem spinal stenosis. The frequency of occurrence is estimated to be as follows:

cervical spine (primarily): 30%
thoracic spine (primarily): rare
lumbar spine (primarily): 40%
cervical and lumbar (combination): 30%

Symptoms due to the more common types of spinal stenosis usually begin in the sixth to eighth decade of life, and are most often associated with degenerative arthritis of the spine. Cervical spinal stenosis will primarily cause symptoms in the neck and upper extremities; occasionally it will cause referred pain into the lower extremities. Lumbar stenosis will cause symptoms in the lower back, buttocks, and lower extremities; it may also affect bladder and rectal functions. If not correctly diagnosed and treated, symptoms grow progressively worse and functional disabilities of the upper and lower extremities develop. Surgical decompression of the spinal cord and/or nerve roots is necessary to prevent irreversible damage and permanent loss of function.

The classical symptom of central spinal stenosis is neurogenic claudication. This is the development of intense and disabling pain in both legs brought on by standing or walking, and relieved only by sitting or lying down; riding a bicycle does not produce this pain. In contrast, the leg pains of vascular (circulatory) claudication do not occur with standing, but begin only after walking for varying periods of time; they promptly subside when walking ceases and the person remains standing; riding a bicycle produces the same pain experienced while walking.

Diagnostic Symptoms and Signs

Not invisible but unnoticed, Watson. You did not know where to look, and so you missed all that was important.

—SHERLOCK HOLMES

Central Stenosis of the Cervical Spine

Congenital deformity (trefoil or clover-leaf canal) may be present high in the cervical spine at birth; this causes an initial degree of stenosis which is usually without symptoms. In later life, degenerative arthritis involving bone (vertebra), intervertebral discs, and spinal ligaments (spondylosis) is the most common cause of cervical stenosis. Large arthritic spurs (osteophytes) can form on the vertebra and, in the course of time, produce increasing pressure on the spinal cord. This chronic compression of the cord at the cervical level eventually damages the nerve fibers within the cord causing a pattern of symptoms known as the "central cord syndrome." The diagnostic features of the central cord syndrome are the following:

Neck pain and stiffness, and referred pain to the lower extremities is *increased* by forcefully tilting the head backward.

Varying degrees of weakness in the muscles of the upper extremities (but no pain or numbness).

Abnormal neurological findings in the hands: positive Hoffmann and/or Wartenberg signs (ask your physician for explanation).

Referred pain and abnormal sensations (paresthesias) felt in both lower extremities—very symmetrical in right and left thighs and lower legs.

Increased knee-jerk reactions (patellar reflexes). This sign is clearly indicative of cervical cord compression.

Normal (not absent) ankle-jerk reactions (Achilles reflexes).

ALERT!

Cervical spinal stenosis can create symptoms in the legs that somewhat resemble those due to lumbar spinal stenosis. This can occur in the absence of lumbar stenosis or in its presence, as in tandem spinal stenosis. The attending physician must be aware of this so that the existence of cervical stenosis with central cord syndrome is recognized and not misdiagnosed.

Lateral Stenosis of the Cervical Spine

When the lateral recesses of the cervical canal are narrowed by degenerative arthritis (or other disease process), the nerve roots that supply the upper extremities may be compressed. Depending upon the nature and degree of compression of the right and left nerve roots, the symptoms felt in the arms and hands may vary in intensity. Characteristic symptoms are the following:

Loss of strength in the muscles of the arms and hands

Diminished dexterity in the fingers

Numbness and diminished sensation in the fingers and hands

Pain and abnormal sensations (paresthesias) in the arms and hands

Decreased reflexes in the arms and hands

Central Stenosis of the Lumbar Spine

When spondylosis occurs in the lumbar spine (usually the lower three vertebras), the combination of arthritic bone enlargement, degenerated discs, and thickened spinal ligaments can cause sufficient narrowing of the spinal canal to produce compression of the spinal cord. This may cause the following symptoms:

Neurogenic claudication: intense pain in the legs as described above

Paresthesias: a variety of abnormal sensations in the legs variously described as burning, tingling, crawling, cramplike, or shocklike; if relief is not sought by sitting or lying down, areas of numbness can develop.

Weakness in the legs; limited ability to stand and walk

Decreased knee and ankle reflexes

Lateral Stenosis of the Lumbar Spine

This is the more common pattern of stenosis at the lumbar level. There are two principal causes for compression of the lumbar nerve roots: (1) arthritic narrowing of the openings (foramina) through which the nerve roots exit the spinal canal to reach the lower back and legs—this process can affect the right or the left or both nerve roots, and at one or more levels; (2) a protruding or ruptured intervertebral disc that compresses the nerve root segment between the cord and the exit tunnel; this is usually limited to one side and causes symptoms in the leg supplied by the compressed nerve. Expected symptoms in the leg (or legs) are the following:

Pain and stiffness originating in the lower back

Sharp pain radiating from the back into the buttock, back of the thigh, and lower leg—the path of the sciatic nerve; this pattern is known as sciatica.

Intermittent paresthesias, but not as intense or constant as those associated with cord compression

Decreased strength of leg muscles

Areas of numbness and impaired sensation

Decreased knee and ankle reflexes

Increased back pain with raising the leg on the affected side: positive straight-leg-raising test

Diagnostic Differences Between Cervical and Lumbar Spinal Stenosis When Leg Symptoms Are Confusing

	Cervical	Lumbar
Leg pain and paresthesia	Equal, symmetrical in both legs	Asymmetrical or one leg only
Pain quality	Constant, diffuse, deep ache, burning	Sharp, radiating, related to movement
Pain location	Front and outer side of thigh	Back of thigh and leg
Knee/patellar reflex	Increased	Decreased
Ankle/Achilles reflex	Normal	Decreased
Tandem walking	Disturbed	Undisturbed

ALERT!

Diagnostic Tips

Congenital narrowing of any segment of the spinal canal may predispose to clinical stenosis in later life. Diagnostic studies should always look for this. If the size of the canal is compromised at birth, lesser degrees of acquired disease may initiate symptoms.

Segmental narrowing of the spinal canal can exist concurrently at two or more levels. This may cause symmetrical manifestations in both legs. All sites of significant stenosis must be found and decompressed to relieve symptoms.

When neurological symptoms begin equally in both legs at the same time and progress symmetrically, the cause of cord compression should be sought at higher rather than lower levels of the spine: (1) cervical stenosis or (2) thoracic or upper lumbar stenosis.

If lumbar decompressive surgery fails to relieve symptoms of spinal stenosis—the "failed back" syndrome—careful examinations of the cervical spine are mandatory before further lumbar surgery is considered.

Pain in the lower back accompanied by loss of sensation in the buttocks, genitalia, or thighs, and disturbance of bladder or bowel function is known as the "cauda equina syndrome." This is caused by compression of nerve roots below the first lumbar vertebra. Early surgical decompression is advisable.

CT scans and myelography are the imaging tests of choice to document central and lateral spinal stenosis. MRI alone is not as accurate and can give false-positive and false-negative results.

Diagnostic Tests and Procedures

Carefully targeted neurological examinations
Conventional nerve conduction studies
Conventional X-ray studies of the spine
CT scans of the spine
MRI studies of the spine
Myelograms of the spinal canal, with and without CT scans
Cerebrospinal fluid examinations
Intraoperative spinal sonography

Diagnostic "Markers" for This Disorder

Unequivocal demonstration of central or lateral stenosis of the spinal canal by CT scan, MRI, or myelogram.

Similar Conditions That May Confuse Diagnosis

Amyotrophic lateral sclerosis
Primary lateral sclerosis

Progressive bulbar paralysis
Spinal muscular atrophy
Vascular intermittent claudication

Causes

Established Causes
Congenital malformation of vertebra
Gout: deposition of uric acid crystals
Ossification of the posterior longitudinal ligament
Osteoarthritis of the spine (degenerative spondylosis)
Paget's disease of bone
Pseudogout: deposition of calcium pyrophosphate crystals
Spinal injury
Spinal tumors

Known Risk Factors for Developing This Disorder
Achondroplasia (developmental failure of joint cartilage formation)
Genetic predisposition to malformation of vertebra
Participation in extremely rough contact sports

Goals of Treatment

Can This Disorder Be Cured?
If a correct diagnosis is made early and adequate decompressive surgery is performed promptly, excellent relief of symptoms can be expected.

Specific Goals
- Early recognition of the disorder and accurate diagnosis
- Optimal decompression of spinal cord and/or nerve roots
- Appropriate postoperative physical therapy and rehabilitation
- Abolition of all pain and discomfort
- Restoration of full function

Health Professionals Who Participate in Managing This Disorder
Family physicians
General internists
Neurologists
Neuroradiologists
Anesthesiologists
Neurosurgeons
Orthopedic surgeons
Physical therapists

Currently Available Therapies for This Disorder

For patients with mild symptoms and tolerable pain; surgery not yet warranted:

- Routine back care training: lifting, stooping, sleeping
- Isometric exercises to strengthen abdominal muscles
- Elastic back support
- Epidural injections of cortisonelike (corticosteroid) preparations
- Nonsteroidal anti-inflammatory drugs (NSAIDs) for pain

For patients with moderate to severe pain and progressive disability; surgery warranted:

- Definitive preoperative imaging studies to document location and nature of stenosis
- Appropriate decompressive surgery, with or without fusion
- Postoperative physical therapy and rehabilitation

Management of Therapy

When symptoms suggest the possibility of spinal stenosis, careful attention must be given to diagnostic imaging studies to ensure that *all sites of stenosis* are identified.

If symptoms are relatively mild and not progressive, a trial of conservative management with close follow-up observation is acceptable.

If symptoms are not relieved by conservative treatment, and pain with disability is progressive, early decompressive surgery is mandatory. Increasing pain is indicative of continuous compression of nerve tissue and potentially irreversible nerve damage. The longer the period of nerve compression, the lesser the benefit from decompressive surgery. Following surgery, appropriate physical therapy and rehabilitation guidance are required for optimal recovery of function. For chronic or permanent neuropathic pain that persists following decompressive surgery, full evaluation by an accredited pain management center is advised.

Treatment Outcomes

The degree of symptom relief following decompressive surgery is related to the duration of symptoms prior to surgery: the longer the period of symptoms, the less the improvement; the shorter the period of symptoms, the greater the improvement. Chronic neuropathic pain induces change in the activities of the central nervous system that may result in permanent pain syndromes, hence the need for accurate diagnosis and timely surgical decompression.

Special Considerations for the Elderly

The elderly patient withstands spine surgery very well. In the absence of other contraindications, consideration of age should not deter appropriate decompressive surgery.

The Role of Prevention in This Disorder

Primary Prevention
- Avoidance of repeated occupational and recreational injuries to the spine.
- Maintenance of normal body weight and good physical conditioning

Secondary Prevention
- Prompt evaluation of recurrent or chronic back pain that does not respond to self-treatment
- Appropriate diagnostic studies followed by timely medical/surgical therapy

Resources

Recommended Reading
   Primer on the Rheumatic Diseases, 10th edition, H.R. Schumacher, Jr., M.D., ed. Atlanta: Arthritis Foundation, 1993.

Additional Information and Services
The Arthritis Foundation
1314 Spring Street, NW
Atlanta, GA 30309
Phone: (404) 872-7100
   Publications available.

Disease Management Expertise
   See Appendix 7, Pain Management Centers.

STROKE

Other Names
Cerebral vascular accident, CVA, ischemic stroke, intracerebral hemorrhage, subarachnoid hemorrhage, cerebral thrombosis, cerebral hemorrhage, cerebral embolism

Prevalence/Incidence in U.S.
Current estimate: approximately 3 million stroke victims are alive today
Estimated new cases annually: 500,000
Estimated deaths annually: 143,000

Age Group 30 to 65+ years

Male-to-Female Ratio Males—54%; Females—46%

Principal Features and Natural History
The term stroke connotes a sudden critical disruption in the structure and function of a portion of the brain that is attributable to interruption of

normal arterial blood flow. The two fundamental mechanisms responsible for strokes are (1) blockage (occlusion) of an artery without rupture of the vessel wall and (2) rupture of a vessel wall permitting hemorrhage into adjacent brain tissue. The former is referred to as an ischemic stroke: brain tissue deprived of essential blood flow. The latter is referred to as a hemorrhagic stroke: brain tissue damaged by extravasation of blood into the surrounding area, and compounded by loss of oxygen and vital nutrients.

Strokes are generally classified according to the nature and causes of interrupted arterial blood flow.

Ischemic strokes (75% of all strokes) are due to the following:

- thrombus formation (blood clot) within the artery that completely blocks the flow of blood (30% of ischemic strokes)
- embolism: a small blood clot that originates inside the heart, breaks loose, and is carried in the bloodstream to the brain where it lodges in a small vessel blocking the flow of blood (20% of ischemic strokes).
- lacunar strokes: small arteries blocked by thrombus formation (20% of ischemic strokes)
- unexplained (cause unknown) strokes (30% of ischemic strokes)

Intracerebral hemorrhagic strokes (15% of all strokes) are due to the following:

- hypertension (high blood pressure) that causes rupture of the vessel wall
- amyloid degeneration of arteries seen in the elderly
- congenital arterial–venous malformations that rupture
- hemorrhage due to anticoagulant drugs or rare bleeding disorders

Subarachnoid hemorrhage around the brain—between the surface of the brain and its covering (10% of all strokes)—are due to the following:

- ruptured congenital ("berry") aneurysm—a small, berrylike bulging in the wall of an artery (80% of subarachnoid hemorrhages)
- amyloid degeneration of arteries seen in the elderly
- inflammatory or infectious diseases that involve brain surface arteries
- abuse of stimulant drugs

Diagnostic Symptoms and Signs

These are directly related to the areas of brain tissue that are damaged by the stroke:

Severe headache, with or without vomiting

Impaired consciousness, restlessness, disorientation, drowsiness, coma

Loss of balance, unsteady gait, dizziness

Double vision, or loss of vision in one eye

Impaired speech or loss of speech

Numbness, abnormal sensations involving face or extremities

Weakness or paralysis of face, upper and/or lower extremities, usually one-sided

Diagnostic Tests and Procedures

Detailed neurological examination

Computed cerebral axial tomography (CAT scan) to be done within 24 hours. This distinguishes between ischemic and hemorrhagic stroke.

Cerebral angiography to visualize arterial defects

Magnetic resonance angiography (MRA)

Carotid artery duplex ultrasonography to detect carotid artery stenosis

Echocardiography to detect thrombus within the heart as a source of embolization to the brain

Similar Conditions That May Confuse Diagnosis

Migraine headache syndromes

Subdural hematoma (blood clot on surface of brain following head trauma)

Brain tumors

Seizure disorders (epilepsy)

Acute arteritis (inflammation of arterial walls)

Multiple sclerosis

Acute infections of the central nervous system

ALERT!

It is mandatory that you, your family, and your associates recognize *transient ischemic attacks (TIAs)* and understand their significance. A TIA is a neurological symptom or sign caused by focal ischemia (reduced blood flow within the brain) that disappears completely within 24 hours. Think of the TIA as a warning, an indicator of a stroke in the making, sooner or later. Most TIAs last between 10 and 20 minutes, the majority less than an hour. The risk of a subsequent stroke following a TIA is 5–10% per year. The highest incidence of stroke is in the first month after the TIA.

The following symptoms may be indicative of a TIA. If you experience any of these, consult your physician promptly regarding the need for evaluation.

Numbness and/or weakness of the face, arm, or hand

Transient loss of the ability to speak or understand spoken or written language

Slurred or inarticulate speech

Numbness or loss of sensation in an arm or leg, or in an arm and leg on the same side

Weakness or paralysis in an arm or leg, or in an arm and leg on the same side

Transient vertigo, loss of balance, or unsteady gait

Double vision or loss of part of the visual field

Acute confusion, disorientation, delirium, or loss of memory

Sudden onset of profound general weakness

Causes

Established Causes
Atherosclerotic cerebral vascular disease
Uncontrolled hypertension
Embolism
Head trauma

Known Risk Factors for Developing This Disorder
Atherogenic blood lipid disorders
Hypertension
Diabetes
Sickle cell disease
Atrial fibrillation (source of embolism)
Concurrent cigarette smoking and use of oral contraceptives
Long-term heavy cigarette smoking
Excessive alcohol consumption

Drugs That Can Cause This Disorder
anabolic steroids
cocaine (intranasal use, smoking "crack")
oral contraceptives
phenylpropanolamine

Goals of Treatment

Can This Disorder Be Cured?
Brain tissue that has been destroyed by stroke cannot be restored.

Can This Disorder Be Treated Effectively?
Rehabilitation programs can improve some residual disabilities following stroke.

Specific Goals
- Recognition of TIAs and prompt intervention to prevent stroke
- Recognition of early established stroke and immediate thrombolytic therapy to minimize brain damage

Health Professionals Who Participate in Managing This Disorder
Family physicians
General internists
Geriatricians
Neurologists
Ophthalmologists
Optometrists

Neurosurgeons
Vascular surgeons
Physiatrists
Behavioral psychologists
Pharmacists
Physician assistants
Nurse practitioners
Occupational therapists
Physical therapists
Rehabilitation specialists
Speech therapists

Currently Available Therapies for This Disorder

Drug Therapy
- aspirin for stroke prevention
- ticlopidine (Ticlid) as aspirin substitute
- heparin or warfarin for anticoagulation as appropriate
- alteplase (tissue plasminogen activator, TPA) for acute ischemic stroke

Nondrug Treatment Methods
- carotid endarterectomy
- carotid artery bypass graft

The Role of Prevention in This Disorder

Since meaningful therapeutic options following established stroke are very limited, emphasis should be placed on the prevention of initial stroke or recurrent stroke. Concentrated efforts by health care providers, patients, and their families should be directed to modifying known risk factors for stroke:
- Maintenance of ideal body weight
- Low-fat, low-cholesterol, high-fiber diet
- Regular aerobic exercise program
- Correction of blood lipid disorders
- Total and permanent cessation of smoking
- Avoidance of excessive alcohol consumption
- Consistent control of hypertension
- Strict control of diabetes

Resources

Recommended Reading

The Johns Hopkins White Paper on Stroke, Simeon Margolis, M.D., Ph.D., and Thomas J. Preziosi, M.D. Baltimore: The Johns Hopkins Medical Institutions, 1996.

Additional Information and Services
American Heart Association
National Center
7272 Greenville Avenue
Dallas, TX 75231-4596
Phone: (214) 373-6300; Fax: (214) 706-1341
   Publications available.

National Stroke Association
300 E. Hampden Avenue, Suite 240
Englewood, CO 80110-2654
Phone: 1-800-787-6537
   Provides information on support networks for stroke victims and their families. Also serves as a clearinghouse of information on stroke, including referrals to local support groups.

TOURETTE SYNDROME
(too RET)

Other Names Gilles de la Tourette's syndrome (or disease), GTS, TS

Prevalence/Incidence in U.S. 100,000 persons have some form of TS, according to current estimates.

Age Group Onset before 18 years of age, usually between 4 and 10 years

Male-to-Female Ratio 3 to 1

Principal Features and Natural History
Tourette syndrome is a genetic, neurological disorder characterized by a spectrum of vocal and/or movement "tics"—spontaneous, involuntary vocal sounds and utterances and jerking movements of facial or body muscles. Vocal sounds may begin as grunts or barklike noises; later manifestations may be the stereotyped repetition of words or phrases spoken by someone else (echolalia), or the compulsive use of obscene and vulgar language (coprolalia). Movement tics may consist of rapid eye blinking, facial grimacing, twitching or jerking of the limbs. The combination of vocal and movement tics can be mild, moderate, or severe in nature. However, contrary to earlier belief, coprolalia occurs in the minority of cases and is not essential to make the diagnosis of TS. Tics can be limited to either vocal or movement forms, and can wax and wane in intensity over time. Some patients are able to suppress their tics for several min-

utes or a few hours. Tics usually increase in frequency and severity as a result of anxiety or stress.

For many individuals with TS the pattern of tics diminishes in their late teens or early twenties. Approximately 30% of TS patients will experience spontaneous remission of tics in adulthood.

Note: Some authorities now believe that Tourette syndrome also includes the abnormal behavioral patterns referred to as Attention Deficit Hyperactivity Disorder (ADHD) and Obsessive-Compulsive Disorder (OCD). They contend that the manifestations of all three disorders are genetically related variants of a common neurologic dysfunction (see the Profiles of ADHD and OCD in this section).

Diagnostic Symptoms and Signs
Both multiple movement and one or more vocal tics have been present at some time during the course of the illness, but not necessarily concurrently.

Tics occur (usually in bouts) many times a day, nearly every day, or intermittently for more than one year without a tic-free period of more than three consecutive months.

The symptoms cause marked distress or significant impairment in social, occupational, or other important areas of functioning.

Symptoms began before 18 years of age.

Symptoms are not due to the direct physiologic effects of stimulant substances or the result of a general medical condition, such as Huntington's disease or postviral encephalitis.

Diagnostic Tests and Procedures
Currently available clinical diagnostic tests reveal no abnormalities. The diagnosis of TS is based on clinical observation of tics.

Some physicians may advise appropriate diagnostic procedures to rule out other disorders: electroencephalogram (EEG), magnetic resonance imaging (MRI), computerized axial tomography (CAT scan) of the brain.

Diagnostic "Markers" for This Disorder
None discovered to date.

Similar Conditions That May Confuse Diagnosis
Heavy metal poisoning (lead, mercury, etc.)
Huntington's disease
Lesch-Nyhan syndrome
Myoclonic seizures
Postviral encephalitis

Subacute sclerosing panencephalitis
Sydenham's chorea
Wilson's disease

Causes

Established Causes
None confirmed to date.

Theoretical Causes
Possible dysfunction of certain neurotransmitters (dopamine, serotonin, endorphins) in the basal ganglia of the brain.

Known Risk Factors for Developing This Disorder
A family history of any of the neurologic behavioral disorders now considered to constitute Tourette syndrome.

Drugs That Can Cause This Disorder

There are no drugs in current use that cause symptoms in accord with the criteria that define TS.

The following drugs may cause abnormal involuntary movements (AIMs); however, these do not conform to the pattern of "tics" that are diagnostic of TS.

amiodarone
amitriptyline
bromocriptine
carbamazepine
chlorpromazine
clozapine
fluphenazine
haloperidol
levodopa/carbidopa
mesoridazine
metoclopramide
molindone
pimozide
prochlorperazine
selegiline
thiothixene
trifluoperazine

Goals of Treatment

Can This Disorder Be Cured?
No curative treatment is available at this time.

Can This Disorder Be Treated Effectively?

Can symptoms be relieved? Yes, but not completely eliminated.

A variety of drugs are available that can reduce the frequency and severity of tics and behavioral abnormalities. Effective drug treatment does not shorten the course of the disorder.

Specific Goals

- To help the patient and family to accept the diagnosis realistically, and to adapt in a positive and helpful manner
- To determine the most effective treatment for control of tics: the drug of choice and its optimal dosing schedule
- To educate members of the family, the patient's teachers and other associates regarding the nature of TS; to guide their responses to the affected individual; to teach appropriate management techniques designed to control behavior and enhance emotional growth and stability

Health Professionals Who Participate in Managing This Disorder

Family physicians
General internists
Neurologists
Clinical psychologists
Psychiatrists
Neuropsychiatrists
Pharmacists
Mental health social workers
Special education teachers

Currently Available Therapies for This Disorder

Nondrug Treatment Methods

- Psychotherapies: insight therapy; supportive therapy; behavioral modification
- Stress management: relaxation techniques; biofeedback procedures

Drug Therapy

There is no medication that is *specific* for TS. Drugs are used to treat (control) symptoms as deemed necessary and appropriate.

For control of Tourette tics:

- clonazepam (Klonopin)
- clonidine (Catapres)
- fluphenazine (Permitil, Prolixin)
- haloperidol (Haldol)
- pimozide (Orap)

For control of Attention Deficit Hyperactivity Disorder (ADHD):
- dextroamphetamine (Dexedrine)
- methylphenidate (Ritalin)
- pemoline (Cylert)

For control of Obsessive-Compulsive Disorder (OCD):
- clomipramine (Anafranil)
- fluoxetine (Prozac)
- fluxoxamine (Luvox)
- paroxetine (Paxil)
- sertraline (Zoloft)

New Drugs in Development for Treating This Disorder

Risperidone (Risperdal), recently approved by FDA for the treatment of schizophrenia, appears to be a good alternative treatment for TS in both children and adults. It has fewer side effects than haloperidol (Haldol) or pimozide (Orap).

Management of Therapy

The majority of individuals with TS do not require medication; their tics and behavioral aberrations are relatively mild and tolerable.

If medications are required to control tics, selection of the drug and dosage schedule must be individualized and carefully monitored to achieve optimal results.

Drug treatment is started with small doses, then gradually increased until maximal relief of symptoms with minimal side effects is obtained.

If satisfactory control is not achieved with a single drug, a combination of an anti-tic drug and a behavioral-modifying drug may be tried.

Therapeutic Drug Monitoring (Blood Levels)

For clonazepam (Klonopin): recommended blood level range is 10–50 ng/ml.

Use of Haloperidol

Reduces tics in 70% of patients; 50% may experience adverse effects; 25% achieve significant improvement without adverse effects. The optimal dose is that which reduces tics by 75%.

Use of Pimozide

This drug can alter the electrical conduction within the heart; periodic electrocardiograms (ECGs) are advisable.

Use of Clonidine

This is a drug of choice for children with TS who also display behavioral evidence of attention-deficit hyperactivity and/or obsessive-compulsive disorder. Approximately 30% of patients respond favorably. A trial of two months is usually necessary to evaluate this drug's effectiveness.

Important Points to Consider

- When tics are mild and not disabling, antianxiety drugs (benzodiazepines) are preferable to more potent antipsychotic (neuroleptic) drugs.
- Neuroleptic drugs, such as haloperidol, carry the risk of drug-induced involuntary movements or tardive dyskinesia (see Glossary). To reduce the frequency and severity of adverse effects, it is advisable to settle for a 50–75% control of tics.
- The natural course of TS is that it improves and worsens unpredictably, with or without treatment.

Ancillary Drug Treatment (as required)

For attention deficit hyperactivity disorder:
    see ADHD Profile
For obsessive-compulsive disorder:
    see OCD Profile
Note: Drug selection, dosage, and administration schedule must be determined by the physician for each patient individually.

Possible Drug Interactions of Significance

Pimozide *taken concurrently* with

- fluoxetine can cause excessive slowing of the heart rate; monitor the combined use of these drugs carefully.

Quality of Life Considerations

Tourette syndrome does not cause physical deterioration and does not shorten normal life span. Therefore, the most important consideration becomes the quality of the individual's life. When movement and/or vocal tics (especially coprolalia) appear to be increasing in frequency and intensity, effective therapy should be started as early as possible. A pattern of bizarre, disruptive tics may persist into adolescence and adulthood, and often become physically and socially disabling. During the entire course of TS, the person's emotional state is directly related to the frequency and severity of tics.

The Role of Prevention in This Disorder

Primary Prevention

No measures are currently available to prevent the inheritance of this genetic predisposition.

Secondary Prevention

Early diagnosis and appropriate treatment can significantly control the manifestations and course of TS.

Helpful Suggestions for Daily Living

Your Environment
Home, school, and workplace should be carefully structured to provide a sense of comfort and protection and to minimize stress.

Your Lifestyle
- Assure sufficient sleep on a regular basis; avoid undue emotional and physical stress.
- Cultivate hobbies that you find interesting and rewarding; avoid activities that cause anxiety, irritation, or frustration.
- Seek and accept the support and encouragement of your family, friends, teachers, and health care providers; comply honestly and cooperatively with all reasonable therapies.

Resources

Recommended Reading
Contact the Tourette Syndrome Association (see below).

Additional Information and Services
Tourette Syndrome Association, Inc.
42-40 Bell Blvd.
Bayside, NY 11361-2874
Phone: 1-800-237-0717, (718) 224-2999; Fax: (718) 279-9596

Provides information about TS to professionals, schools, and the general public: brochures, films, and videotapes. Operates the National Service Response Team (NASRET) to provide extensive information and referral services to anyone in need of helpful resources.

Disease Management Expertise
The National Service Response Team (NASRET) maintains a state-by-state list of physicians who diagnose and treat TS. Use the above telephone numbers to obtain a referral.

TUBERCULOSIS

Other Names TB, bovine tuberculosis, phthisis

Prevalence/Incidence in U.S.
Current estimate: 10 million persons infected
Estimated new cases annually: 20,000
Estimated deaths annually: 1,700

Age Group

Age	% of Total
0–4	3.6
5–9	1.4
10–14	1.2
15–19	2.2
20–24	5.0
25–34	19.2
35–44	18.7
45–54	13.0
55–64	11.9
65+	23.8

Male-to-Female Ratio Male cases: 67%; Female cases: 33%

Principal Features and Natural History

Tuberculosis is a chronic, recurrent infection that usually begins in the lungs, but can involve any organ system or tissue in the body. Following initial infection by inhaling the causative bacteria (tubercle bacillus), symptoms may develop within a few months or be delayed for years. The natural history of tuberculosis can vary greatly from one person to another, depending upon the virulence of the bacteria and the general health of the individual. The full scope of tuberculous infection can be divided into three stages: (1) primary or initial infection (formerly referred to as childhood infection); (2) latent or dormant infection; and (3) recrudescent or adult-type infection.

Primary Stage Infection

Initial infection occurs almost exclusively by inhaling mucous droplets (containing tubercle bacilli) that are dispersed by an individual with active (open) TB of the lungs when coughing. A small area of inflammation develops at the sites of bacterial invasion in lung tissue, initiating the formation of tubercles—localized foci of infection. This occurrence causes no symptoms, and 90–95% of primary TB infections are not recognized. However, the presence of live tubercle bacilli within the body provokes the production of reactive antibodies that yield a positive result on future skin testing for TB infection. If the infecting bacteria possess high virulence, and/or the resistance of the individual is low, 5–10% of those infected may gradually develop active, progressive disease within a few months. Symptoms of early infection include low-grade fever, fatigue, weight loss, and cough. Black Americans are more susceptible to primary infection than whites. In healthy individuals, most primary infections are self-limited.

Latent Stage Infection

Following initial infection, the large majority of individuals will experience an extended period of latent infection ranging from many years to lifetime. During this period, the infecting tubercle bacilli are alive but dormant. An effective immune system holds them "in check" but does not destroy them. The TB is not "active" and no clinical symptoms develop. However, the potential for "reactivation" of infection is ever present.

Recrudescent Stage Infection

At the time of primary infection in the lung, some tubercle bacilli may gain access to the bloodstream and be disseminated throughout the body. This "seeding" can result in scattered foci of infection in many organs and tissues. However, as in the lung, some of these organisms are not destroyed and can remain dormant and cause no symptoms to indicate their presence. Should some later circumstance suppress the immune system sufficiently, latent infection can reactivate and produce a variety of manifestations. Factors that appear to precipitate "active" TB include: the onset of diabetes, extended use of corticosteroid drugs, aging (over 70 years), HIV infection, and partial removal of the stomach (subtotal gastrectomy). Most commonly the upper portions of the lungs are the site of disease reactivation—pulmonary tuberculosis. Untreated disease will lead to low-grade fever, fatigue, cough, and sputum production—at first yellow or green, later blood-streaked. Complications of progressive lung infection include cavity formation, pleurisy, and lung collapse (pneumothorax).

In the United States about 82% of tuberculous infections are primarily in the lung (pulmonary TB). The remaining infections (18%) occur in other organs and tissues (extrapulmonary TB). The predominant distribution of the latter is as follows:

Site	Percent
Lymph glands	29.9
Pleura	24.2
Bone and/or joint	10.2
Genitourinary	8.7
Generalized	7.8
Meninges	6.2
Abdominal cavity	3.4
Other	9.6

Tuberculosis and HIV Infection (AIDS)

The continuous spread of HIV infection has resulted in (1) a marked increase in the incidence of TB (up 30% in New York State in one year, for instance), and (2) the development of strains of *M. tuberculosis* (tubercle bacilli) that are resistant to all first-line drugs. The progressive decline of immunity that characterizes AIDS is responsible for increasing numbers of both primary TB infection and reactivation of latent disease.

In addition to lung infection, AIDS predisposes to numerous sites of tuberculous infection throughout the body. This is most apparent among black American and Hispanic intravenous drug users, most commonly men 25 to 44 years old. The course of TB in the HIV-infected patient is significantly different from classical tuberculosis. It progresses quite rapidly and is usually resistant to treatment. The sputum of those with AIDS may contain both *M. tuberculosis* and organisms of the *M. avium* complex (MAC). Infections due to MAC organisms occur in 60% of those with AIDS. Disease manifestations and treatment differ significantly from classical pulmonary TB (see the Profile of AIDS in this section).

Drug-Resistant Tuberculosis

The incidence of primary drug-resistant TB has been relatively low in the United States, but current statistics indicate that outbreaks of it will continue to increase. The present incidence is approximately 3.1%. Those at risk for this type of infection include recent immigrants and HIV-infected drug abusers. The highest incidence is found in settings such as prisons, homeless shelters, and hospitals treating patients with AIDS. Extraordinary measures to prevent spread of infection and intensive drug treatment programs will be required to abort an epidemic.

Diagnostic Symptoms and Signs

Malaise, fatigability, weakness
Loss of appetite and weight
Low-grade fever, night sweats
Chronic cough productive of sputum
Eventual production of bloody sputum
Chest pain with breathing
Shortness of breath with extensive disease

Diagnostic Tests and Procedures

Acid-fast stain of sputum smears for identification of tubercle bacilli; minimum of three separate samples
Sputum cultures by BACTEC procedure for positive identification of tubercle bacilli
Drug susceptibility studies on first isolation of tubercle bacilli
Chest X-ray examinations

Diagnostic "Marker" for This Disorder

Positive identification of *Mycobacterium tuberculosis* obtained by culture of sputum.

Similar Conditions That May Confuse Diagnosis

Sarcoidosis of lung
Fungal infections of lung: coccidioidomycosis, histoplasmosis

Other mycobacterial infections:
M. abscessus
M. avium-intracellulare
M. bovis
M. kansasii
M. scrofulaceum

Causes

Established Cause

The term "tuberculosis" is used to designate only those infections caused by *Mycobacterium tuberculosis*, *M. bovis*, or *M. africanum*.

Known Risk Factors for Developing This Disorder

Exposure to a person with active pulmonary tuberculosis
Acquired immunodeficiency virus infection (AIDS)

Drugs That Can Cause This Disorder

Tuberculosis is an infection caused by certain species of mycobacteria. There are no drugs that can cause TB. However, the extended use of cortisonelike drugs (corticosteroids) and immunosuppressive drugs can suppress the immune system sufficiently to induce "reactivation" of latent (dormant) tuberculous infection.

Goals of Treatment

Can This Disorder Be Cured?

Early diagnosis and prompt initiation of appropriate drug therapy can eradicate infection.

Specific Goals

- To individualize the initial selection of drug regimens for maximal response
- To produce early, maximal bactericidal (bacteria kill) effect
- To follow with maximal sterilizing effect so as to prevent relapse
- To prevent the development of drug-resistant tubercle bacilli
- To initiate preventive drug treatment at the optimal time to prevent latent disease from progressing to active infection

Health Professionals Who Participate in Managing This Disorder

Family physicians
General internists
Infectious disease specialists
Pulmonologists
Thoracic surgeons
Pharmacists

Physician assistants
Nurse practitioners
Medical social workers

Currently Available Therapies for This Disorder

Drug Therapy
First-line drugs:
- isoniazid (INH; Laniazid, Nydrazid)
- rifampin (RIF; Rifadin, Rimactane)
- pyrazinamide (PZA)
- ethambutol (EMB; Myambutol)
- streptomycin (SM)

Second-line drugs:
- amikacin (Amikin)
- aminosalicylic acid
- capreomycin (Capastat)
- ciprofloxacin (Cipro)
- cycloserine (Seromycin)
- ethionamide (ETA; Trecator S.C.)
- kanamycin (Kantrex)
- ofloxacin (Floxin)

Management of Therapy

The successful treatment of tuberculosis depends upon (1) initiating treatment with the optimal combination of drugs, and (2) obtaining full compliance of the patient regarding the proper use of medications. The majority of patients with pulmonary TB can be treated satisfactorily on an outpatient basis. However, regular periodic follow-up evaluation is essential.

Drug treatment is carried out in two successive phases:

> Phase One: The initial "intensive" phase, using multiple drugs concurrently in adequate dosage to achieve a maximal kill rate and prevent the development of drug-resistant organisms.

> Phase Two: The "continuation" phase, designed to destroy any remaining organisms and achieve a near-sterile state to the greatest extent possible.

Optional Drug Regimens
- Isoniazid and rifampin daily for nine months
- Isoniazid and rifampin and pyrazinamide daily for two months, followed by isoniazid and rifampin for four months—total treatment period of six months
- Isoniazid and rifampin daily for one month, followed by supervised twice-a-week treatment for eight months—to ensure compliance with medications

- If primary drug-resistance to either isoniazid and/or rifampin is suspected, add ethambutol daily to the regimen

Regimens for Drug-Resistant TB
- If primary or secondary resistance to isoniazid *or* rifampin is likely, use isoniazid plus rifampin plus ethambutol; or isoniazid plus rifampin plus pyrazinamide plus streptomycin.
- If resistance to isoniazid *and* rifampin is suspected, use ethionamide plus pyrazinamide plus streptomycin; or ethionamide plus pyrazinamide plus ethambutol.
- If resistance to streptomycin is known, use amikacin, capreomycin, or kanamycin to replace it.
- If full compliance is not expected with self-administered treatment, a supervised intermittent regimen is recommended.

Therapeutic Drug Monitoring (Blood Levels)
- Recommended blood level range for amikacin: peak: 12–25 mcg/ml; trough: 5–10 mcg/ml
- Recommended blood level range for kanamycin: 25–35 mcg/ml

Ancillary Drug Treatment (as required)
For prevention of peripheral neuropathy with use of isoniazid:
- pyridoxine (vitamin B_6), dosage range from 6 mg to 25 mg daily; give 50 mg twice a week with intermittent isoniazid therapy

For malnutrition:
- high caloric diet with mineral and vitamin supplements

Note: Drug selection, dosage, and administration schedule must be determined by the physician for each patient individually.

Current Controversies in Management
The question of preventive medication to reduce the risk of acquiring active tuberculous infection has become more pertinent and pressing since the advent of AIDS. Risk assessment involves the likelihood of developing active TB and the possibility of experiencing serious liver toxicity while taking the preventive drug (isoniazid). The following considerations are helpful in deciding whether or not it is advisable to take preventive medication.

In decreasing order of risk, the following are candidates for preventive treatment:
- Household members and close associates of anyone recently diagnosed to have active pulmonary tuberculosis
- Individuals whose tuberculin skin test converted from negative to positive within the past two years
- Individuals with a positive tuberculin skin test and chest X-ray findings consistent with inactive pulmonary TB, but without a positive bacteriological culture and no prior course of adequate drug therapy

- HIV-infected individuals with a high risk of prior exposure to active TB
- Individuals with a positive tuberculin skin test and any of the following: extended corticosteroid drug use, immunosuppressive drug therapy, leukemia, lymphoma, diabetes, silicosis, gastrectomy
- Individuals under 35 years of age with a positive tuberculin skin test

The possibility of isoniazid-induced hepatitis is apparently age-related.

   Under 20 years old: rare liver damage

   20 to 24 years old: 0.3% liver damage

   Over 50 years old: 2.3% liver damage

Preventive drug therapy consists of isoniazid in a dose of 300 mg daily for adults and 10 mg per kilogram of body weight daily for children (not to exceed 300 mg daily). If tolerated, this is taken for periods ranging from 6 to 12 months. This procedure has reduced the incidence of active TB by 75% during the first year and by 50–66% in subsequent years. Contraindications to the use of isoniazid are any form of active liver disease or a history of previous adverse reaction to it.

Important Points to Consider

Individuals in high-risk groups for HIV exposure and who are newly diagnosed to have tuberculosis should be tested for HIV infection.

Patient compliance with a prescribed treatment regimen is critical to the elimination of tuberculous infection. Studies show that 20% to 50% of those who start drug therapy do not complete it. This failure to comply has serious consequences: the infected patient remains a threat for further spread of TB; the infected patient is at increased risk for relapse of disease; eventual curative drug treatment becomes more prolonged and expensive; the causative strains of tubercle bacilli have a greater chance to develop resistance to drugs.

There are many valid reasons that make it difficult for some patients to fully comply with medication regimens. Each patient should explain the problems encountered in daily living that interfere with the regular use of drugs as prescribed. Patients and caregivers—working together—should develop strategies that best accommodate the patient's lifestyle with regard to the effective use of medications. Patients know best what will and what will not work for them. Close cooperation is most important during the first eight weeks of treatment to ensure good compliance.

Possible Drug Interactions of Significance

Because of the number and nature of drugs that may be used to manage this disorder, adequate consideration of the volume and complexity of potential drug interactions is beyond the scope of this book. Consult *The Essential Guide to Prescription Drugs*, or a similar drug reference book for possible interactions of significance (see Appendix 17, Drug Information Sources).

Special Considerations for Women

Rifampin can reduce the effectiveness of oral contraceptives. A barrier method of contraception is recommended during rifampin therapy.

Pregnancy

Kanamycin and streptomycin are designated Pregnancy Category D drugs. Their use during pregnancy could be harmful to the fetus. Discuss this with your physician (see Appendix 15, FDA Pregnancy Categories).

Breast-Feeding

Consult your physician regarding the compatibility of nursing and any drugs you are taking.

Special Considerations for the Elderly

Approximately 30% of newly diagnosed cases of tuberculosis occur in persons over 65 years of age. Those who are institutionalized are at greater risk for developing TB. In older individuals the initial symptoms of active infection may be quite vague: fatigue, weight loss, and cough without fever or night sweats. This pattern of symptoms should arouse suspicion and prompt appropriate evaluation.

The Role of Prevention in This Disorder

Primary Prevention

The Centers for Disease Control and Prevention of the Public Health Service issued the following statements on April 26, 1996, regarding the role of BCG vaccine in the prevention and control of tuberculosis in the United States:

- The risk for *M. tuberculosis* infection in the overall population is low. The primary strategy for preventing and controlling TB is to minimize the risk for transmission by the early identification and treatment of patients who have active infectious TB.
- The second most important strategy is the identification of persons who have latent *M. tuberculosis* infection and, if indicated, the use of preventive therapy with isoniazid to prevent the latent infection from progressing to active TB disease.
- The use of BCG vaccine has been limited because (1) its effectiveness in preventing infectious forms of TB is uncertain, and (2) the reactivity of tuberculin that occurs after vaccination interferes with the management of persons who are possibly infected with *M. tuberculosis*.
- The use of BCG vaccination as a TB prevention strategy is reserved for selected persons who meet specific criteria. BCG vaccination should be considered for infants and children who reside in settings in which

the likelihood of *M. tuberculosis* transmission and subsequent infection is high.

- BCG vaccination may be considered for health care workers who are employed in settings in which the likelihood of transmission and subsequent infection with *M. tuberculosis* strains resistant to isoniazid and rifampin is high, provided comprehensive TB infection-control precautions have been implemented in the workplace and have not been successful.
- BCG vaccination is not recommended for children and adults who are infected with human immunodeficiency virus (HIV) because of the potential adverse reactions associated with the use of the vaccine in these persons.
- In the United States, the use of BCG vaccination is rarely indicated. BCG vaccination is not recommended for inclusion in immunization or TB control programs, and it is not recommended for most health care workers.

Secondary Prevention

- Close monitoring of anyone known to have latent TB infection for indications of reactivation
- Prompt initiation of appropriate drug therapy as indicated and careful follow-up to ensure compliance

Resources

Recommended Reading

Facts About Tuberculosis and *TB: What You Should Know*, two booklets available from the American Lung Association. For copies call 1-800-LUNG-USA (1-800-586-4872).

Additional Information and Services

American Lung Association
1740 Broadway
New York, NY 10019-4374
Phone: 1-800-LUNG-USA, (212) 315-8700; Fax: (212) 265-5642

State groups: 59. Local groups: 72. Publications and videotapes available.

ULCERATIVE COLITIS

Other Names Idiopathic proctocolitis, inflammatory bowel disease

Prevalence/Incidence in U.S. 1 million (including 100,000 children); 15,000 new cases annually

Age Group Peak incidence occurs between 19 and 49 years of age; 75% of cases develop before the age of 40.

Male-to-Female Ratio Same incidence in men and women

Principal Features and Natural History

Ulcerative colitis is a chronically recurrent disorder of the colon (large intestine) and rectum characterized by inflammation and ulceration. Its course follows a pattern of frequent spontaneous remissions and recurrences without apparent cause. It may be associated with disease in other organs of the body, notably the skin, joints, eye, liver, and blood vessels, making it a multiple system disorder. The principal symptoms of the diseased colon are abdominal cramping and bloody diarrhea; associated symptoms include fatigue, weakness, occasional low-grade fever, weight loss, anemia, and dehydration.

The more severe forms of ulcerative colitis can be very difficult to control. When repeated trials of adequate medicinal therapy fail to induce and maintain remission and the patient experiences life-threatening complications, surgical removal of the entire colon (colectomy) can be an acceptable resolution. Circumstances that warrant surgical intervention include:

Urgent management of complications: bowel obstruction, bowel perforation, uncontrollable hemorrhage, toxic megacolon (a nonfunctional, dilated colon filled with toxic waste)

Elective management of unresponsive, long-standing disease in a patient whose condition progressively deteriorates

Preventive management of the patient with a 10-year history of recurrently active ulcerative colitis and recent biopsy findings of precancerous or cancerous tissue in the colon or rectum

Total colectomy is a curative procedure. The colon is not essential to survival. With appropriate rehabilitative therapy, satisfactory well-being and a good quality of life can be achieved.

Diagnostic Symptoms and Signs

Abdominal cramping
Recurrent episodes of diarrhea
Bloody stools
Loss of appetite, loss of weight
Fever, fatigue (in severe cases)
Involvement of other tissues (45% of cases):
Skin rashes and ulcerations on extremities
Burning and redness of eyes, blurred vision
Migratory pain and swelling in large joints

Diagnostic Tests and Procedures
Complete blood cell counts
Red blood cell sedimentation rate (see Glossary): an indicator of inflammation; useful in monitoring response to treatment
Appropriate blood chemistries, liver function tests
Stool examinations for pathogenic (disease-causing) bacteria or parasites
X-ray studies of the colon: barium enemas with air contrast
Colonoscopy for direct inspection of the colon and to obtain biopsy specimens

Diagnostic "Markers" for This Disorder
There are no specific markers for this disease. The diagnosis of ulcerative colitis is made by exclusion.

Similar Conditions That May Confuse Diagnosis
Irritable bowel syndrome
Subacute or chronic bacterial or parasitic infections of the colon
Drug-induced colitis: an adverse effect of some antibiotics
Diverticulitis
Colon or rectal cancer
Crohn's disease
AIDS-associated diarrhea

Causes

Established Causes
The definitive cause is unknown at this time.

Theoretical Causes
The clinical and pathological features of ulcerative colitis suggest that it is an autoimmune disorder (see Appendix 5, The Immune System).

Known Risk Factors for Developing This Disorder
Genetic predisposition. There is a familial pattern and frequent occurrence in twins.

Drugs That Can Cause This Disorder
No drugs initiate true ulcerative colitis. However, the following anti-infective drugs can cause pseudomembranous colitis, a disorder that closely resembles an acute episode of ulcerative colitis:
    amoxicillin
    ampicillin
    cephalosporins (see Appendix 16, Drug Classes)
    chloramphenicol

clindamycin
lincomycin
penicillin
tetracycline
trimethoprim and sulfamethoxsazole in combination

Goals of Treatment

Can This Disorder Be Cured?
There are no medications that can cure ulcerative colitis. However, a total colectomy is curative.

Can This Disorder Be Treated Effectively?
Mild to moderate cases respond reasonably well to medications designed to induce remission and prevent recurrence of active disease.

Severe and unresponsive cases with life-threatening complications often require surgery.

Specific Goals
- Control of pain and diarrhea
- Prompt control of acute episodes; suppression of inflammation and ulceration
- Induction of a lasting remission
- Prevention of recurrence of acute episodes
- Detection of early colon or rectal cancer; curative surgery

Health Professionals Who Participate in Managing This Disorder
Family physicians
General internists
Gastroenterologists
Inflammatory bowel disease specialists
Clinical immunologists
General surgeons
Colon/Rectal surgeons
Psychiatrists
Pharmacists
Dietitians/Nutritionists

Currently Available Therapies for This Disorder

Drug Therapy
Anti-inflammatory drugs:
- mesalamine (Asacol, Pentasa, Rowasa)
- olsalazine (Dipentum)
- sulfasalazine (Azulfidine)

Cortisonelike steroids:
- ACTH (adrenocorticotropic hormone): by intramuscular injection
- prednisone, prednisolone (generic): by mouth
- hydrocortisone enemas (Cortenema)
- hydrocortisone foam (Cortifoam)
- hydrocortisone suppositories (Anusol-HC)
- methylprednisolone enema (Medrol Enpak)

Antidiarrheals:
- diphenoxylate (Lomotil)
- loperamide (Imodium)

Antispasmodics:
- dicyclomine (Bentyl)
- propantheline (Pro-Banthine)

Immunosuppressive drugs:
- azathioprine (Imuran)
- cyclosporine (Sandimmune)
- 6-mercatopurine (Purinethol)

Nondrug Treatment Methods

DIETARY MANAGEMENT
- Avoidance of spicy and highly seasoned foods, caffeine, and raw fruits and vegetables during acute episodes of diarrhea
- Nutritional supplements are required
- Periods of bowel rest and total parenteral (intravenous) nutrition during severe attacks

SURGICAL PROCEDURES
- Total proctocolectomy (removal of colon and rectum) with ileostomy (surgical creation of an opening between the small intestine and the surface of the abdomen to facilitate defecation).
- Subtotal colectomy with ileal pouch anal anastomosis: surgical connection of the terminal ileum to a preserved anus, allowing anal defecation and avoiding ileostomy. Postoperative inflammation within the pouch is well controlled with metronidazole.

New Drugs in Development for Treating This Disorder
- balsalazide (Colazide): provides a more colon-specific delivery of mesalamine
- budesonide (Entocort): effective corticosteroid enema preparation that lacks the systemic adverse effects of other products

Management of Therapy
- The majority (up to 90%) of cases of active ulcerative colitis respond well to medical treatment or have a spontaneous remission. Approximately 20% have a prolonged remission after the first acute attack.

Studies indicate that 55% of individuals who experience ulcerative coli-tis remain in remission at any given time during the course of the dis-order. To minimize the risks of long-term drug use, the smallest dose of maintenance drugs (Azulfidine and prednisone) that prevents recur-rence should be determined.

- It is essential that every recurrence of acute colitis (relapse) be treated promptly and vigorously. Chronically active ulcerative colitis predis-poses to a higher than normal incidence of cancer of the colon and rectum. Estimates are 3% after the first 10 years of disease, increasing to 20% per decade thereafter. Everyone subject to ulcerative colitis should have a thorough examination of the colon and rectum annually regardless of the status of the disorder.
- Antidiarrheal drugs should be used with extreme caution. Excessive use can induce a paralysis of colon activity and increase the risk of developing toxic megacolon—a massive distention of the colon with air and toxic waste; perforation constitutes a surgical emergency.
- Iron preparations for anemia should not be taken during a period of acute inflammation or active ulceration. Iron therapy should be with-held until a remission is established.

Use of Sulfasalazine

- This effective and reliable drug is used to treat acute attacks of active colitis and to prevent relapse during periods of remission. It is used con-currently with cortisonelike steroids during acute attacks to control inflammation and ulceration and to induce remission. During the quies-cent phase of colitis, it is used in small doses (up to 2 grams/day) for the long-term maintenance of remission. It may be taken indefinitely.
- This drug is best taken with or following food to reduce stomach irrita-tion.
- The long-term use of this drug can impair folic acid absorption and may cause a folic acid deficiency. Consult your physician regarding the need for a supplement.
- During long-term use, it is advisable to monitor blood cell counts to detect the development of anemia or abnormally low white blood cells.
- Mesalamine, the active derivative of sulfasalazine, is used in the form of a rectal suspension (retention enema), taken at bedtime for night-long action. The initial course of treatment is from three to six weeks. Carefully read and follow the printed instructions that are provided with this drug.

Use of Cortisonelike Steroids

- Steroids should be used when there are obvious symptoms of disease activity: diarrhea, bloody stools, nocturnal bowel movements, anemia, weight loss, etc. They are also of value in treating the systemic mani-festations of this disorder: dermatitis, arthritis, iritis, etc.

- These drugs are the mainstay of treatment for acute, active ulcerative colitis. They can induce remission in 70–80% of cases.
- To ensure prompt and adequate control of acute inflammation, initial dosage should be high. Response usually occurs within 10 to 14 days. After a remission has been induced, steroid dosage is reduced to a minimum that will stabilize the colon and prevent relapse. The long-term maintenance use of steroids is controversial. If individual circumstances warrant the continual use of low-dose steroids, it is preferable to use alternate-day dosage—a single morning dose every 48 hours. This is effective in preventing recurrence for some patients and it carries a lower risk of causing adverse effects.
- When the inflammation and ulceration are limited to the rectum, steroids can be administered in the form of enemas, foams, and suppositories for local application. This minimizes systemic effects.
- The long-term use of prednisone (even in small doses) can cause significant adverse effects (see Appendix 6, Long-Term Corticosteroid Therapy).

Therapeutic Drug Monitoring (Blood Levels)
Cyclosporine (Sandimmune): recommended range: 100–150 ng/ml

Ancillary Drug Treatment (as required)
For abdominal cramps:
- dicyclomine (Bentyl)
- propantheline (Pro-Banthine)
  To be used sparingly.
For diarrhea:
- diphenoxylate (Lomotil)
- loperamide (Imodium)
  To be used sparingly.
For anxiety:
- buspirone (Buspar), nonsedating
- diazepam (Valium), sedating
For depression:
  see Profile of depression in this section
For anemia:
- iron preparations (not during acute stage of colitis)
- folic acid (if appropriate for type of anemia)
  Note: Drug selection, dosage, and administration schedule must be determined by the physician for each patient individually.

Possible Drug Interactions of Significance
Allopurinol may *increase* the effects of
- azathioprine (Imuran) and 6-mercaptopurine (Purinethol), making it necessary to reduce their dosages.

Sulfasalazine may *increase* the effects of
- sulfonylureas and increase the risk of hypoglycemia (see Appendix 16, Drug Classes).

Allopurinol *taken concurrently* with
- cyclosporine (Sandimmune) may result in cyclosporine toxicity.

Prednisone *taken concurrently* with
- cyclosporine (Sandimmune) may increase the blood levels of both drugs; dose reductions of both drugs may be needed.

Special Considerations for Women

Pregnancy

Effective contraception is strongly advised.

Azathioprine (Imuran) and 6-mercaptopurine (Purinethol) are both designated Pregnancy Category D drugs. Their safe use during pregnancy is questionable (see Appendix 15, FDA Pregnancy Categories).

Quality of Life Considerations

If you have severe, protracted ulcerative colitis that has failed to respond to the best medicinal therapy available, you should be fully informed regarding surgical options. You may not realize that total colectomy is curative; that the colon is not essential to survival; and that modern surgical techniques can provide totally acceptable ileostomies that are easily managed and amenable to a normal pattern of living.

The Role of Prevention in This Disorder

Primary Prevention

There is no known way to prevent the initial development of ulcerative colitis.

Secondary Prevention

Every effort should be made to determine the therapeutic program that is most effective for each patient individually. If disease activity persists in spite of adequate medicinal therapy, surgical options are available to manage life-threatening complications and to prevent the development of colon or rectal cancer.

Resources

Recommended Reading

The Angry Gut: Coping with Colitis and Crohn's Disease, W. Grant Thompson. New York: Plenum Press, 1993.

Additional Information and Services

American Digestive Disease Society

60 East 42nd Street, Room 411
New York, NY 10165
Telecommunications services: Gutline, available to the public every Tuesday evening from 7:30 to 9:00 P.M. Publications available.

Crohn's and Colitis Foundation of America
386 Park Avenue South, 17th Floor
New York, NY 10016
Phone: 1-800-343-3637, (212) 685-3440; Fax: (212) 779-4098
Local groups: 73. Publications available.

ZOLLINGER-ELLISON SYNDROME
(ZOL in jer EL i son)

Other Names ZES, Z-E syndrome, gastrinomas, pancreatic ulcerogenic tumor syndrome

Age Group Can begin in childhood. Usual time of diagnosis is between ages of 20 and 70 years, with mean age of 50 years.

Male-to-Female Ratio Males and females are affected equally.

Principal Features and Natural History
The Zollinger-Ellison syndrome can be thought of as a severe form of peptic ulcer disease, but with significant differences in cause, diagnosis, disease course, and management. The principal features of ZES include: (1) unusually severe and intractable peptic ulcers, (2) excessive production of stomach acid (hyperacidity), and (3) the presence of one or more tumors that produce the hormone "gastrin," hence the name gastrinomas. Gastrin stimulates the production of stomach acid. The gastrinomas may be single or multiple, small or large, benign or malignant (cancerous). They are usually located in the pancreas or duodenum (small intestine), but may also be found in the spleen and abdominal lymph nodes. During surgery for removal of gastrinomas, 35% of patients are found to have a localized tumor; 31% have malignant tumors with spread to the liver, lungs, or bones; and in 34% no tumor can be found.

Early symptoms of ZES may be diarrhea and light-colored stools containing fat-like substances. These are followed by the onset of intense abdominal pain, acid indigestion, and heartburn—acid reflux into the esophagus. With the development of peptic ulcers, the patient may experience any of the consequent complications that characterize peptic ulcer disease: bleeding, perforation, or obstruction.

ALERT!

Peptic ulcers associated with ZES may be refractory to any type of treatment for years. Due to lack of recognition of the syndrome, there is often a delay of three to five years from the onset of symptoms to the diagnosis of ZES. All patients with recurrent peptic ulcer disease should be tested for high blood levels of gastrin, a significant diagnostic marker. In view of the life-threatening nature of this disorder, early diagnosis is critical. No patient with chronic peptic ulcer disease should have surgery without first testing the fasting blood level of gastrin.

Diagnostic Symptoms and Signs

The symptoms of ZES are those of recurrent peptic ulcer disease as described above. There are no specific diagnostic signs to be found on physical examination (see the Profile of peptic ulcer disease in this section).

Diagnostic Tests and Procedures

Measurement of fasting blood gastrin levels
Measurements of stomach acid secretion
Provocative test for gastrinoma: secretin stimulation test
X-ray studies of upper gastrointestinal tract (stomach and duodenum)
Gastroscopic visualization of esophagus and stomach
Computed axial tomography (CT scanning) for detection of gastrinomas
Endoscopic ultrasonography for detection of gastrinomas
    Note: All drugs that suppress stomach acid production should be discontinued for several days prior to testing.

Diagnostic "Markers" for This Disorder

Fasting blood gastrin level of 1000 pg/ml or higher
An increased basal stomach acid secretion
Markedly increased rates of stomach acid secretion: basal to peak acid
    output ratio greater than 0.5:1.0
A positive secretin stimulation test result: a marked increase in fasting
    blood gastrin levels following an intravenous injection of secretin
X-ray findings of large, thickened folds of lining in the stomach and duo-
    denum, with or without peptic ulcers

Similar Conditions That May Confuse Diagnosis

Classical peptic ulcer disease (without gastrinomas)
Multiple endocrine neoplasias type I (MEN-I syndrome)

Causes

Established Causes

None known at this time.

Theoretical Causes
Genetic predisposition.

Known Risk Factors for Developing This Disorder
Family history of peptic ulcer disease in parent or sibling.

Drugs That Can Cause This Disorder
There are no drugs that can cause true ZES. See the Profile of peptic ulcer disease in this section for the names of drugs that can initiate stomach or duodenal ulcers.

Goals of Treatment

Can This Disorder Be Cured?
Complete cure by surgical removal of gastrinomas is possible in 20–30% of ZES patients.

Can This Disorder Be Treated Effectively?
Excessive stomach acid secretion can be controlled effectively with available medications, providing excellent relief of symptoms.

Specific Goals
- Control of stomach acid secretion to relieve symptoms and deter ulcer formation
- Detection and removal of gastrinomas to produce a cure whenever possible
- Control of malignant tumors that cannot be removed

Health Professionals Who Participate in Managing This Disorder
Family physicians
General internists
Gastroenterologists
Diagnostic radiologists
Clinical pathologists
Medical oncologists
Surgical oncologists
Abdominal surgeons
Pharmacists

Currently Available Therapies for This Disorder

Drug Therapy
- omeprazole (the drug of choice)
- lansoprazole
- histamine-blocking drugs: cimetidine, famotidine, nizatidine, ranitidine

- antacids: aluminum and magnesium hydroxide preparations

Nondrug Treatment Methods
- Surgical removal of gastrinoma; 30% of gastrinomas are amenable to surgical resection.
- Surgical vagotomy (severing the vagus nerve to the stomach) following resection of gastrinoma.

Management of Therapy
Initial treatment is designed to control excessive production of stomach acids, arrest development of peptic ulcers, and promote healing. After stomach acid production is reasonably controlled, definitive tests are performed to establish the diagnosis of ZES. If diagnostic tests are indicative of ZES, detection studies are performed to demonstrate the presence of gastrinoma.

Consultation with a surgical oncologist is sought to devise an optimal strategy for managing each patient individually. Localized gastrinomas with no evidence of malignant spread are removed. Optional vagotomy may be performed at the surgeon's discretion. Malignant gastrinomas that are amenable to resection may be removed. Consultation with a medical oncologist is sought to determine the advisability of chemotherapy to suppress tumor spread (metastases).

It should be noted that 25% of gastrinomas are associated with the multiple endocrine neoplasia type I syndrome (MEN-I); this includes hyperparathyroidism, which requires concurrent therapy.

Ancillary Drug Treatment (as required)
Gastrinoma metastasis to liver, etc.:
- chemotherapy: streptozotocin, fluorouracil, doxorubicin

Note: Drug selection, dosage, and administration schedule must be determined by the physician for each patient individually.

Possible Drug Interactions of Significance
Omeprazole may *increase* the effects of
- diazepam
- phenytoin
- warfarin

Special Considerations for Women
Observe the following precautions.

Pregnancy
See Appendix 15, FDA Pregnancy Categories.

Omeprazole: Pregnancy Category C. However, there have been sporadic reports of congenital abnormalities in infants born to women who received omeprazole during pregnancy. Omeprazole should be used during pregnancy only if the potential benefit justifies the potential risk to the fetus.

Breast-Feeding

Omeprazole: omit drug or refrain from nursing.

The Role of Prevention in This Disorder

Primary Prevention

No means of prevention known at this time.

Secondary Prevention

Early recognition of the true nature of ZES and prompt treatment.

Resource for Additional Information and Services

National Digestive Diseases Information Clearinghouse
Two Information Way
Bethesda, MD 20892-3570
Phone: (301) 654-3810

Provides educational materials and refers callers to relevant organizations for services to patients with digestive diseases and disorders.

SECTION FOUR

Terminal Illness:
The Dying Patient

For many of us who have lived for months or years with one or more chronic disorders, our condition may deteriorate gradually to a state of terminal illness. We come to realize that we are in the process of dying—the ultimate chronic disorder. It now becomes important for us to understand that this, too, is a manageable part of living, just as everything that has gone before. Appropriate adjustments are in order for all concerned: patient, family, friends, caregivers, health care professionals. Adjustments in attitude and perspective, in treatment goals and therapeutic procedures are incumbent upon all to help the patient—to the greatest extent that circumstances allow—experience a "good death." While every situation of this nature is somewhat unique, and some aspects are often beyond our control, there are reasonable actions to consider that may lessen the physical and emotional suffering of the patient and calm the anguish felt by those in attendance.

Who Are the Terminally Ill?

The patient who is considered to be terminally ill is suffering from a disease or disorder that is known to be fatal, has reached a level of irreversible deterioration for which there is no curative therapy, and whose life expectancy is judged to be no more than six months.

Of all natural causes of death, 75–80% are attributable to chronic disorders. The following disorders are the current leading causes of terminal illness and death in the United States:

Disorder	Annual Deaths
Heart diseases (all)	717,000
Coronary artery disease	480,000
Congestive heart failure	39,000
Hypertension	35,800
Cancer	538,000
Stroke	150,000
Alzheimer's disease	100,000
Chronic obstructive lung disease	91,000
Diabetes	50,000
AIDS	32,900
Suicide (often depression-related)	30,000
Liver diseases	26,000
Kidney diseases	21,700

Historical Perspectives

The Past

Historically it was the Christian monastic orders of the Middle Ages that first established the "hospice"—a place of charitable refuge that offered rest and refreshment to travelers and provided compassionate care for the elderly, the infirm, and the sick. Although not serving the terminally ill exclusively, the early hospice clearly created the model and defined the mission of its present day counterpart.

A century ago, some hospitals were used exclusively to care for the terminally ill. This reflected a cultural blind spot in the psyche of the time—a reluctance to acknowledge the inevitability of death and a desire to avoid the subject as much as possible. The idea of death was somehow toxic. The hospital provided a place to hide death when it intruded upon the home and family.

During the early decades of this century, the practice of medicine was a "cottage industry." The physician functioned independently and with nearly complete autonomy. Medical science provided very little (by today's standards) to manage chronic disorders and postpone terminal illness. Most practitioners were primary care physicians—the family doctor. The doctor–patient relationship was usually strong and genuine, built on mutual respect and trust. The management of terminal illness and approaching death was a very important element in the art of medicine. The physician, well aware of the attitudes and feelings of the patient and family, usually took the lead in tactfully reaching a consensus as to when the time had come to "let go." Honoring the conscience and wishes of all involved, the physician (when circumstances warranted) would quietly and respectfully take appropriate action to end suffering and ease the way to a peaceful death. This was America before the age of advanced medical technology—the home was the hospice in miniature.

The Present

The truly remarkable achievements of medical science and technology over the past 100 years have contributed greatly to our current longevity and our ability to manage beneficially many diseases and disorders. However, the number and nature of successes made possible by modern medicine have fueled some unrealistic and inappropriate expectations and demands. It is generally recognized that American medical practice, when compared with that of other advanced countries, is significantly more aggressive. Our ability to actually "do something"—such as prolonging life artificially in a brain-dead individual—has clouded our reasoning and deranged our judgment regarding the justification and morality of "doing it." The more brilliant and gratifying our technological accomplishments (e.g., organ transplantation), the more oblivious we choose to be regarding short-term costs and long-term consequences for society. Our fervor for medical progress and its abundant rewards ("miracles") has imprinted our societal consciousness with the notion that "death is the enemy," to be defeated at all costs. Our collective focus has been skewed to favor consideration of how long we can live rather than how well we are living while still alive—the quality of life. On occasion, the consequence of "medical progress" is the intensification of pain and suffering and the prolongation of dying, as with chemotherapy pursued beyond the point of salvage.

This is not to be construed as an argument against appropriate and rational medical research. It is a plea for the acknowledgment of some fundamental realities that part of our culture appears reluctant to address:

- Death is inevitable, a normal event in everyone's span of life. Its character and timing are ultimately determined by natural forces, with and without medical intervention.
- Death is not our enemy. Physical and emotional pain and suffering are our enemies. Let us conquer these.
- The goal of medical science should not be the myopic and near-fanatical prolongation of life that is useless and without meaning.
- The primary focus of medical science should be the optimal enhancement of the quality of life for the duration that natural forces permit.
- The fundamental obligation of all health care professionals is first to help their patients achieve a "good life," and, when the time comes, to facilitate a "good death."

Management Strategies

Self-Education

Once you know your diagnosis and prognosis, try to do your homework as soon as you can. If your condition and circumstances allow, obtain pertinent information about your disorder and its management. This will enable you to communicate with your physicians more effectively; you will be better prepared to make judgments and decisions regarding treatments that are recommended. For many at this critical time, awareness and understanding of their condition can lessen anxiety and uncertainty, improving their ability to accept their situation and cope with it.

Personal Philosophy

If you have not already done so, now is the time to examine your true feelings and attitudes about life, death, and dying. During our healthy years, many of us find that the business of daily living leaves little time for reflective thought of this nature. Engage in quiet contemplation about your life. Discuss your conclusions with a receptive member of your family or a close friend. Some find a pastoral counselor can be helpful in analyzing their feelings and resolving conflicts. What you are seeking is a persuasive and satisfying conclusion that fits you and your life. This is what you need now for acceptance of what is happening to you—and for a peaceful closure.

Palliative Medical Care

You have been told that your attending physicians have exhausted all modes of therapy available to them for your disorder, that there is no curative or stabilizing treatment that can prevent your death. Unfortunately, many highly skilled physicians (in their specialties) look upon this as a medical failure that they do not wish to acknowledge—so they just disappear. Fortunately, we now have other highly skilled physicians to take over—specialists in palliative medicine, trained to properly treat all aspects of the terminally ill.

In the United States, the Academy of Hospice Physicians is the national organization that fosters formal training in the knowledge and skills of palliative medicine. Its membership consists of over 1,600 physicians from a variety of medical specialties now practicing in the United States and 17 other countries. The Academy's mission is dedicated to the comprehensive treatment of the terminally ill as set forth in the following Position Statement:

> We stand in fellowship with all those who are striving to diminish the pain and suffering of the dying.
>
> As hospice physicians involved in the compassionate care of the terminally ill, we have observed that competent palliative care usually relieves the pain and suffering of terminally ill persons and their families.
>
> In the current debate we oppose the legalization of euthanasia (mercy killing) and assisted suicide. We call instead for public policy changes

that ensure genuine access to comprehensive hospice services for all dying patients regardless of socioeconomic status, age or diagnosis.

The Academy's administrative office is located in Gainesville, Florida, and can be reached by calling (904) 377-8900 for further information and referral to palliative-care physicians in your area.

In the United Kingdom, the Association for Palliative Medicine of Great Britain and Ireland is the official organization representing palliative medicine as a "sole subject specialty." Its membership consists of 540 specialist physicians and 87 doctors in training. Palliative-medicine physicians work together with acute care specialists in medicine, surgery, and oncology to provide comprehensive care to the terminally ill. Like their American counterpart (above), the Association is fully committed to the provision of meticulous palliative care for the terminally ill, and is firmly opposed to physician-assisted death. The experience of the Association's staff physicians confirms that the quality of life of the dying can be significantly enhanced by effective intervention.

Hospice Care

The first hospice in this century was the St. James Hospice established in London by the Sisters of Charity in 1905. The birth of the modern hospice movement occurred in 1967 with the founding of St. Christopher's Hospice in London by Dr. Cicely Saunders. It was she who recognized that our modern medical system fails to provide the special types of supportive care so desperately needed by the terminally ill and dying patient. The obvious validity of the hospice concept was soon widely recognized, and the movement has spread throughout England, Europe, North America, and Australia. The first American hospice was started in New Haven, Connecticut, in 1974. As I write this there are more than 1,900 operational hospice programs and 115,000 persons involved in the provision of hospice care in the United States. Communities that provide hospice services can be found in every state in the union.

The typical hospice organization is a relatively small, community-based group of citizens who share a commitment to provide medical and social services to the terminally-ill patient and family who request help. Administrative functions are provided by a small nucleus of permanent staff. Many of the actual hospice services are provided by volunteers. The majority of hospices are independent entities, some are a division of a hospital, and some are part of a home health agency. Hospice care is usually rendered in the patient's home; alternative sites are nursing homes and hospice centers. The hospice staff, working as an interdisciplinary team, orchestrates the mix of personnel and services provided to patients and families as individual circumstances require. Hospice teams can include doctors, nurses, home health aids, physical and occupational therapists, social workers, coordinators of volunteers, counselors, and members of the clergy. Major emphasis is placed on optimizing the patient's quality of life: effective management of pain, relief of disease-induced symptoms, assistance with daily activities of living, response to emotional and spiritual needs, support and respite for caregivers. In addition, hospices help provide medications, supplies, equipment, and hospital services if required. Following the death of the patient, hospice continues to provide support for family and close friends for at least a year.

Note: When a patient is accepted by hospice to receive palliative care, the hospice team responds appropriately and offers its "gift of caring." However, the patient and family remain in charge; they do not surrender control. The hospice team respects the privacy and wishes of the patient and family. Hospice is not intrusive; no attempt is made to "take over." The sole focus of hospice care is the provision of comfort, in all its forms, and no attempt is made to delay or hasten the patient's death.

The National Hospice Organization located in Arlington, Virginia, is the principal source of hospice information in the United States. To inquire about the availability of hospice in your community, call the National Hospice Helpline: 1-800-658-8898.

Recommendations

- It is advisable to give some thought to the issues of death and dying while one is in good health. Considerations should include the use of advanced life-support measures in the event of sudden, life-threatening injury or illness and one is unable to communicate their wishes.
- After carefully formulating one's attitudes, beliefs, and decisions regarding life-support procedures, these should be put in writing and made known to family, friends, clergy, and personal physicians.
- In addition, such conclusions, decisions, and directions should be incorporated in legal documents known as "advance directives." These should be prepared by a lawyer who is fully informed regarding the legal aspects of such documents in the jurisdiction of your residence. Advance directives include:
  - The Living Will: a legal document that allows one to state, in advance, specific wishes regarding the use of life-sustaining procedures, should the person be in a terminal condition or persistent vegetative state and unable to communicate with caregivers.
  - The Durable Power-of-Attorney for Medical Affairs: sometimes called a Health Care Proxy, a legal document that empowers a specific individual to make health care decisions on behalf of the patient. This power-of-attorney need not be limited to terminal illness; it can be as broad and inclusive as the grantor wishes to make it.

- Copies of both advance directives should be distributed as follows:
  - safe-deposit box
  - spouse/family members
  - designated power-of-attorney
  - personal physician
  - personal attorney
  - community hospital
  - member of the clergy
- Should hospitalization be required, the patient's advocate (spouse, family member, physician, etc.) should confirm that the hospital has a copy of the advance directives and that they are strictly implemented.
- Eighty percent of deaths in the United States occur in the hospital. If a patient with a chronic disorder is judged to be terminally ill while hospitalized, and if it is feasible to do so, consideration should be given to the following:
  - obtaining the services of a specialist in palliative medicine, if the attending physician(s) cannot or will not provide equivalent care
  - obtaining the services of a licensed operational hospice program in the community
  - moving the patient to home, nursing home, or equivalent facility
- A "good death" has been described as one in which pain and suffering—physical and emotional—do not exceed what can be decently endured. Regardless of the setting in which the terminally ill patient is dying, every possible measure should be used to ensure that pain is prevented or adequately controlled (see Appendix 3, Cancer Pain Management).

The Ongoing Debate Regarding Assisted Death

As with most issues that focus on critical aspects of the human condition, the spectrum of beliefs and opinions concerning assisted death is very wide. At one end is the Judeo-Christian ethic that proscribes murder: Thou shalt not kill. At the other end is the model proposed by Dr. Jack Kevorkian: the somewhat hasty accommodation by a physician in response to a suffering patient's plea for assisted suicide, with questionable evaluation for treatable depression and lack of appropriate peer review for justification. Spread between the ends of the spectrum are a variety of defendable positions—some that are strongly opposed to physician-assisted death; some that would sanction the practice when performed in accordance with valid, enforceable guidelines. After reviewing the writings of numerous knowledgeable and sincere workers in the field of death and dying, it is apparent that no reasonable consensus has been reached regarding assisted death, nor does it appear that general agreement will be achieved in the near future.

Arguments for Physician-Assisted Death

- The archaic attitude that the physician's first responsibility is to maintain life (prevent death) at all costs is no longer tenable in the high-tech world of modern medicine. It is now possible to maintain meaningless "life" in brain-dead bodies for years.
- A fundamental principle of the doctor–patient relationship is that the patient can trust the physician to perform in the patient's best interest—to provide appropriate and *compassionate* care throughout their relationship. Many physicians genuinely believe that their primary responsibility to the patient is to relieve unrelenting suffering and to respect the competent patient's thoughtful choices.
- Physician-assisted death can be handled rationally on a case-by-case basis. In those rare cases when all available palliative measures fail to relieve the terminally ill patient's pain and suffering, and the patient voluntarily states that continued living is truly unendurable and he chooses to die, assisting death is a rational and obligatory humane consideration. It is morally reprehensible for a physician to be indifferent to the patient's final, uncontrollable suffering and to deliberately refuse to provide compassionate relief.
- It is preferable to sanction a small number of legally controlled, justifiable physician-assisted deaths than to tacitly concede that such practices frequently occur secretly and without regulation.

Arguments Against Physician-Assisted Death

- A physician's integrity prohibits participation in any activity that is designed to cause a patient's death. Under no circumstances should a physician use his medical skills to implement the process of dying. The role of the physician is to heal.
- Meticulous palliative care of the dying patient who requests assisted death often results in satisfactory control of pain, suffering, and distressing symptoms. Many patients are restored to a quality of life that they find acceptable, and the request for assisted death is withdrawn.
- Reactive depression is a common manifestation of chronic disorders. Deepening depression in terminal illness may well motivate the request for physician-assisted death. Effective treatment of this associated depression may dispel the desire to die.
- The legalization of physician-assisted death could lead to unmanageable exploitation of vulnerable, terminally ill patients who are desperate for relief that conventional medical care has not provided. The possible emergence of "death specialists and clinics" is totally unacceptable.

Toward a Reasonable Resolution?

Over the past 20 years we have seen the patient's right to die—to refuse medical treatment—legally sanctioned and affirmed by use of advance directives, and now public support for legalizing physician-assisted death is increasing. According to all available opinion polls, a clear majority of Americans favor the right of the patient to request a physician's assistance in dying, if rational and terminally ill with an incurable disease. In a poll conducted by the newspaper *USA WeekEnd* in February 1995, over 23,000 readers responded to the question, "If you were terminally ill, would you want the right to end your life with a doctor's help?" The responses were published in the March 10–12, 1995 issue: Yes: 81%, No: 19%. In November 1994, Oregon voters approved the Death with Dignity Act legalizing regulated physician-assisted suicide. Sixty percent of Oregon physicians believe that physician-assisted suicide is ethical and should be legal in appropriate cases. Similar proposals in Washington and California were defeated. Studies carried out in Michigan in 1994 and 1995 found that 66% of the public and 56% of physicians supported carefully defined legalization of physician-assisted suicide. Oregon's law is now being challenged and is under legal review. It is anticipated that eventually the Supreme Court will be asked to rule on the constitutionality of physician-assisted death.

As this crucial debate escalates, many of us will engage in thoughtful soul-searching in attempting to reach a personal conclusion. After reviewing the thoughts and opinions of numerous scholars in this field, this author has selected the following passages from the writings of two eminent physicians for you, the reader, to ponder. In my opinion, they represent the best understanding I have found on the subject of managing terminal illness and dying: insightful, circumspect, rational, and practical.

With permission of the author, Dr. Sherwin B. Nuland, the following passage is taken from his book *How We Die: Reflections on Life's Final Chapter*. It is a consoling, transcendent perspective for each of us to consider as we contemplate our eventual death.

> Nature has a job to do. It does its job by the method that seems most suited to each individual whom its powers have created. It has made this one susceptible to heart disease and that one to stroke and yet another to cancer, some after a long time on this earth and some after a time much too brief, at least by our own reckoning. The animal economy has formed the circumstances by which each generation is to be succeeded by the next. Against the relentless forces and cycles of nature there can be no lasting victory.

With permission of the author, Dr. Howard Brody of Michigan State University, the following excerpts are taken from his article, "Assisted Death—A Compassionate Response to a Medical Failure," published in the *New England Journal of Medicine*, Volume 327, Number 19, November 5, 1992. The passages chosen illustrate his rational and feasible approach that gives due consideration to legal constraints, the physician's ethical responsibilities, and the patient's apprehension regarding terminal care.

What should be the stance of the law toward physician-assisted death?—I argue here that an adjudication of assisted death might follow from viewing it as a compassionate response to one sort of medical failure, rather than as something to be prohibited outright or as something to be established as a standard policy. This would seem to translate, in law, into allowing compassionate and competent medical practice to serve as a defense against a charge of homicide or of assisting a suicide.

Medicine produces a good death when it uses life-prolonging interventions as long as they produce a reasonable quality of life (defined in terms of the patient's own life goals) and when it then employs the highest quality of hospice-style terminal care.

Modern medicine has come to see a patient's death as a failure, and the unavoidable approach of death as a reason to back off rather than as a call for even more intensive medical engagement (albeit palliative rather than curative). But all our patients eventually die, and it is wrongheaded to see death itself as a sign of medical failure. Rather, we should acknowledge failure when the ravages of disease or ill-constructed medical interventions produce a "bad" death. A good death, as described above, should be hailed as a medical success story.

I wish to argue that walking away [from the dying patient], denying that medicine can do anything to help in the patient's plight, is an immoral abrogation of medical power, especially in cases in which the prior exercise of the medical craft has extended the patient's life and resulted in the complications that have brought the patient to the present state of suffering.

It follows that if assisting a death is to be morally defensible, it can be so only on the merits of the specific case, assuming that a failure of medical care has occurred despite competent practice and that only an extraordinary action can produce a reasonably compassionate outcome for the suffering patient who voluntarily requests assistance.—Assisted death ought to be seen as a last resort.

The details of this system should be left to legal experts. There is, however, one other condition that humane legal management of assisted death ought to meet. A good death occurs as much as possible among caring and supportive people. If the law forces already suffering patients to die alone—for fear that seeking the supportive presence of others might implicate them in an illegal act—then the law undermines important social values of family and community.

Those on both sides of the debate over assisted death can agree that all patients should be confident that physicians will aid them with the latest palliative care to relieve terminal suffering and will respect their right to refuse life-prolonging treatment and to execute advance health care directives. One hopes that this view, if fully and effectively implemented, would considerably reduce the number of patients who will request a physician's aid in dying.

Unfortunately, far too many American physicians still think that neglect of symptom control and a "never say die" attitude in the face of worsening illness constitute good medical care. That these instead constitute inappropriate medical practice is a position that must be argued vigorously if the American public is ever to regain the trust in physician's compassion that we have all too nearly lost.

Recommended Additional Reading

How We Die: Reflections on Life's Final Chapter, Sherwin B. Nuland, M.D. New York: Alfred A. Knopf, 1994.

The Troubled Dream of Life: Living with Mortality, Daniel Callahan. New York: Simon & Schuster, 1993.

"Assisted Death—A Compassionate Response to a Medical Failure," Howard Brody, M.D., Ph.D. *The New England Journal of Medicine,* Vol. 327, No. 19, Nov. 5, 1992.

Arguing Euthanasia: The Controversy Over Mercy Killing, Assisted Suicide, and the "Right to Die," J.D. Moreno, Ph.D., ed. New York: Simon & Schuster, 1995.

Carpe Diem: Enjoying Every Day with a Terminal Illness, Ed Madden. National Hospice Organization, South Deerfield, MA 01373-0200. Phone: 1-800-646-6460.

The Hospice Handbook, Larry Beresford. National Hospice Organization, South Deerfield, MA 01373-0200. Phone: 1-800-646-6460.

Resources for Additional Information and Services

Academy of Hospice Physicians
Dale C. Smith, Executive Director
408 West University Avenue
P.O. Box 14288
Gainesville, FL 32604-2288
Phone: (352) 377-8900

National Hospice Organization
1901 North Moore Street, Suite 901

Arlington, VA 22209
Phone: (703) 243-5900

Operates the Hospice Helpline: 1-800-658-8898, 8:30 A.M.–5:30 P.M. ET, Monday–Friday. Provides information on hospice programs available in the caller's area.

Hospice Education Institute
5 Essex Square
P.O. Box 713
Essex, CT 06246
Phone: 1-800-544-2213, 9:00 A.M.–4:30 P.M. ET, Monday–Friday

Provides information and counseling on death and dying and the role of hospice. Makes referrals to local agencies and publishes a directory of hospices.

SECTION FIVE

Chronic Disorders in the Elderly: Special Considerations

Who Are the Elderly?

Our culture has long recognized the age of 65 years to be the appropriate time to retire. But the vast majority of us are not truly "old" at 65. Geriatricians, those physicians who specialize in treating the elderly, generally recognize 75 years of age as a reasonable transition point from "middle age" to the "older" segment of society. Gerontologists, those who study the processes of aging, currently hold that 120 years is the maximal life span for the human species. So the elderly are those between the ages of 75 and 120 years. They consist of a growing group of Americans, currently 6% of the population. The oldest segments within this group are growing at the fastest rate of all.

It is important to understand that individually we all age at different rates and in different ways. One's physiological age is much more significant than one's chronological age. The quality of life depends largely on physiological age—how well our body systems continue to function as we grow older. Those who are genetically programmed to develop premature coronary artery disease may, while in their fifth or sixth decade of life, experience serious heart disorders that are common (and expected) in the eighth and ninth decades—a 75-year-old heart in a 50-year-old body. On the other hand, those who derive from a gene pool endowed with longevity may live to be 100, still alert and reasonably active. Thus we have the relatively young who are already "old" in some respects, and the truly old who are still relatively "young."

How Do the Elderly Differ from the Young?

Gerontology teaches that we begin to age (actually die) the moment we are born. It is postulated that all body cells have a built-in clock that governs their longevity and programs the time of their death. Although there is marked variation among individuals in the rate of aging, there are patterns of age-related change that we all share. These are referred to as the processes of "normal aging." They involve the steady decline in organ system functions and the subtle alterations in mechanisms that control the integrated balance of body activities necessary to maintain health, a process called homeostasis.

Changes in Body Composition
- The water content of the body decreases, predisposing to dehydration.
- The sodium content of the body decreases, predisposing to lethargy, muscle cramps, loss of appetite, nausea, confusion, disorientation, seizures.
- The lean body mass decreases from about 130 pounds (at age 25) to 105 pounds (at age 75 to 80). The main loss of tissue occurs from muscle.
- The fat content of the body doubles, increasing from 14% to 30% of total body weight.

Changes in Organ System Functions
- Reduction in brain size and permanent loss of nerve cells; age-related memory loss
- Impaired perception of thirst, leading to inadequate fluid intake and dehydration
- Impaired vision: decreases in visual acuity, near vision, peripheral vision, and night vision, predisposing to falls
- Impaired balance reflexes and slowed reaction time, predisposing to falls
- Gradual decline in the heart's response to exercise, resulting in decreased exercise heart rate
- Stiffening of arterial walls, resulting in increased systolic blood pressure (isolated systolic hypertension)
- Gradual weakening of the muscles of breathing and stiffening of the chest wall, resulting in decreased ventilation and gas exchange within the lungs; this predisposes to airway obstruction
- Reduction in liver size and blood flow, causing some delay in drug elimination
- Significant decline in kidney function (beginning at 35 years), requiring downward adjustments in dosages of drugs excreted by the kidney

- Gradual decline of immune system functions, resulting in decreased resistance to infections, increased susceptibility to cancer, and predisposition to autoimmune disorders
- Cessation of estrogen production (menopause), resulting in fragility of bone (osteoporosis)
- Reduced tolerance for dietary sugar, predisposing to diabetes mellitus

Health Maintenance by the Elderly

Studies of aging indicate that most body organs can continue to function reasonably well in elderly individuals who maintain healthy lifestyles and have no overt manifestations of chronic disorders. Undoubtedly such individuals (1) would be endowed genetically with good health and longevity and (2) would have adopted health maintenance practices early in life that constitute primary prevention—preventing the initial development of disease. Unfortunately, the "diseases of aging" are time-related. Many of them have their onset in midlife and progress silently for varying periods of time before producing recognizable symptoms. Therefore, those in the seventh decade of life must employ the strategies of secondary prevention—arresting or reversing the progression of diseases that, in all likelihood, have already started. There are two practical approaches to take: (1) the adoption of a lifestyle that eliminates or reduces the known risks for disease development; (2) the use of screening procedures that can detect the presence of silent (asymptomatic) disease while in its early stages and amenable to treatment.

Preventive Lifestyles

The following can be started at any age—the earlier in life, the better:
- Regular exercise: walking, bicycling, swimming for 20 to 30 minutes, two or three times a week
- Sound nutrition: a balanced diet that includes fruits, vegetables, adequate fiber, and the full recommended daily allowances of vitamins and minerals, with fat limited to 30% of total calories. Avoid "megadoses" of vitamins.
- Maintenance of normal weight for body build, sex, and age
- Moderate alcohol intake: one or two drinks daily, if there is no history of alcoholism. The choice of alcoholic beverage is irrelevant; alcohol in any form raises levels of HDL cholesterol that deters atherosclerosis.
- Complete abstention from all forms of tobacco
- Total avoidance of habit-forming substances
- Maintenance of a positive, optimistic attitude
- Pursuit of meaningful activities
- Adequate restful sleep: approximately seven to eight hours daily

- Regular immunization with influenzal and pneumococcal vaccines, as appropriate, is recommended.

Routine Screening Procedures

The following can be included in periodic health maintenance examinations at intervals deemed appropriate by your personal physician:

- Body weight: to be monitored closely. Obesity is a risk factor for the development of hypertension, heart disease, diabetes, gallstones, osteoarthritis, and breast cancer; unexplained weight loss can be an early sign of hyperthyroidism or cryptic malignancy.
- Blood pressure: elevated blood pressure (hypertension) is a risk factor for coronary artery disease, stroke, and kidney failure; proper treatment providing continuous control of blood pressure can modify these developments.
- Internal eye pressure: elevated intraocular pressure is the cause of glaucoma—irreversible damage to the optic nerve that can lead to blindness. During the early stages, there are no symptoms to indicate its presence; early detection can prevent loss of vision.
- Skin changes: inspection of skin lesions can detect early skin cancers; it is essential that malignant melanoma be recognized and treated as early as possible.
- Mouth examination: inspection of mouth and throat for abnormal tissues that could be precancerous or cancerous. 15,000 new cases of oral cancer occur annually in those over 65 years of age; risk factors include heavy use of tobacco and alcohol.
- Breast examination (manual): early detection and biopsy of significant breast tissue changes (in both women *and* men) can lead to curative surgery for breast cancer.
- Mammography: this imaging of breast tissue can detect early, minute cancers that cannot be felt by manual examination, greatly improving chances for cure.
- Lung function test: a measurement of the ability to exhale air from the lungs; used to detect early evidence of airway obstruction that could progress to chronic obstructive pulmonary disease (COPD), a common cause of death in the elderly.
- Fecal examination for occult blood: the finding of blood in a stool specimen could lead to the detection of asymptomatic rectal or colon cancer.
- Digital rectal examination: in women, this can detect cancer of the rectum; in men, it can detect rectal cancer and enlargement and/or cancer of the prostate gland.
- Cervical smear with Papanicolaou staining (Pap test): this can detect precancerous and cancerous cells in the uterine cervix, permitting complete cure.

- Complete blood cell count: for the detection of significant anemias, polycythemia, and leukemias.
- Blood lipids: measurements of total cholesterol, HDL cholesterol, LDL cholesterol, and triglycerides to evaluate risk factors for atherosclerotic heart disease, cerebrovascular disease, and peripheral vascular disease; provides essential information for recommending dietary and drug therapies.
- Blood glucose: measurements of blood sugar levels to detect and manage diabetes mellitus.
- Blood TSH and T_4: measurements of the thyroid-stimulating hormone (TSH) and thyroxine (T_4) to detect thyroid gland dysfunctions. Hypothyroidism is quite common in the elderly, but often not diagnosed; hyperthyroidism in the elderly presents symptoms quite different than those seen in young individuals, making the diagnosis difficult.
- Blood PSA: measurement of the prostate-specific antigen, a protein made by the prostate gland that can serve as a marker for prostate cancer.

Common Disorders in the Elderly

For the elderly who are found to have a chronic disorder of significant dimensions, the management strategy becomes one of tertiary prevention—the achievement and maintenance of functional capacity by preventing progression of the disease and resultant deterioration of health. This may require a variety of diagnostic and therapeutic procedures: laboratory and imaging tests, drug therapy, surgery, radiation, physical therapy, etc. The following points regarding the more common disorders are worthy of consideration.

Note: It is mandatory that any plan of treatment be individualized in accord with each patient's unique circumstances and requirements. Consult your physician for guidance regarding any of the following suggestions.

Hypertension
- Restrict the use of salt.
- Maintain a normal body weight.
- Ask your physician for a program of regular, moderate exercise.
- Comply fully with the regimen of antihypertensive medications prescribed and monitored by your physician.
- If practical, obtain an automated blood pressure instrument and monitor your own blood pressure at home and work setting; keep records for your physician.

- *Caution:* The elderly tend to be more sensitive to the actions of anti-hypertensive drugs. Initial doses should be small. Your blood pressure should be reduced gradually; rapid and excessive drops in pressure can predispose to stroke and heart attack (myocardial infarction). Your blood pressure should be maintained in the high-normal range to accommodate age-related changes in your blood vessels.
- Read the Profile of hypertension in Section Three.

Coronary Artery Disease and Cerebrovascular Disease

The consequences of coronary heart disease and stroke are among the most common causes of death in the elderly.

- Maintain a normal body weight.
- Ask your physician for a program of regular, moderate exercise.
- Cease tobacco smoking completely and permanently.
- Reduce dietary saturated fats and cholesterol.
- If warranted by blood lipid levels, a trial of cholesterol-lowering drugs may be considered. At age 70, an elevated total cholesterol is not considered to be a risk factor. However, if HDL cholesterol is markedly low or LDL cholesterol is markedly high, a trial of drug therapy may be warranted.
- Monitor blood pressure every six months. If hypertension develops, obtain adequate treatment.
- Read the Profile of coronary artery disease (CAD) in Section Three. Understand that angina pectoris (chest pain) is a manifestation of CAD; learn the numerous variations of anginal pain. Be aware that anginal pain is often absent in the elderly. Over 50% of elderly individuals who have a heart attack (myocardial infarction) do not experience chest pain—they have a "silent coronary:" instead of pain, initial manifestations may be sudden shortness of breath, weakness, confusion, and fainting.
- If you do experience classical episodes of angina, comply fully with the regimen of antianginal medications prescribed by your physician.
- Read the Profile of stroke in Section Three. Understand the significance of transient ischemic attacks (TIAs) and the kind of medical attention you should seek.
- Consider the use of prophylactic low-dose aspirin—one tablet of 81 mgs daily (generally thought of as a "baby" aspirin); its anticoagulant effect may provide some protection against stroke and heart attack. *Be sure to ask your physician for guidance before starting this.*

Lung Cancer

- Cease tobacco smoking completely and permanently.
- Maintain a well-balanced, highly nutritious diet.

- Obtain influenzal and pneumococcal vaccinations at appropriate intervals.
- Treat lower respiratory tract infections promptly and vigorously.
- Read the Profile of lung cancer in Section Three.

Diabetes Mellitus

- Maintain a normal body weight.
- Maintain a low-fat, low-cholesterol diet to arrest atherosclerosis.
- Understand that the threshold for the passage of sugar from blood to urine is higher in the elderly; a negative urine sugar test will occur with higher blood sugar levels.
- If practical, monitor your blood sugar levels with an automated instrument at home.
- It is not always feasible for the elderly to attempt "tight" control of blood sugar. This practice significantly increases the risk of hypoglycemia, a reaction not well tolerated by the older brain. Learn to recognize the early symptoms of developing hypoglycemia.
- Read the Profile of diabetes mellitus in Section Three.

Obesity

- Recognize that chronic obesity is a definite risk factor for several disorders that commonly affect the elderly: coronary artery disease, cerebrovascular disease, peripheral vascular disease, hypertension, type II diabetes mellitus, gallstones, breast and uterine cancer.
- Of the two major types of obesity—central (the "middle-age spread" of abdominal obesity) and peripheral (lower body obesity)—it is central obesity that is linked with coronary artery disease.
- Those individuals with longstanding central obesity who also have a family history of cholesterol disorders and type II diabetes are at greatest risk for the development of atherosclerotic heart and vascular diseases.
- An aggressive treatment program emphasizing a low-calorie diet and exercise (within tolerance) is strongly recommended. This should be carefully prescribed and supervised for the elderly.

Chronic Obstructive Lung Diseases

These diseases include asthma, chronic bronchitis, and emphysema; all are common chronic disorders in the elderly, and each has its own profile in Section Three.

- Cease tobacco smoking completely and permanently.
- Treat asthma aggressively; attempt to reduce the frequency and duration of episodes.
- Treat attacks of acute bronchitis promptly and effectively with antibiotics and expectorants.

- Obtain influenzal and pneumococcal vaccinations at appropriate intervals.
- Read the Profiles of asthma, chronic bronchitis, and emphysema in Section Three.

Colon Cancer

- Increase consumption of fruits, vegetables, and whole grain cereals, especially those high in carotene and vitamin C.
- Avoid salt-cured, salt-pickled, and smoked foods.
- Restrict intake of high-fat and high-cholesterol foods.
- Use alcoholic beverages sparingly.
- Prevent constipation, establish regular bowel movements by daily intake of fiber.
- Be alert for any changes in the pattern of bowel movements: change in size of stool, persistent looseness, presence of blood.
- Read the Profile of colon cancer in Section Three.

Hypothyroidism (Underactive Thyroid Gland)

- This is a very common condition in the elderly. However, less than half of the cases are recognized and treated. The symptoms of mild to moderate thyroxine (thyroid hormone) deficiency closely resemble the features of aging: lethargy, fatigability, increased requirement for sleep, weight gain, dry skin, impaired concentration, etc. If your physician does not consider this possibility, request appropriate blood tests to evaluate your thyroid status.
- The elderly are very sensitive to thyroxine. Treatment of hypothyroidism must begin with very small doses; small increments can be made every two to three weeks until the optimal dose is reached.
- Be aware that the administration of thyroxine can unmask latent coronary artery disease and result in the emergence of angina. Report promptly any development of chest pain, with or without physical exertion.
- Read the Profile of hypothyroidism in Section Three.

Hyperthyroidism (Overactive Thyroid Gland)

- Although not as common as hypothyroidism in the elderly, hyperthyroidism (excessive thyroxine) can be a more serious disorder—more difficult to recognize and treat.
- In the elderly patient, hyperthyroidism often produces quite a different pattern of symptoms from those seen in younger adults. Only 25% of patients over 65 years of age exhibit the "typical" features of hyperthyroidism. Instead of nervousness, irritability, excessive activity, and increased appetite, the patient may be apathetic, listless, weak, and anorexic.

- In the absence of classical features of hyperthyroidism, the dominant symptoms may suggest coronary artery disease: angina, heart rhythm abnormalities, and heart failure; or gastrointestinal malignancy: weight loss, anorexia, indigestion, abdominal distress, alternating diarrhea and constipation.
- If the patient does not respond to treatment and the correct diagnosis is not apparent, the patient's family should request an evaluation of thyroid status.

Osteoporosis

- Osteoporosis affects about 25 million Americans and is associated with 1,300,000 fractures annually. It is a major cause of illness and disability in the elderly. Effective treatments are available.
- If your physical condition permits, weight-bearing exercise on a regular basis is advisable: walking 45 to 60 minutes three to five times per week.
- If you have not always eaten high-calcium foods or taken a calcium supplement, ask your pharmacist or physician to recommend an appropriate product. The optimal dosage is 1500 mg per day for those without a history of kidney stones or excessive calcium in the urine. Calcium citrate is the preferred form of calcium for the elderly.
- Use of vitamin D: limit the dose to the recommended daily allowance (RDA) of 400 IU found in one-a-day vitamin tablets.
- Use of estrogen replacement therapy (ERT): if you have been taking estrogen since menopause, do not discontinue it without your physician's advice. It most certainly has had some preventive influence regarding the development of osteoporosis. However, if you now have osteoporosis and are not taking estrogen, discuss the benefits and risks of estrogen therapy with your physician. Current opinion holds that benefits—prevention of both osteoporosis and coronary artery disease—outweigh the minimal (and uncertain) risk of developing breast cancer.
- Use of calcitonin: this drug increases bone mass in postmenopausal osteoporosis. Formerly given only by injection, it is now available as a nasal spray. Its use is reserved for women who will not or cannot use estrogen replacement therapy. Concurrent use of calcium and vitamin D (as above) is necessary.
- Use of fluoride: an old drug in a new slow-release formulation stimulates the formation of new bone. It is given together with calcium citrate.
- Use of alendronate: this is a newly released nonhormonal drug that increases new bone formation and decreases fractures associated with osteoporosis. Concurrent use of calcium and vitamin D (as above) is necessary. Concurrent use of estrogen is not recommended.

- Osteoporosis greatly increases the risk of fractures, both spontaneous fractures and those resulting from falls. Appropriate caution should be used at all times to prevent falls. Numerous drugs in common use can cause unsteadiness in the elderly and contribute to falling. See "The Use of Medicinal Drugs by the Elderly" below.
- Read the Profile of osteoporosis in Section Three.

The Use of Medicinal Drugs by the Elderly

The prevalence of chronic disorders in the elderly—often two or more concurrently in the same individual—leads unavoidably to the simultaneous use of more than one drug. Quite often the patient's disorders may require the services of several physicians, each prescribing medications with little or no communication among them (polypharmacy). It has been estimated that older Americans take an average of 4.5 drugs at any one time. Nursing home residents are given from three to eight drugs daily. The elderly experience three times more adverse drug reactions than younger segments of the population. Studies reveal that this is not due primarily to age, but is directly related to the number of drugs the patient is taking concurrently.

The age-related changes in body composition and function, as discussed in the previous part, significantly alter the way the elderly respond to many medications. This makes it necessary to carefully individualize every drug selection and dosage schedule to accommodate the patient's unique characteristics and the features of the disorder(s). Also, it is imperative to closely monitor the patient's response so that timely adjustments can be made to enhance benefit or avert toxicity.

General Principles

- Be certain that drug therapy is necessary. Have reasonable alternatives been ineffective?
- Use the fewest drugs possible to achieve the treatment goal. If feasible, limit concurrent use to three drugs.
- Keep dosage schedules simple; use single-daily dosage forms when possible.
- Begin treatment with small doses; increase doses with small increments (as needed) and at a slow rate.
- Maintenance doses for the elderly are often smaller than for younger persons.
- Avoid large tablets and capsules if other dosage forms are available. Liquid preparations are easier for the elderly to swallow, and they permit finer dosage adjustments.

- All drug container labels should include (1) the drug name; (2) directions for use; (3) the name of the disorder for which the drug is prescribed. Many medication errors occur among the elderly because item (3) is not provided.
- For use by the elderly, drugs should be packaged in easy-to-open containers; avoid "childproof" caps and stoppers.
- No drug should be taken in the dark; identify every drug in adequate light to verify that the intended drug is taken.
- Only drugs for emergency use should be kept on the bedside table: nitroglycerin for Prinzmetal's angina; a fast-acting bronchodilator for bronchial asthma attacks. These two disorders characteristically occur between 2:00 and 4:00 A.M.
- Ask your physician to periodically review all drugs you are taking and discontinue those you no longer need.
- Learn all you can about the drugs you are taking—how they work, possible adverse effects and interactions with foods and other drugs, precautions for use, etc. (see Appendix 17 for sources of drug information).

Optimal Timing of Medications: Chronotherapeutics

Most of us are aware of "biological clocks"—the circadian wake–sleep cycles that are disrupted by jet air travel across time zones and the need to periodically shift work schedules from day to night. The science of biological rhythms—chronobiology—has established that many biological functions of the body occur at set points throughout the 24-hour day. Also, it is now recognized that several serious chronic disorders manifest their dominant features at approximately the same time during the day or night. This has major implications for the timing of medications if the goal of therapy is optimal effectiveness and control of symptoms. The following examples illustrate this new aspect of drug therapy: timing the administration of drugs to increase their efficacy and decrease their toxicity.

- Hypertension and related events: blood pressure increases 20% immediately after awakening in the morning and may continue to rise over the next few hours. This is the peak time for the occurrence of the cluster of serious events associated with hypertension: classical angina, heart attack (myocardial infarction), sudden cardiac death, thrombotic stroke. Many long-acting antihypertensive drugs (usually taken after breakfast) lose their effectiveness after 18 to 20 hours—before the morning surge of blood pressure. A new formulation of verapamil, taken at bedtime, exerts its peak antihypertensive action between 5 A.M. and noon, the critical period.
- Asthma: the peak period for attacks of bronchial asthma is between 3 and 5 A.M. Oral prednisone given at 3 P.M. (instead of in the morning)

and once-a-day formulations of theophylline given at 6 to 7 P.M. (instead of divided doses throughout the day) provide better control of nocturnal asthma.

- Migraine headache: recurrent migraine headaches frequently begin on arising at about 7 A.M. Preventive medications, such as long-acting propranolol, should be most effective if taken at bedtime.
- Rheumatoid arthritis: the joint pain and disability of rheumatoid arthritis peak about 6 A.M. Nonsteroidal anti-inflammatory drugs (NSAIDs) relieve morning pain more effectively if taken late at night on retiring.
- Osteoarthritis: the joint pain and disability of osteoarthritis peak about 7 to 8 P.M. NSAIDs relieve evening pain more effectively if taken at noon.
- Peptic ulcer: the peaks of stomach acid secretion are in the evening and again late at night. Suppression of stomach acid is essential for ulcer healing. Histamine-blocking drugs are more effective in controlling stomach acid when taken once daily at 6 to 7 P.M.
- Chronic pain: it has long been recognized that chronic pain intensifies and becomes more resistant to treatment (intractable) at night, usually peaking between 11 P.M. and midnight. The timing of analgesic drug administration should assure that the peak action of the drug coincides with the peak intensity of pain.

Pain Management in the Elderly

Providing relief of pain in elderly patients is usually more complex than it is in younger individuals. Quite often the source of the pain is an incurable disease, so the primary cause cannot be removed; the pain is chronic in nature and sometimes progressively worsens. Age-related changes in the elderly influence the selection and administration of pain medications, and the elderly may respond differently to the drugs of choice for pain relief.

Pain is quite common in the elderly: 25–50% of the community-dwelling population over age 60 report some form of pain; 71% of nursing home residents experience pain—34% of them claim constant pain and 66% describe intermittent pain. Among elderly cancer patients, 33% in treatment programs and 66% with advanced disease have significant pain.

Pain specialists classify pain into three major types: somatic, visceral, and neuropathic. The elderly patient usually experiences one or more of the three forms.

1. Somatic pain: originates in the skin and deeper tissues; pain is usually well localized, and is aching or gnawing in character; examples are joint and musculoskeletal pains. Responds well to nonopioid and opioid analgesics (see drug lists below).

2. Visceral pain: originates in the viscera (organs) located within the chest and abdominal cavities; pain is not always well localized, and is described as deep-seated, squeezing, and pressurelike. It may be referred to areas on the surface somewhat remote from the point of origin; examples are heart pain, gallbladder pain, and kidney stone pain. Responds well to opioid analgesics.
3. Neuropathic pain: originates in injured tissues of the nervous system—brain, spinal cord, or peripheral nerves. Pain is often severe and of a different quality than somatic or visceral pain; it is described as a constant, dull ache, with vicelike, burning, tingling, or shocklike features; examples are spinal stenosis (compression of the spinal cord), carpal tunnel syndrome (compression of the median nerve), diabetic peripheral neuropathy. Responds very poorly to opioid (morphinelike) analgesics but does respond to adjuvant drug therapy (see below).

Any pain that lasts longer than three months is considered to be chronic pain. The majority of pain patterns experienced by the elderly are of a chronic nature, and consist of three types:
1. Chronic pain associated with a medical disease or disorder—cancer, diabetes, etc. (see also Appendix 3)
2. Chronic noncancer pain that is part of a specific pain syndrome—osteoarthritis, spinal stenosis, etc.
3. Chronic noncancer pain associated with a neuropsychiatric disorder—dementia, depression, etc.

It is obvious that many elderly patients will experience chronic pain patterns of different types and from various origins. A very careful assessment is necessary in each case to ensure accurate diagnosis and effective management of the pain component.

ALERT!

Be aware of the referral pattern of some pain syndromes; a referred pain in the arm or leg can represent cancer spread to the brachial or lumbar nerve plexus; referred pain sites can be tender to pressure and cause an erroneous diagnosis of local disease in the arm or leg.

Pain in the elderly is most often due to organic disease; it is rarely due to a psychological disorder alone. However, a masked depression may well be a part of the total pain experience. If this is not recognized and appropriately treated, the overall result of pain management will be unsatisfactory.
General principles for the use of analgesic drugs:
• A specific drug that is best suited for the type of pain, its intensity, and the patient's overall status is recommended.

- Remember that the elderly are more sensitive to all analgesic drugs; start with small doses and increase cautiously as necessary.
- After the optimal dose of a drug has been determined for adequate pain control, it should be given on a regular basis.
- Drug combinations, as warranted to enhance pain relief or reduce side effects, are recommended.
- It is advisable to monitor for side effects and treat appropriately:
  - Excessive sedation
  - Depression of breathing
  - Nausea and vomiting
  - Constipation
  - Retention of urine
  - Muscle twitching, seizures
- It is advisable to discontinue opioid drugs gradually to prevent acute withdrawal symptoms.

ANALGESIC DRUGS SUITABLE FOR USE IN THE ELDERLY

Mild analgesics:
- nonopioid drugs: acetaminophen, aspirin, nonsteroidal anti-inflammatory drugs (NSAIDs) (see also Appendixes 8 and 16)
- weak opioid drugs: codeine, oxycodone, propoxyphene, pentazocine (not preferred)

Strong analgesics:
- strong opioids: morphine, levorphanol, hydromorphone, oxymorphone, methadone, fentanyl, nalbuphine, butorphanol
- *ALERT!* meperidine (Demerol) should be avoided in the elderly.

Adjuvant analgesics—used to relieve neuropathic pain:
- tricyclic antidepressants: amitriptyline
- anticonvulsants: phenytoin, carbamazepine, valproic acid
- baclofen
- mexiletine

Drugs Metabolized Primarily by the Liver

It is advisable to reduce the dosage of the following drugs for patients with impaired liver function:

alprazolam
amitriptyline
barbiturates (see Appendix 16)
carbamazepine
chlordiazepoxide
desipramine
diazepam
diphenhydramine

flurazepam
ibuprofen
imipramine
lidocaine
meperidine
nitrazepam
nortriptyline
phenytoin
propranolol
quinidine
theophylline
tolbutamide
warfarin

Drugs Eliminated Primarily by the Kidneys

It is advisable to reduce the dosage of the following drugs for patients with impaired kidney function:

aminoglycoside antibiotics (see Appendix 16)
atenolol
captopril
clonidine
digoxin
disopyramide
diuretics (see Appendix 16)
enalapril
famotidine
lisinopril
lithium
nadolol
NSAIDs (see Appendixes 8 and 16)
procainamide
ranitidine
tocainide

Possible Complications of Diuretic Therapy

The age-related alterations of critical body functions in the elderly predisposes them to possible adverse reactions to diuretic drugs:

- Excessive dehydration can predispose to uremia (kidney failure).
- Reduced blood volume can predispose to hypotension (low blood pressure), with dizziness, fainting, and falling.
- Reduced sugar tolerance can predispose to diabetes.
- Excessive loss of blood potassium can predispose to digitalis toxicity and heart rhythm disturbances.

- Increased levels of blood uric acid can predispose to gout.
- Increased urine volumes can predispose to impaired bladder function—urine retention or incontinence.

Symptoms and Signs of Adverse Drug Reactions in the Elderly

Adverse drug reactions occur most frequently in the elderly, especially older white women. This is generally attributed to the greater use of drugs by this group. Drug reactions in the elderly may differ significantly from patterns seen in younger persons. It is often difficult to distinguish an adverse drug effect from an early manifestation of a new disorder. Both physician and patient must maintain a high index of suspicion to make this distinction correctly. If any of the following symptoms or signs develop, consider first the possibility that they may be drug-induced.

Bladder or bowel incontinence
Confusion
Constipation
Depression
Memory loss
Parkinson-like features
Restlessness
Tardive dyskinesia (see Glossary)
Unsteadiness, falls

Drugs Most Likely to Cause Adverse Drug Reactions in the Elderly

Note: Consult Appendix 16 to learn the generic names of the drugs within each of the following drug classes:

analgesics
antibiotics
anticoagulants
antidepressants
antihypertensives
antiparkinsonism drugs
antipsychotics
bronchodilators
digitalis/digoxin
diuretics
NSAIDs
oral hypoglycemics
sedative/hypnotics

Drugs That May Cause Orthostatic Hypotension (see Glossary)

Excessive drops in blood pressure on arising from a lying or sitting position can cause fainting. The resultant fall can cause serious injury in an elderly, frail individual.

Note: Consult Appendix 16 to learn the generic names of the drugs within each of the following drug classes:

    antiarrhythmics: drugs for heart rhythm disorders
    antihypertensives
    beta-blockers: drugs for angina and hypertension
    calcium blockers: drugs for angina and hypertension
    digoxin
    diuretics
    nitrates: drugs for angina
    psychotropics: drugs for mental disorders

Drugs That May Cause Sluggishness, Unsteadiness, and Falling in the Elderly

Note: Consult Appendix 16 to learn the generic names of the drugs within each of the following drug classes:

    barbiturates
    benzodiazepines
    beta-blockers
    sedative/hypnotics

Drugs That May Cause Confusion and Behavioral Disturbances in the Elderly

Note: Consult Appendix 16 to learn the generic names of the drugs within each of the following drug classes:

    anticholinergics
    anticonvulsants
    antidepressants
    antidiabetic drugs
    antihistamines
    antiparkinsonism drugs
    barbiturates
    benzodiazepines
    cimetidine
    digitalis preparations
    diuretics
    ergoloid mesylates
    meprobamate
    methocarbamol
    methyldopa
    narcotic/opioid drugs
    NSAIDs
    reserpine
    sedative/hypnotics
    thiothixene

Drugs That May Cause Parkinson-like Symptoms in the Elderly

ALERT! This is most important to know: It is not uncommon for a patient who is taking any of the following drugs to be told that he has "early Parkinson's Disease"—an erroneous diagnosis.

amitriptyline
amodiaquine
chloroquine
chlorprothixene
diazoxide
diphenhydramine
droperidol
haloperidol
imipramine
lithium
methyldopa
metoclopramide
phenothiazines (see Appendix 16)
reserpine
thiothixene
trifluoperidol

Drugs That May Cause Urinary Retention and/or Constipation in the Elderly

Note: Consult Appendix 16 to learn the generic names of the drugs within the following drug classes:

amantadine
androgens
antidepressants
antiparkinsonism drugs
atropinelike drugs
epinephrine
ergoloid myselates
isoetharine
narcotic/opioid drugs
phenothiazines
terbutaline

Drugs That May Cause Loss of Bladder Control (Urinary Incontinence) in the Elderly

Note: Consult Appendix 16 to learn the generic names of the drugs within each of the following drug classes:

diuretics
sedatives/hypnotics
tranquilizers

Drugs That May Predispose the Elderly to the Development of Hypothermia

Note: Consult Appendix 16 to learn the generic names of the drugs within the following drug classes:

alcohol

sedatives/hypnotics

tranquilizers

Recommended Reading

The American Geriatrics Society's Complete Guide to Aging & Health, Mark E. Williams, M.D. New York: Harmony Books, Crown Publishers, 1995.

SECTION SIX

Drug-Induced
Chronic Disorders

TABLE 1

DRUGS THAT MAY CAUSE BLOOD CELL DYSFUNCTION OR DAMAGE

All blood cells originate and develop in the bone marrow. They arise from self-renewing "stem" cells that have the capacity to differentiate into specific cell lines that produce fully developed, distinctive blood cell forms: erythrocytes (red blood cells), leukocytes (white blood cells), and thrombocytes (blood platelets). The leukocytes include three varieties: granulocytes, monocytes (macrophages), and lymphocytes. Drugs that adversely affect the formation and development of blood cells can (1) act on any stage of cell production; (2) impair the production of one cell line; (3) influence the production of all cell lines.

Through a variety of mechanisms, some medicinal drugs can adversely affect mature cells circulating in the bloodstream. Examples can be found in the tables that follow.

Drugs That Cause Inevitable (Dose-Dependent) *Aplastic Anemia*‡

actinomycin D	cytarabine	mercaptopurine
azathioprine	doxorubicin	methotrexate
busulphan	epirubicin	mitomycin
carboplatin	etoposide	mitozantrone
carmustine	fluorouracil	plicamycin
chlorambucil	hydroxyurea	procarbazine
cisplatin	lomustine	thioguanine
cyclophosphamide	melphalan	thiotepa

Drugs That May Cause Idiosyncratic (Dose-Independent) *Aplastic Anemia*

amodiaquine	indomethacin	prothiaden
benoxaprofen	mepacrine	pyrimethamine
carbimazole	oxyphenbutazone	sulfonamides*
chloramphenicol	penicillamine	sulindac
chlorpromazine	phenylbutazone	thiouracils
felbamate	phenytoin	ticlopidine
gold	piroxicam	trimethoprim/
		sulfamethoxazole

Drugs That May *Impair Red Blood Cell Production* (only)

azathioprine	isoniazid	sulfasalazine
carbamazepine	methyldopa	sulfathiazide
chloramphenicol	penicillin	sulfonamides*
chlorpropamide	pentachlorophenol	sulfonylureas*
dapsone	phenobarbital	thiamphenicol
fenoprofen	phenylbutazone	tolbutamide
gold	phenytoin	trimethoprim/
halothane	pyrimethamine	sulfamethoxazole

Drugs That May Significantly *Reduce Granulocyte Cell Counts* (various mechanisms)

acetaminophen	chlorothiazide	gold
acetazolamide	chlorpromazine	hydralazine
allopurinol	chlorpropamide	hydrochlorothiazide
amitriptyline	chlorthalidone	imipramine
amodiaquine	cimetidine	indomethacin
benzodiazepines*	clindamycin	isoniazid
captopril	dapsone	levamisole
carbamazepine	desipramine	meprobamate
carbimazole	disopyramide	methimazole
cephalosporins*	ethacrynic acid	methyldopa
chloramphenicol	fansidar	oxyphenbutazone
chloroquine	gentamicin	penicillamine

penicillins*
pentazocine
phenacetin
phenothiazines*
phenylbutazone
phenytoin
procainamide
propranolol
propylthiouracil

pyrimethamine
quinidine
quinine
ranitidine
rifampin
sodium aminosalicylate
streptomycin
sulfadoxime

sulfonamides*
tetracyclines*
ticlopidine
tocainide
tolbutamide
trimethoprim/
   sulfamethoxazole
vancomycin

Drugs That May Significantly *Reduce Blood Platelet Counts*

acetazolamide
actinomycin
allopurinol
alpha-interferon
amiodarone
ampicillin
aspirin
carbamazepine
carbenicillin
cephalosporins*
chenodeoxycholic acid
chloroquine
chlorothiazide
chlorpheniramine
chlorpropamide
chlorthalidone
cimetidine
cyclophosphamide
danazol
desferrioxamine

diazepam
diazoxide
diclofenac
digoxin
diltiazem
furosemide
gentamicin
gold
hydrochlorothiazide
imipramine
isoniazid
isotretinoin
levamisole
meprobamate
methyldopa
mianserin
minoxidil
morphine
nitrofurantoin
oxprenolol

oxyphenbutazone
penicillamine
penicillin
phenylbutazone
phenytoin
piroxicam
procainamide
quinidine
quinine
ranitidine
rifampin
sodium aminosalicylate
sulfasalazine
sulfonamides*
thioguanine
ticlopidine
trimethoprim/
   sulfamethoxazole
valproate
vancomycin

Drugs That Cause Significant *Hemolytic Anemia* Due to Glucose-6-Phosphate Dehydrogenase (G6PD) Deficiency of Red Blood Cells

acetanilid
methylene blue
nalidixic acid
naphthalene
niridazole
nitrofurantoin

pamaquine
phenazopyridine
phenylhydrazine
primaquine
sulfacetamide

sulfamethoxazole
sulfanilamide
sulfapyridine
thiazosulfone
toluidine blue

Drugs That May Cause *Hemolytic Anemia* by Other Mechanisms

antimony
chlorpropamide
cisplatin
mephenesin

methotrexate
para-aminosalicylic acid
penicillamine
phenazopyridine

quinidine
quinine
rifampin
sulfasalazine

Drugs That May Cause *Megaloblastic Anemia*

acyclovir	metformin	primidone
alcohol	methotrexate	pyrimethamine
aminopterin	neomycin	sulfasalazine
azathioprine	nitrofurantoin	tetracycline
colchicine	nitrous oxide	thioguanine
cycloserine	oral contraceptives	triamterene
cytarabine	para-aminosalicylic acid	trimethoprim
floxuridine	pentamidine	vinblastine
fluorouracil	phenformin	vitamin A
hydroxyurea	phenobarbital	vitamin C (large doses)
mercaptopurine	phenytoin	zidovudine

Drugs That May Cause *Sideroblastic Anemia*

alcohol	isoniazid	phenacetin
chloramphenicol	penicillamine	pyrazinamide
cycloserine		

Drugs That May Cause *Leukemia*

actinomycin	cyclophosphamide	phenylbutazone
anthracyclines	epipodophyllotoxins	procarbazine
chlorambucil	melphalan	sulfinpyrazone
chloramphenicol	nitrosoureas	thioTEPA

*See Appendix 16, Drug Classes
‡See Glossary

TABLE 2

DRUGS THAT MAY CAUSE HEART DYSFUNCTION OR DAMAGE

Drugs of very diverse classes can adversely affect both the function and structure of the heart. Disorders of the heart (that require drug therapy) often determine the nature of adverse effects induced by drugs. Some adverse effects are due to direct pharmacological actions of a drug on heart tissues (as with antiarrhythmic drugs); other reactions are caused indirectly by altering biochemical balances that influence heart function (as with excessive loss of potassium due to diuretics that results in abnormal heart rhythms and digitalis toxicity).

Drugs That May Cause or Contribute to *Abnormal Heart Rhythms* (arrhythmias)

aminophylline	beta-adrenergic-blocking	chlorpromazine
amiodarone	drugs*	cimetidine
amitriptyline	beta-adrenergic bron-	digitoxin
antiarrhythmic drugs*	chodilators*	digoxin
bepridil	carbamazepine	diltiazem

disopyramide
diuretics*
doxepin
encainide
fentolterol
flecainide
isoproterenol
ketanserin
lidocaine

maprotiline
methyldopa
mexiletine
milrinone
phenothiazines*
prenylamine
procainamide
quinidine
ranitidine

sotalol
terbutaline
theophylline
thiazide diuretics*
thioridazine
trazodone
tricyclic antidepressants*
verapamil

Drugs That May *Depress Heart Function* (reduce pumping efficiency)

beta-adrenergic-blocking
   drugs*
cocaine
daunorubicin
diltiazem

disopyramide
doxorubicin
epinephrine
flecainide

fluorouracil
isoproterenol
nifedipine
verapamil

Drugs That May *Reduce Coronary Artery Blood Flow* (reduce oxygen supply to heart muscle)

amphetamines*
beta-adrenergic-blocking
   drugs* (abrupt
   withdrawal)
cocaine

ergotamine
fluorouracil
nifedipine
oral contraceptives

ritodrine
vasopressin
vinblastine
vincristine

Drugs That May *Impair Healing of Heart Muscle* Following Heart Attack (myocardial infarction)

adrenocortical steroids*

nonsteroidal anti-inflammatory drugs (NSAIDs)*

Drugs That May Cause *Heart Valve Damage*

ergotamine

methysergide

minocycline (blue–black
   pigmentation)

Drugs That May Cause *Pericardial Disease*

actinomycin D
anthracyclines
bleomycin
cisplatin
cyclophosphamide

cytarabine
fluorouracil
hydralazine
methysergide
minoxidil

phenylbutazone
practolol
procainamide
sulfasalazine

*See Appendix 16, Drug Classes

TABLE 3

DRUGS THAT MAY CAUSE LUNG DYSFUNCTION OR DAMAGE

Adverse drug reactions that directly affect the lung are often difficult to distinguish from natural diseases or disorders that commonly involve lung function or structure. As with other organ systems, the lung is subject to both principal types of drug reactions: Type A—those due to known and expected pharmacological drug actions; Type B—those due to unexpected and unpredictable allergic or idiosyncratic reactions on the part of the drug user.

Drugs That May Adversely Affect *Blood Vessels of the Lung*

Drugs That May Cause Pulmonary Hypertension
amphetamines*
fenfluramine
oral contraceptives
tryptophan

Drugs That May Cause Vasculitis (blood vessel damage) with or without Hemorrhage
aminoglutethimide
amphotericin
cocaine
febarbamate
nitrofurantoin
penicillamine
phenytoin

Drugs That May Cause Thromboembolism
estrogens*
oral contraceptives (high estrogen type)

Drugs That May Cause Adult Respiratory Distress Syndrome (ARDS)
bleomycin
codeine
cyclophosphamide
dextropropoxyphene
heroin
hydrochlorothiazide
methadone
mitomycin
naloxone
ritodrine
terbutaline
vinblastine

Drugs That May Adversely Affect the *Bronchial Tubes*

Drugs That May Cause Bronchoconstriction (asthma)
acetaminophen
aspirin
beta-adrenergic-blocking drugs*
carbachol
cephalosporins*
chloramphenicol
deanol
demeclocycline
erythromycin
griseofulvin
maprotiline
methacholine
methoxypsoralen
metoclopramide

morphine
neomycin
neostigmine
nitrofurantoin
nonsteroidal anti-inflammatory drugs*
penicillins*
pilocarpine
propafenone
pyridostigmine
streptomycin
tartrazine (coloring agent)

Drugs That May Cause Bronchiolitis (with permanent obstruction of small bronchioles)
penicillamine
sulfasalazine

Drugs That May *Damage Lung Tissues*

Drugs That May Cause Acute Allergic-Type Pneumonitis

ampicillin
bleomycin
cephalexin
chlorpropamide
gold
imipramine
mephenesin
mercaptopurine
metformin
methotrexate
metronidazole
mitomycin
nalidixic acid
nitrofurantoin
nomifensine
nonsteroidal anti-inflammatory drugs*
para-aminosalicylic acid
penicillamine
penicillin
phenylbutazone
phenytoin
procarbazine
sulfonamides*
tetracycline
vinblastine

Drugs That May Cause Chronic Pneumonitis and Fibrosis (scarring)

amiodarone
bleomycin
bromocriptine
busulfan
carmustine
chlorambucil
cyclophosphamide
ergotamine
gold
hexamethonium
mecamylamine
melphalan
methysergide
nitrofurantoin
pentolinium
practolol
sulfasalazine
tocainide
tolfenamic acid

Drugs That May *Damage the Pleura*

bromocriptine   methysergide   practolol

*See Appendix 16, Drug Classes

TABLE 4

DRUGS THAT MAY CAUSE LIVER DYSFUNCTION OR DAMAGE

The liver is the principal organ that is capable of converting drugs into forms that can be readily eliminated from the body. Given the diversity of drugs in use today and the complex burdens they impose upon the liver, it is not surprising that a broad spectrum of adverse drug effects on liver functions and structures has been documented. The reactions range from mild and transient changes in the results of liver function tests to complete liver failure with death of the host. Many drugs may affect the liver adversely in more than one way, as cited below in several listings. The use of the following drugs requires careful monitoring of their effects on the liver during the entire course of treatment.

Drugs That May Cause *Acute Dose-Dependent Liver Damage* (resembling acute viral hepatitis)

acetaminophen (over-dosage)   salicylates (doses over 2 grams daily)

Drugs That May Cause *Acute Dose-Independent Liver Damage* (resembling acute viral hepatitis)

acebutolol
allopurinol
atenolol
carbamazepine
chlorzoxazone
cimetidine
dantrolene
diclofenac
diltiazem
disulfiram
enflurane
ethambutol
ethionamide
felbamate
halothane
ibuprofen
indomethacin
isoniazid
ketoconazole
labetalol
maprotiline
metoprolol
mianserin
naproxen
nifedipine
para-aminosalicylic acid
penicillins*
phenelzine
phenindione
phenobarbital
phenylbutazone
phenytoin
piroxicam
probenecid
pyrazinamide
quinidine
quinine
ranitidine
rifampin
sulfonamides*
sulindac
tricyclic antidepressants*
valproic acid
verapamil

Drugs That May Cause *Acute Fatty Infiltration of the Liver*

adrenocortical steroids*
antithyroid drugs
isoniazid
methotrexate
phenothiazines*
phenytoin
salicylates*
sulfonamides*
tetracyclines*
valproic acid

Drugs That May Cause *Cholestatic Jaundice*

actinomycin D
amoxicillin/clavulanate
azathioprine
captopril
carbamazepine
carbimazole
cephalosporins*
chlordiazepoxide
chlorpropamide
cloxacillin
cyclophosphamide
cyclosporine
danazol
diazepam
disopyramide
enalapril
erythromycin
flecainide
flurazepam
flutamide
glyburide
gold
griseofulvin
haloperidol
ketoconazole
mercaptopurine
methyltestosterone
nifedipine
nitrofurantoin
nonsteroidal anti-
    inflammatory drugs*
norethandrolone
oral contraceptives
oxacillin
penicillamine
phenothiazines*
phenytoin
propoxyphene
propylthiouracil
sulfonamides*
tamoxifen
thiabendazole
tolbutamide
tricyclic antidepressants*
troleandomycin
verapamil

Drugs That May Cause *Liver Granulomas* (chronic inflammatory nodules)

allopurinol
aspirin
carbamazepine
chlorpromazine
chlorpropamide
diltiazem
disopyramide
gold
hydralazine
isoniazid
methyldopa
nitrofurantoin
penicillin
phenylbutazone
phenytoin
procainamide
quinidine
ranitidine
sulfonamides*
tolbutamide

Drugs That May Cause *Chronic Liver Disease*

Drugs That May Cause Liver Cirrhosis or Fibrosis (scarring)
methotrexate
nicotinic acid

Drugs That May Cause Chronic Cholestasis (resembling primary biliary cirrhosis)
chlorpromazine/valproic
   acid (combination)

chlorpropamide/
   erythromycin
   (combination)
imipramine
phenothiazines*
phenytoin
thiabendazole
tolbutamide

Drugs That May Cause Active Chronic Hepatitis
acetaminophen (chronic
   use, large doses)
dantrolene
isoniazid
methyldopa
nitrofurantoin

Drugs That May Cause *Liver Tumors* (benign and malignant)

anabolic steroids
danazol

oral contraceptives
testosterone

thorotrast

Drugs That May Cause *Damage to Liver Blood Vessels*

adriamycin
anabolic steroids
azathioprine
carmustine

cyclophosphamide/cyclo-
   sporine (combination)
dacarbazine
mercaptopurine
methotrexate

mitomycin
oral contraceptives
thioguanine
vincristine
vitamin A (excessive doses)

*See Appendix 16, Drug Classes

TABLE 5

DRUGS THAT MAY CAUSE KIDNEY DYSFUNCTION OR DAMAGE

With regard to medicinal drugs, the kidneys perform two major functions: (1) the alteration (biotransformation) of the drug to facilitate its processing; (2) the elimination of the drug from the body via the excretion of urine. As with drug effects on the liver, many drugs may adversely affect the kidneys in several ways. This is illustrated in the following tables by the appearance of some drug names in more than one listing. The kidneys are quite sensitive to the toxic effects of medicinal drugs. Vigilance and careful monitoring are always advisable during the course of treatment with any of the drugs cited below.

Drugs That May Primarily *Impair Kidney Function* (without damage)

amphotericin
angiotensin-converting
   enzyme inhibitors*
   (with renal artery
   stenosis; with conges-
   tive heart failure)
beta-adrenergic-blocking
   drugs*
colchicine

demeclocycline
diuretics/NSAIDs* (avoid
   this combination)
glyburide
isofosfamide
lithium/tricyclic anti-
   depressants* (avoid
   this combination)

methoxyflurane
nifedipine
nitroprusside
nonsteroidal anti-
   inflammatory drugs*
rifampin
vinblastine

Drugs That May Cause *Acute Kidney Failure* (due to kidney damage)

Drugs That May Damage the Kidney Filtration Unit (the nephron)
acetaminophen (excessive dosage)
allopurinol
aminoglycoside antibiotics*
amphotericin
bismuth thiosulfate
carbamazepine
cisplatin
cyclosporine
enalapril
ergometrine
hydralazine
metronidazole
mitomycin
oral contraceptives
penicillamine
phenytoin
quinidine
rifampin
streptokinase
sulfonamides*
thiazide diuretics*

Drugs That May Cause Acute Interstitial Nephritis
allopurinol
amoxicillin
ampicillin
aspirin
azathioprine
aztreonam
captopril
carbamazepine
carbenicillin

cefaclor
cefoxitin
cephalexin
cephalothin
cephapirin
cephradine
cimetidine
ciprofloxacin
clofibrate
cloxacillin
diazepam
diclofenac
diflunisal
ethacrynic acid
fenoprofen
foscarnet
furosemide
gentamicin
glafenine
ibuprofen
indomethacin
ketoprofen
mefenamate
methicillin
methyldopa
mezlocillin
minocycline
nafcillin
naproxen
oxacillin
penicillamine
penicillin
phenindione
phenobarbital
phenylbutazone
phenytoin
piroxicam
pirprofen

pyrazinamide
rifampin
sodium valproate
sulfamethoxazole
sulfinpyrazone
sulfonamides*
sulindac
thiazide diuretics*
tolmetin
triamterene
trimethoprim
vancomycin
warfarin

Drugs That May Cause Muscle Destruction and Associated Acute Kidney Failure
adrenocortical steroids*
alcohol
amphetamines*
amphotericin
carbenoxolone
chlorthalidone
clofibrate
cocaine
cytarabine
fenofibrate
haloperidol
halothane
heroin
lovastatin
opioid analgesics*
pentamidine
phenothiazines*
streptokinase
suxamethonium

Drugs That May Cause *Kidney Damage Resembling Glomerulonephritis or Nephrosis*

captopril
fenoprofen
gold
ketoprofen

lithium
mesalamine
penicillamine
phenytoin

practolol
probenecid
quinidine

Drugs That May Cause *Chronic Interstitial Nephritis and Papillary Necrosis* (analgesic kidney damage)

acetaminophen	aspirin	phenacetin
(all with long-term use)		

Drugs That May Cause or Contribute to *Urinary Tract Crystal or Stone Formation*

acetazolamide	methoxyflurane	uricosuric drugs
acyclovir	phenylbutazone	vitamin A
cytotoxic drugs	probenecid	vitamin C
dihydroxyadenine	salicylates*	vitamin D
magnesium trisilicate	sulfonamides*	warfarin
mercaptopurine	thiazide diuretics*	zoxazolamine
methotrexate	triamterene	

*See Appendix 16, Drug Classes

TABLE 6

DRUGS THAT MAY CAUSE NERVE DYSFUNCTION OR DAMAGE

Medicinal drugs may adversely affect any segment of the nervous system from the brain to endpoint distribution of peripheral nerves. There is wide variability in the patterns of response to drugs among individuals in both therapeutic effects and unwanted adverse effects. Individual variability is determined largely by genetic programming of drug metabolism and responsiveness. The following scheme of classification groups drugs according to the familiar clinical syndromes that represent drug-induced neurological disorders.

Drugs That May Cause *Significant Headache*

amyl nitrate	indomethacin	sulindac
bromocriptine	labetalol	terbutaline
clonidine	naproxen	tetracyclines*
ergotamine (prolonged	nifedipine	theophylline
use)	nitrofurantoin	tolmetin
etretinate	nitroglycerin	trimethoprim/
hydralazine	perhexiline	sulfamethoxazole
ibuprofen	propranolol	

Drugs That May Cause *Seizures* (convulsions)

ampicillin	cimetidine	halothane
atenolol	ciprofloxacin	indomethacin
carbenicillin	cycloserine	isoniazid
cephalosporins*	disopyramide	lidocaine
chloroquine	ether	lithium

(cont.)

mefenamic acid
nalidixic acid
oxacillin
penicillins* (synthetic)

phenothiazines*
pyrimethamine
terbutaline
theophylline

ticarcillin
tricyclic antidepressants*
vincristine

Drugs That May Cause *Stroke*

anabolic steroids
cocaine

oral contraceptives

phenylpropanolamine

Drugs That May Cause Features of *Parkinsonism*

amitriptyline
amodiaquine
chloroquine
chlorprothixene
desipramine
diazoxide

diphenhydramine
droperidol
haloperidol
imipramine
levodopa
lithium

methyldopa
metoclopramide
phenothiazines*
reserpine
thiothixene
trifluoperidol

Drugs That May Cause *Acute Dystonias* (acute involuntary movement syndromes—AIMS)

carbamazepine
chlorzoxazone
haloperidol

metoclopramide
phenothiazines*
phenytoin

propranolol
tricyclic antidepressants*

Drugs That May Cause *Tardive Dyskinesia*‡

haloperidol

phenothiazines*

thiothixene

Drugs That May Cause *Neuroleptic Malignant Syndrome (NMS)*†

Drugs That May Cause *Peripheral Neuropathy*‡

amiodarone
amitriptyline
amphetamines*
amphotericin
anticoagulants*
carbutamide
chlorambucil
chloramphenicol
chloroquine
chlorpropamide
cimetidine
clioquinol
clofibrate
colchicine

colistin
cytarabine
dapsone
disopyramide
disulfiram
ergotamine
ethambutol
glutethimide
gold
hydralazine
imipramine
indomethacin
isoniazid
methaqualone

methimazole
methysergide
metronidazole
nalidixic acid
nitrofurantoin
nitrofurazone
penicillamine
penicillin
perhexiline
phenelzine
phenylbutazone
phenytoin
podophyllin
procarbazine

propranolol	sulfonamides*	tolbutamide
propylthiouracil	sulfoxone	vinblastine
streptomycin	thalidomide	vincristine

Drugs That May Cause a *Myasthenia Gravis* Syndrome

| aminoglycoside antibiotics* | penicillamine | polymixin B |
| beta-adrenergic-blocking drugs* | phenytoin | trihexyphenidyl |

*See Appendix 16, Drug Classes
†See this term in the Glossary for a list of causative drugs
‡See Glossary

TABLE 7

DRUGS THAT MAY INTERACT WITH ALCOHOL

Beverages containing alcohol may interact unfavorably with a wide variety of drugs. The most important (and most familiar) interaction occurs when the depressant action on the brain of sedatives, sleep-inducing drugs, tranquilizers, and narcotic drugs is intensified by alcohol. Alcohol may also reduce the effectiveness of some drugs, and it can interact with certain other drugs to produce toxic effects. Some drugs may increase the intoxicating effects of alcohol, producing further impairment of mental alertness, judgment, physical coordination, and reaction time.

Although drug interactions with alcohol are generally predictable, the intensity and significance of these interactions can vary greatly from one individual to another and from one occasion to another. This is because many factors influence what happens when drugs and alcohol interact. These factors include individual variations in sensitivity to drugs (including alcohol), the chemistry and quantity of the drug, the type and amount of alcohol consumed, and the sequence in which drug and alcohol are taken. If you need to use any of the drugs listed in the following tables, you should ask your physician for guidance concerning the use of alcohol.

Drugs with Which It Is Advisable to Avoid Alcohol Completely

Drug Name or Class	Possible Interaction with Alcohol
amphetamines	excessive rise in blood pressure with alcoholic beverages containing tyramine**
antidepressants*	excessive sedation, increased intoxication
barbiturates*	excessive sedation
bromides	confusion, delirium, increased intoxication
calcium carbamide	disulfiramlike reaction**
carbamazepine	excessive sedation
chlorprothixene	excessive sedation
chlorzoxazone	excessive sedation
disulfiram	disulfiram reaction**
ergotamine	reduced effectiveness of ergotamine
fenfluramine	excessive stimulation of nervous system with some beers and wines

furazolidone	disulfiramlike reaction**
haloperidol	excessive sedation
MAO inhibitor drugs*	excessive rise in blood pressure with alcoholic beverages containing tyramine**
meperidine	excessive sedation
meprobamate	excessive sedation
methotrexate	increased liver toxicity and excessive sedation
metronidazole	disulfiramlike reaction**
narcotic drugs	excessive sedation
oxyphenbutazone	increased stomach irritation and/or bleeding
pentazocine	excessive sedation
pethidine	excessive sedation
phenothiazines*	excessive sedation
phenylbutazone	increased stomach irritation and/or bleeding
procarbazine	disulfiramlike reaction**
propoxyphene	excessive sedation
reserpine	excessive sedation, orthostatic hypotension**
sleep-inducing drugs (hypnotics):	excessive sedation
carbromal	
chloral hydrate	
ethchlorvynol	
ethinamate	
glutethimide	
flurazepam	
methaqualone	
methyprylon	
temazepam	
triazolam	
thiothixene	excessive sedation
tricyclic antidepressants*	excessive sedation, increased intoxication
trimethobenzamide	excessive sedation

Drugs with Which Alcohol Should Be Used Only in Small Amounts
(use cautiously until combined effects have been determined)

Drug Name or Class	Possible Interaction with Alcohol
acetaminophen (Tylenol, etc.)	increased liver toxicity
amantadine	excessive lowering of blood pressure
antiarthritic/ anti-inflammatory drugs	increased stomach irritation and/or bleeding
anticoagulants (coumarins)*	increased anticoagulant effect
antidiabetic drugs (sulfonylureas)*	increased antidiabetic effect, excessive hypoglycemia**
antihistamines*	excessive sedation
antihypertensives*	excessive orthostatic hypotension**
aspirin (large doses or continuous use)	increased stomach irritation and/or bleeding
benzodiazepines*	excessive sedation
carisoprodol	increased alcoholic intoxication

diethylpropion	excessive nervous system stimulation with alcoholic beverages containing tyramine**
dihydroergotoxine	excessive lowering of blood pressure
diphenoxylate	excessive sedation
dipyridamole	excessive lowering of blood pressure
diuretics*	excessive orthostatic hypotension**
ethionamide	confusion, delirium, psychotic behavior
fenoprofen	increased stomach irritation and/or bleeding
griseofulvin	flushing and rapid heart action
ibuprofen	increased stomach irritation and/or bleeding
indomethacin	increased stomach irritation and/or bleeding
insulin	excessive hypoglycemia**
iron	excessive absorption of iron
isoniazid	decreased effectiveness of isoniazid, increased incidence of hepatitis
lithium	increased confusion and delirium (avoid all alcohol if any indication of lithium overdosage)
methocarbamol	excessive sedation
methotrimeprazine	excessive sedation
methylphenidate	excessive nervous system stimulation with alcoholic beverages containing tyramine**
metoprolol	excessive orthostatic hypotension**
nalidixic acid	increased alcoholic intoxication
naproxen	increased stomach irritation and/or bleeding
nicotinic acid	possible orthostatic hypotension**
nitrates* (vasodilators)	possible orthostatic hypotension**
nylidrin	increased stomach irritation
orphenadrine	excessive sedation
phenelzine	increased alcoholic intoxication
phenoxybenzamine	possible orthostatic hypotension**
phentermine	excessive nervous system stimulation with alcoholic beverages containing tyramine**
phenytoin	decreased effect of phenytoin
pilocarpine	prolongation of alcohol effect
prazosin	excessive lowering of blood pressure
primidone	excessive sedation
propranolol	excessive orthostatic hypotension**
sulfonamides*	increased alcoholic intoxication
sulindac	increased stomach irritation and/or bleeding
tolmetin	increased stomach irritation and/or bleeding
tranquilizers (mild):	excessive sedation
chlordiazepoxide	
clorazepate	
diazepam	
hydroxyzine	
meprobamate	
oxazepam	
phenaglycodol	
tybamate	
tranylcypromine	increased alcoholic intoxication

Drugs Capable of Producing a Disulfiramlike Reaction** When Used Concurrently with Alcohol

antidiabetic drugs (sulfony- lureas)*	disulfiram	procarbazine
calcium carbamide	furazolidone	quinacrine
chloral hydrate	metronidazole	sulfonamides*
chloramphenicol	nifuroxine	tinidazole
	nitrofurantoin	tolazoline

*See Appendix 16, Drug Classes

**See Glossary

SECTION SEVEN

Glossary

abuse Used in the context of substance abuse, this term refers to the recurrent use of a substance that results in major lack of responsibility in fulfilling the normal obligations of domestic, scholastic, occupational, or social life. Persistent use of the substance continues in spite of serious interpersonal, social, or legal consequences. The behavior pattern of substance abuse does not constitute substance dependence; the features of tolerance and withdrawal symptoms are absent.

addiction Although this term has long been a part of our language and its meaning is clearly understood by all, it is not officially accepted by the psychiatric community. With the intent of coining more precise definitions, the term addiction has been replaced by the terms *abuse* and *dependence*. However, current authorities in this field still use the term addiction to indicate a state of intense dependence (upon a drug) that is characterized by uncontrolled drug-seeking behavior, tolerance for the drug's effects, and withdrawal manifestations when the drug is withheld (see also the terms ABUSE, DEPENDENCE, TOLERANCE, and WITHDRAWAL SYNDROME).

adverse effect or reaction An abnormal, unexpected, infrequent, and usually unpredictable injurious response to a drug. Used in this restrictive sense, the term *adverse reaction* does *not* include effects of a drug which are normally a part of its pharmacological action, even though such effects may be undesirable and unintended (see SIDE EFFECT). Adverse reactions are of three basic types: those due to drug *allergy,* those caused by individual *idiosyncrasy,* and those representing *toxic* effects of drugs on tissue structure and function (see also ALLERGY, IDIOSYNCRASY, and TOXICITY).

allergy, drug An abnormal mechanism of drug response that occurs in individuals who produce injurious antibodies that react with foreign substances—in this instance, a drug. The person who is allergic by nature and has a history of hay fever, asthma, hives, or eczema is more likely to develop drug allergies. Allergic reactions to drugs take many forms: skin eruptions of various kinds, fever, swollen glands, painful joints, jaundice, interference with breathing, acute collapse of circulation, etc. Drug allergies can develop gradually over a long period of time, or they can appear with dramatic suddenness and require life-saving intervention (see also Appendix 5, The Immune System).

analgesic A drug that is used primarily to relieve pain. Analgesics are of three basic types: (1) simple, nonnarcotic analgesics that relieve pain by suppressing the local production of prostaglandins and related substances; examples are acetaminophen, aspirin, and the large group of nonsteroidal anti-inflammatory drugs known as NSAIDs or aspirin substitutes (Motrin, Advil, Naprosyn, etc.). (2) Narcotic analgesics or opioids ("like opium" derivatives) that relieve pain by suppressing its perception in the brain; examples are morphine, codeine, and hydrocodone (natural derivatives of opium), and meperidine or pentazocine (synthetic drug products). (3) Local anesthetics that prevent or relieve pain by rendering sensory nerve endings insensitive to painful stimulation; an example is the urinary tract analgesic phenazopyridine (Pyridium).

anaphylactic (anaphylactoid) reaction A group of symptoms which represent (or resemble) a sometimes overwhelming and dangerous allergic reaction due to extreme hypersensitivity to a drug. Anaphylactic reactions, whether mild, moderate, or severe, often involve several body systems. Mild symptoms consist of itching, hives, nasal congestion, nausea, abdominal cramping and/or diarrhea. Sometimes these precede more severe symptoms such as choking, shortness of breath, and sudden loss of consciousness (usually referred to as anaphylactic shock).

Characteristic features of anaphylactic reaction must be kept in mind. It can result from a very small dose of drug; it develops suddenly, usually within a few minutes after taking the drug; it can be rapidly progressive and can lead to fatal collapse in a short time if not reversed by appropriate treatment. A developing anaphylactic reaction is a true medical emergency. Any adverse effect that appears within 20 minutes after taking a drug should be considered the early manifestation of a possible anaphylactic reaction. Obtain medical attention immediately! (See also ALLERGY, DRUG, and HYPERSENSITIVITY.)

antihypertensive A drug used to lower excessively high blood pressure. The term *hypertension* denotes blood pressure above the normal range. It does not refer to excessive nervous or emotional tension. The term *antihypertensive* is sometimes used erroneously as if it had the same meaning as *antianxiety* (or tranquilizing) drug action.

Today there are more than 80 drug products in use for treating hypertension. Those most frequently prescribed for long-term use fall into three major groups:
1. Drugs that increase urine production (the diuretics)
2. Drugs that relax blood vessel walls
3. Drugs that reduce the activity of the sympathetic nervous system

Regardless of their mode of action, all these drugs share an ability to lower the blood pressure. It is important to remember that many other drugs can interact with antihypertensive drugs: some add to their effect and cause excessive reduction in blood pressure; others interfere with their action and reduce their effectiveness. Anyone who is taking medications for hypertension should consult with his or her physician whenever drugs are prescribed for the treatment of other conditions as well (see also Appendix 16, Drug Classes).

aplastic anemia A form of bone marrow failure in which the production of all three types of blood cells is seriously impaired (also known as pancytopenia). Aplastic anemia can occur spontaneously from unknown causes, but about one-half of reported cases are induced by certain drugs or chemicals. The offending drug may be difficult to identify; a delay of from one to six months may occur between the use of a causative drug and the detection of anemia. The symptoms reflect the consequences of inadequate supplies of all three blood cell types: deficiency of red blood cells (anemia) results in fatigue, weakness, and pallor; deficiency of white blood cells (leukopenia) predisposes to infections; deficiency of blood platelets (thrombocytopenia) leads to spontaneous bruising and hemorrhage. Treatment is difficult and the outcome unpredictable. Even with the best of care, approximately 50% of cases end fatally.

Although aplastic anemia is a rare consequence of drug treatment (3 in 100,000 users of quinacrine, for example), anyone taking a drug capable of inducing it should have complete blood cell counts periodically if the drug is to be used over an extended period of time. For a listing of causative drugs, see also Section Six, Table 1.

atherosclerosis A form of hardening of the arteries in which the inner layers of artery walls become thick and rough due to localized deposits (plaque) of fat, cholesterol, and cellular debris; these are referred to as atheromas. As their inner walls become lined with atheromas, arteries are progressively narrowed and blood flow is significantly reduced. Atherosclerosis is the principal cause of cerebral vascular disease and stroke, coronary artery disease and heart attack (myocardial infarction), and peripheral vascular disease.

blood platelets The smallest of the three types of blood cells produced by the bone marrow. Platelets are normally present in very large numbers. Their primary function is to assist the process of normal blood clotting so as to prevent excessive bruising and bleeding in the event of injury. When present in proper numbers and functioning normally, platelets preserve the retaining power of the walls of the smaller blood vessels. By initiating appropriate clotting processes in the blood, platelets seal small points of leakage in the vessel walls, thereby preventing spontaneous bruising or bleeding (that which is unprovoked by trauma).

Certain drugs and chemicals may reduce the number of available blood platelets to abnormally low levels. Some of these drugs act by suppressing platelet formation; other drugs hasten their destruction. When the number of functioning platelets falls below a critical level, blood begins to leak through the thin walls of smaller vessels. The outward evidence of this leakage is the spontaneous appearance of scattered bruises in the skin of the thighs and legs. This is referred to as purpura. Bleeding may occur anywhere in the body, internally as well as superficially into the tissues immediately beneath the skin (see also Section Six, Table 1).

bone marrow depression A serious reduction in the ability of the bone marrow to carry on its normal production of blood cells. This can occur as an adverse reaction to the toxic effect of certain drugs and chemicals on bone marrow components. When functioning normally, the bone marrow produces the majority of the body's blood cells. These consist of three types: the red blood cells (erythrocytes), the white blood cells (leukocytes), and the blood platelets (thrombocytes). Each type of cell performs one or more specific functions, all of which are indispensable to the maintenance of life and health.

Drugs that are capable of depressing bone marrow activity can impair the production of all types of blood cells simultaneously or of only one type selectively. Periodic examinations of the blood can reveal significant changes in the structure and number of the blood cells that indicate a possible drug effect on bone marrow activity.

Impairment of the production of red blood cells leads to anemia, a condition of abnormally low red cells and hemoglobin. This causes weakness, loss of energy and stamina, intolerance of cold environments, and shortness of breath on physical exertion. A reduction in the formation of white blood cells can impair the body's immunity and lower its resistance to infection. These changes may result in the development of fever, sore throat, or pneumonia. When the formation of blood platelets is suppressed to abnormally low levels, the blood loses its ability to quickly seal small points of leakage in blood vessel walls. This may lead to episodes of unusual and abnormal spontaneous bruising or to prolonged bleeding in the event of injury.

Any of these symptoms can occur in the presence of bone marrow depression. They should alert both patient and physician to the need for prompt studies of blood and bone marrow (see also Section Six, Table 1).

cause-and-effect relationship A possible causative association between a drug and an observed biological event, most commonly a side effect or an adverse effect. Knowledge of a drug's full spectrum of effects, both wanted and unwanted, is highly desirable when weighing its benefits and risks in any treatment situation. However, it is often impossible to establish with certainty that a particular drug is the primary agent responsible for a suspected adverse effect. In the evaluation of every cause-and-effect relationship, therefore, meticulous consideration must be given to such factors as the time sequence of drug administration and possible reaction, the use of multiple drugs, possible interactions among these drugs, the effects of the disease under treatment, the physiological and psychological characteristics of the patient and the possible influence of unrecognized disorders and malfunctions.

The majority of adverse drug reactions occur sporadically, unpredictably, and infrequently in the general population. A *definite* cause-and-effect relationship between drug and reaction is established when (1) the adverse effect immediately follows administration of the drug; or (2) the adverse effect disappears after the drug is discontinued (dechallenge) and promptly reappears when the drug is used again (rechallenge); or (3) the adverse effects are clearly the expected and predictable toxic consequences of drug overdosage.

In contrast to the obvious "causative" (definite) relationship, there exists a large gray area of "probable," "possible," and "coincidental" associations that are clouded by varying degrees of uncertainty. These classifications usually apply to alleged drug reactions that require a relatively long time to develop, are of low incidence, and for which there are no clear-cut objective means of demonstrating a causal mechanism that links drug and reaction. Clarification of cause-and-effect relationships in these uncertain groups requires carefully designed observation over a long period of time, followed by sophisticated statistical analysis. Occasionally the public is alerted to a newly found "relationship" based upon suggestive but incomplete data. Though early warning is clearly in the public interest, such announcements should make clear whether the presumed relationship is based upon definitive criteria or is simply inferred because the use of a drug and an observed event were found to occur together within an appropriate time frame.

The most competent techniques for evaluating cause-and-effect relationships of adverse drug reactions have been devised by the Division of Tissue Reactions to Drugs, a research unit of the Armed Forces Institute of Pathology. Based upon a highly critical examination of all available evidence, the Division's study of 2,800 drug-related deaths yielded the following levels of certainty regarding cause-and-effect relationship:

No association	5.0%
Coincidental	14.5%
Possible	33.0%
Probable	30.0%
Causative	17.5%

It is significant that expert evaluation of 2,800 drug-related cases concluded that only 47.5% could be substantiated as definitely or probably causative.

contraindication A condition or disease that precludes the use of a particular drug. Some contraindications are *absolute,* meaning that the use of the drug would expose the patient to extreme hazard and therefore cannot be justified. Other contraindications are *relative,* meaning that the condition or disease does not entirely bar the use of the drug but requires that before the decision to use the drug is made, special consideration be given to factors which could aggravate existing disease, interfere with current treatment, or produce new injury.

dementia A group of mental disorders characterized by a general loss of intellectual abilities, including memory, judgment, and abstract thinking, but not due to delirium. Dementias result from a variety of causes. They may be transient, relatively stable, or progressive.

dependence Current synonyms for this term are *compulsive use* and *habituation.* Dependence implies a psychological and/or physical "need" for an addictive drug. Thus a distinction may be made between *psychological dependence* and *physical dependence.*

Psychological dependence may occur with any drug that has a potential for abuse. It is a subjective feeling that the drug is necessary to achieve an optimal level of functioning, an enhanced sense of well-being, or a highly pleasurable state. It is characterized by little or no tendency to increase the dose (see also TOLERANCE) and no or only minor physical manifestations on withdrawal. Some authorities choose to broaden their definition of addiction to include psychological dependence.

Physical dependence occurs after the body undergoes physiological changes to adapt to the constant presence of the drug. Physical dependence includes two features: *tolerance* and *withdrawal* manifestations. Addictive drugs provide relief from anguish and pain swiftly and effectively; they also induce a physiological tolerance that requires increasing dosage or repeated use if they are to remain effective. These two actions foster the continued need for the drug and lead to its becoming a functioning component in the biochemistry of the brain. As this occurs, the drug assumes an "essential" role in ongoing chemical processes (thus some authorities prefer the term *chemical dependence*). Sudden removal of the drug from the system causes a major upheaval in brain chemistry and provokes a withdrawal syndrome—the intense mental and physical pain experienced by the user when intake of the drug is stopped—the hallmark of physical dependence.

Note: Some authorities maintain that many individuals with a substance dependence experience a blend of psychological and physical dependence.

disulfiramlike (Antabuse-like) reaction The symptoms that result from the interaction of alcohol and any drug that is capable of provoking the pattern of response typical of the "Antabuse effect." The interacting drug interrupts the normal decomposition of alcohol by the liver and thereby permits the accumulation of a toxic by-product that enters the bloodstream. When sufficient levels of both alcohol and drug are present in the blood the reaction occurs. It consists of intense flushing and warming of the face, a severe throbbing headache, shortness of breath, chest pains, nausea, repeated vomiting, sweating, and weakness. If the amount of alcohol ingested has been large enough, the reaction may progress to blurred vision, vertigo, confusion, marked drop in blood pressure, and loss of consciousness. Severe reactions may lead to convulsions and death. The reaction can last from 30 minutes to several hours, depending upon the amount of alcohol in the body. As the symptoms subside, the individual is exhausted and usually sleeps for several hours (see also Section Six, Table 7).

diuretic A drug that alters kidney function to increase the volume of urine. Diuretics use several different mechanisms to increase urine volume, and these, in turn, have different effects on body chemistry. Diuretics are used primarily to (1) remove excess water from the body (as in congestive heart failure and some types of liver and kidney disease), and (2) treat hypertension by promoting the excretion of sodium from the body (see also Appendix 16, Drug Classes).

drug class A group of drugs that are similar in chemistry, method of action, and use in treatment. Because of their common characteristics, many drugs within a class will produce the same side effects and have similar potential for provoking related adverse reactions and interactions. However, significant variations among members within a drug class can occur. This sometimes allows the physician an important degree of selectivity in choosing a drug if certain beneficial actions are desired or particular side effects are to be minimized (see also Appendix 16, Drug Classes).

drug fever The elevation of body temperature that occurs as an unwanted manifestation of drug action. Drugs can induce fever by several mechanisms; these include allergic reactions, drug-induced tissue damage, acceleration of tissue metabolism, constriction of blood vessels in the skin with resulting decrease in loss of body heat, and direct action on the temperature-regulating center in the brain.

The most common form of drug fever is that associated with allergic reactions. It may be the only allergic manifestation apparent, or it may be part of a complex of allergic symptoms that can include skin rash, hives, joint swelling and pain, enlarged lymph glands, hemolytic anemia, or hepatitis. The fever usually appears about 7 to 10 days after starting the drug and may vary from low-grade to alarmingly high levels. It may be sustained or intermittent, but it usually persists for as long as the drug is taken. In previously sensitized individuals drug fever may occur within one or two hours after taking the first dose of medication.

Although many drugs are capable of producing fever, the following are more commonly responsible:

allopurinol
antihistamines
atropinelike drugs
barbiturates
coumarin anticoagulants
hydralazine
iodides
isoniazid
methyldopa
nadalol
novobiocin
para-aminosalicylic acid
penicillin
pentazocine
phenytoin
procainamide
propylthiouracil
quinidine
rifampin
sulfonamides

generic name The official, common, or public name used to designate an active drug entity, whether in pure form or in dosage form. Generic names are coined by committees of officially appointed drug experts and are approved by governmental agencies for national and international use. Thus they are nonproprietary. Many drug products are marketed under the generic name of the principal active ingredient and bear no brand name of the manufacturer.

hemolytic anemia A form of anemia (deficient red blood cells and hemoglobin) resulting from the premature destruction (hemolysis) of circulating red blood cells. Several mechanisms can be responsible for the development of hemolytic anemia; among these is the action of certain drugs and chemicals. Some individuals are susceptible to hemolytic anemia because of a genetic deficiency in the makeup of their red blood cells. If such people are given certain antimalarial drugs, "sulfa" drugs, or numerous other drugs, some of their red cells will disintegrate on contact with the drug. About 10% of American blacks have this genetic trait.

Another type of drug-induced hemolytic anemia is a form of drug allergy. Many drugs in wide use (including quinidine, methyldopa, levodopa, and chlorpromazine) are known to cause hemolytic destruction of red cells as a hypersensitivity (allergic) reaction.

Hemolytic anemia can occur abruptly (with evident symptoms) or silently. The acute form lasts about seven days and is characterized by fever, pallor, weakness, dark-colored urine, and varying degrees of jaundice (yellow coloration of eyes and skin). When drug-induced hemolytic anemia is mild, involving the destruction of only a small number of red blood cells, there may be no symptoms to indicate its presence. Such episodes are detected only by means of laboratory studies (see also IDIOSYNCRASY and ALLERGY, DRUG).

For listings of causative drugs, see Section Six, Table 1.

hepatitislike reaction Changes in the liver, induced by certain drugs, which closely resemble those produced by viral hepatitis. The symptoms of drug-induced hepatitis and virus-induced hepatitis are often so similar that the correct cause cannot be established without precise laboratory studies.

Hepatitis due to drugs may be a form of drug allergy (as in reaction to many of the phenothiazines), or it may represent a toxic adverse effect (as in reaction to some of the monoamine oxidase inhibitor drugs). Liver reactions of significance usually result in jaundice and represent serious adverse effects (see also JAUNDICE) (see Section Six, Table 4).

HMO Abbreviation for Health Maintenance Organization: a managed health care delivery system that provides a broad spectrum of medical therapies and services by a collective group of practitioners within a common organization.

hypersensitivity This term has been subject to varying usages for many years. One common use has been to identify the trait of overresponsiveness to drug action, that is, an intolerance to even small doses. Used in this sense, the term indicates that the nature of the response is appropriate but the degree of response is exaggerated.

The term is more widely used today to identify a state of allergy. To have a *hypersensitivity* to a drug is to be *allergic* to it (see ALLERGY, DRUG).

For instance, the patient was known to be *hypersensitive* (allergic) by nature, having a history of seasonal hay fever and asthma since childhood. During a recent illness, he was given tetracycline to combat infection and became sensitized (allergic) to this drug. As treatment for a subsequent infection, he was given doxycycline (a related drug of the same class). His *hypersensitivity* to all drugs of the tetracycline class manifested itself as a diffuse, measleslike rash.

hypnotic A drug that is used primarily to induce sleep. There are several classes of drugs that have hypnotic effects: antihistamines, barbiturates, benzodiazepines, and several unrelated compounds. Within the past 15 years the benzodiazepines, because of their relative safety and lower potential for inducing dependence, have largely replaced the barbiturates as the most commonly used hypnotics. The body usually develops a tolerance to the hypnotic effect after several weeks of continual use. To maintain their effectiveness, hypnotics should be used intermittently for short periods of time.

hypoglycemia A condition in which the amount of glucose (a sugar) in the blood is below the normal range. Since normal brain function is dependent upon an adequate supply of glucose, reducing the level of glucose in the blood below a critical point causes serious impairment of brain activity. The resulting symptoms are characteristic of the hypoglycemic state. Early indications are headache, a sensation resembling mild drunkenness, and an inability to think clearly. These may be accompanied by hunger. As the level of blood glucose continues to fall, nervousness and confusion develop. Varying degrees of weakness, numbness, trembling, sweating, and rapid heart action follow. If sugar is not provided at this point and the blood glucose level drops further, impaired speech, incoordination, and unconsciousness, with or without convulsions, will follow.

Hypoglycemia in any stage requires prompt recognition and treatment. Because of the potential for injury to the brain, the mechanisms and management of hypoglycemia should be understood by all who use drugs capable of producing it.

hypothermia A state of the body characterized by an unexpected decline of internal body temperature to levels significantly below the norm of 98.6 degrees F or 37 degrees C. By definition, hypothermia means a body temperature of less than 95 degrees F or 35 degrees C. The elderly and debilitated are more prone to develop hypothermia if clothed inadequately and exposed to cool environments. Most episodes are initiated by room temperatures below 65 degrees F or 18.3 degrees C. The condition often develops suddenly, can mimic a stroke, and has a mortality rate of 50%. Some drugs, such as phenothiazines, barbiturates, and benzodiazepines, are conducive to the development of hypothermia in susceptible individuals.

idiosyncrasy An abnormal mechanism of drug response that occurs in individuals who have a peculiar defect in their body chemistry (often hereditary) which produces an effect totally unrelated to the drug's normal pharmacological action. Idiosyncrasy is not a form of allergy. The actual chemical defects responsible for certain idiosyncratic drug reactions are well understood; others are not. There are many examples. Here are two:

1. Approximately 100 million people in the world (including 10% of American blacks) have a specific enzyme deficiency in their red blood cells that causes these cells to disintegrate when exposed to drugs such as sulfonamides (Gantrisin, Kynex), nitrofurantoin (Furadantin, Macrodantin), probenecid (Benemid), quinine, and quinidine. As a result of this reaction, these drugs (and others) can cause a significant anemia in susceptible individuals.

2. Approximately 5% of the population of the United States is susceptible to the development of glaucoma on prolonged use of cortisone-related drugs.

immunosuppressive A drug that significantly impairs (suppresses) the functions of the body's immune system. In some instances immunosuppression is an intended drug effect, as in the use of cyclosporine to prevent the immune system from rejecting a transplanted heart or kidney. In other instances it is an unwanted side effect, as in the long-term use of cortisonelike drugs (to control chronic asthma) that suppresses the immune system sufficiently to permit reactivation of a dormant tuberculosis. Immunosuppressant drugs are being used to treat several chronic disorders that are thought to be autoimmune diseases, notably advanced rheumatoid arthritis, ulcerative colitis, and systemic lupus erythematosus (see Appendix 5, The Immune System).

incidence The number of new and recurrent cases of a disease or disorder that develops in a population during a specified period of time, such as a year.

interaction An unwanted change in the body's response to a drug that results when a second drug that is capable of altering the action of the first is administered at the same time. Some drug interactions can enhance the effect of either drug, producing an overresponse similar to overdosage. Other interactions may reduce drug effectiveness and cause inadequate response. A third type of interaction can produce a seemingly unrelated toxic response with no associated increase or decrease in the pharmacological actions of the interacting drugs.

Theoretically, many drugs can interact with one another, but in reality significant drug interactions are comparatively infrequent. Many interactions can be anticipated, and the physician can make appropriate adjustments in dosage to prevent or minimize unintended fluctuations in drug response.

jaundice A yellow coloration of the skin (and the white portion of the eyes) that occurs when excessive bile pigments accumulate in the blood as a result of impaired liver function. Jaundice can be produced by several mechanisms: It may occur as a manifestation of a wide variety of diseases, or it may represent an adverse reaction to a particular drug. At times it is difficult to distinguish between disease-induced jaundice and drug-induced jaundice.

Jaundice due to a drug is always a serious adverse effect. Anyone taking a drug that is capable of causing jaundice should watch closely for any significant change in the color of urine or feces. Dark discoloration of the urine and paleness (lack of color) of the stool may be early indications of a developing jaundice. Should either of these symptoms occur, it is advisable to discontinue the drug and notify the prescribing physician promptly. Diagnostic tests are available to clarify the nature of the jaundice (see Section Six, Table 4).

metastasis The spread of cancerous cells from the original site of development to other parts of the body. This occurs by transport of cells through the bloodstream or lymph vessels. Cancer cells in the metastatic (secondary) tumor are like those in the original (primary) tumor. Thus biopsy examination of metastatic tissue, such as a lymph node, can identify the specific cell type of the original cancer.

mortality The total number of deaths due to a given disease or disorder in a population during a specified interval of time, usually a year.

necrosis When tissue cells are damaged beyond repair, they undergo progressive, irreversible degeneration, and ultimate death. This is referred to as tissue necrosis.

neuroleptic malignant syndrome (NMS) A rare, serious, sometimes fatal idiosyncratic reaction to the use of neuroleptic (antipsychotic) drugs. The principal features of the reaction are hyperthermia (temperatures of 102 to 104 degrees F), marked muscle rigidity, and coma. Other symptoms include rapid heart rate and breathing, profuse sweating, tremors, and seizures. Two-thirds of reported cases occur in men, one-third in women. The mortality rate is 15–20%.

The following drugs have a potential for inducing this reaction:
amitriptyline + perphenazine (Triavil)
amoxapine (Asendin)
chlorpromazine (Thorazine)
chlorprothixene (Taractan)
clomipramine (Anafranil)
fluphenazine (Permitil, Prolixin)
haloperidol (Haldol)
imipramine (Tofranil, etc.)
levodopa + carbidopa (Sinemet)
loxapine (Loxitane)
metoclopramide (Reglan, Octamide)
molindone (Moban)
perphenazine (Etrafon, Trilafon)
pimozide (Orap)
prochlorperazine (Compazine)
thioridazine (Mellaril)
thiothixene (Navane)
trifluoperazine (Stelazine)
trimeprazine (Temaril)

neurotransmitter Throughout the body, the nervous system conveys messages (electrical impulses) along nerve fibers that connect nerve cells to each other and to various tissues and organs. At the connecting points of nerve fibers, referred to as synapses, there is a very small gap—the sending and receiving ends are not physically joined. To facilitate the transmission of the nerve impulse across the gap, the sending nerve releases a chemical substance that stimulates the receiving cell to respond. This chemical is referred to as a *neurotransmitter*. The principal neurotransmitters include acetylcholine, dopamine, endorphins, enkephalins, epinephrine, gamma-aminobutyric acid, glutamic acid, glycine, norepinephrine, serotonin, and substance P.

oncogene A gene which, under certain conditions, can initiate and perpetuate the conversion of normal tissue cells into cancer cells. An oncogene can be a normal constituent of a virus (v-onc) or an altered cellular gene of a body tissue (c-onc).

orthostatic hypotension A type of low blood pressure that is related to body position or posture (also called postural hypotension). The individual who is subject to orthostatic hypotension may have a normal blood pressure while lying down, but on sitting upright or standing he will experience sudden sensations of lightheadedness, dizziness, and a feeling of impending faint that compel him to return quickly to a lying position. These symptoms are manifestations of inadequate blood flow (oxygen supply) to the brain due to an abnormal delay in the rise in blood pressure that normally occurs as the body adjusts the circulation to the erect position.

Many drugs (especially the stronger antihypertensives) may cause orthostatic hypotension. Individuals who experience this drug effect should report it to their physician so that appropriate dosage adjustment can be made to minimize it. Failure to correct or to compensate for these sudden drops in blood pressure can lead to severe falls and injury.

The tendency to orthostatic hypotension can be reduced by avoiding sudden standing, prolonged standing, vigorous exercise, and exposure to hot environments. Alcoholic beverages should be used cautiously until their combined effect with the drug in use has been determined.

Parkinson-like disorders (parkinsonism) A group of symptoms that resembles those caused by Parkinson's disease, a chronic disorder of the nervous system also known as shaking palsy. The characteristic features of parkinsonism include a fixed, emotionless facial expression (masklike in appearance); a prominent trembling of the hands, arms, or legs; and stiffness of the extremities that limits movement and produces a rigid posture and gait.

Parkinsonism is a fairly common adverse effect that occurs in about 15% of all patients who take large doses of strong tranquilizers (notably the phenothiazines) or use them over an extended period of time. If recognized early, the Parkinson-like features will lessen or disappear with reduced dosage or change in medication. In some instances, however, Parkinson-like changes may become permanent, requiring appropriate medication for their control (see the Disorder Profile of Parkinson's disease in Section Three).

peripheral neuritis (peripheral neuropathy) A group of symptoms that results from injury to nerve tissue in the extremities. A variety of drugs and chemicals are capable of inducing changes in nerve structure or function. The characteristic pattern consists of a sensation of numbness and tingling that usually begins in the fingers and toes and is accompanied by an altered sensation to touch and vague discomfort ranging from aching sensations to burning pain. Severe forms of peripheral neuritis may include loss of muscular strength and coordination.

A relatively common form of peripheral neuritis is that seen with the long-term use of isoniazid in the treatment of tuberculosis. If vitamin B_6 (pyridoxine) is not given concurrently with isoniazid, peripheral neuritis may occur in sensitive individuals. Vitamin B_6 can be both preventive and curative in this form of drug-induced peripheral neuritis.

Since peripheral neuritis can also occur as a late complication following many viral infections, care must be taken to avoid assigning a cause-and-effect relationship to a drug which is not responsible for the nerve injury (see CAUSE-AND-EFFECT RELATIONSHIP).

See Section Six, Table 6 for further discussion of drug-induced nerve damage.

placebo effect The literal translation of placebo is "I will please." A placebo is an inactive, harmless substance made to look like a medication that is given to evaluate a patient's psychological response to treatment. If a placebo relieves the patient's symptoms, the favorable response is attributed to the power of suggestion—the patient's anticipation of benefit.

porphyria The porphyrias are a group of hereditary disorders characterized by excessive production of prophyrins, essential respiratory pigments of the body (one porphyrin is a component of hemoglobin, the pigment of red blood cells). Two forms of porphyria—acute intermittent porphyria and cutaneous porphyria—can be activated by the use of certain drugs. Acute intermittent porphyria involves damage to the nervous system; an acute attack can include fever, rapid heart rate, vomiting, pain in the abdomen and legs, hallucinations, seizures, paralysis, and coma. Twenty-three drugs (or drug classes) can induce an acute attack; among these are the barbiturates, "sulfa" drugs, chlordiazepoxide (Librium), chlorpropamide (Diabinese), methyldopa (Aldomet), and phenytoin (Dilantin). Cutaneous porphyria involves damage to the skin and liver. An episode can include reddening and blistering of the skin, followed by crust formation, scarring, and excessive hair growth; repeated liver damage can lead to cirrhosis. This form of porphyria can be precipitated by chloroquine, estrogen, oral contraceptives, and excessive iron.

prevalence The total number of cases of a disease or disorder that exist in a population at a specific time.

priapism The prolonged, painful erection of the penis, usually unassociated with sexual arousal or stimulation. It is caused by obstruction to the outflow (drainage) of blood through the veins at the root of the penis. Erection may persist for 30 minutes to a few hours and then subside spontaneously; or it may persist for up to 30 hours and require surgical drainage of blood from the penis for relief. More than half of the episodes of priapism induced by drugs result in permanent impotence. Sickle cell anemia (or trait) may predispose to priapism; individuals with this disorder should avoid all drugs that may induce priapism.

Drugs reported to induce priapism include the following:

anabolic steroids (male hormonelike drugs: Anadrol, Anavar, Android, Halotestin, Metandren, Oreton, Testred, Winstrol)
chlorpromazine (Thorazine)
cocaine
guanethidine (Ismelin)
haloperidol (Haldol)
heparin
levodopa (Sinemet)
molindone (Moban)
prazosin (Minipress)
prochlorperazine (Compazine)
trazodone (Desyrel)
trifluoperazine (Stelazine)
warfarin (Coumadin)

prostaglandins A very diverse group of chemical substances derived from arachidonic acid and found in numerous tissues throughout the body. When first discovered, they were thought to originate in the prostate gland, hence their name; however, this is not true. Prostaglandins are found in certain blood cells and in many body tissues. They are involved in normal functions of the lungs, stomach, kidneys, uterus, and blood vessels; they are also involved in allergic, inflammatory, and pain-producing tissue reactions.

prostatism This term refers to the difficulties associated with an enlarged prostate gland. As the prostate enlarges (a natural development in aging men), it constricts the urethra (outflow passage) where it joins the urinary bladder and impedes urination. This causes a reduction in the size and force of the urinary stream, hesitancy in starting the flow of urine, interruption of urination, and incomplete emptying of the bladder. Atropine and drugs with atropinelike effects can impair the bladder's ability to compensate for the obstructing prostate gland, thus intensifying all of the above symptoms.

Raynaud's phenomenon This term refers to intermittent episodes of reduced blood flow into the fingers or toes, with resulting coldness, paleness, discomfort, numbness, and tingling. It is due to an exaggerated constriction of the small arteries that supply blood to the digits. Characteristically an attack is precipitated either by emotional stress or exposure to cold. It can occur as part of a systemic disorder (lupus erythematosus, scleroderma), or it can occur without apparent cause (Raynaud's disease). Some widely used drugs, notably beta-adrenergic blockers and products that contain ergotamine, are conducive to the development of Raynaud-like symptoms in predisposed individuals.

Reye (Reye's) syndrome An acute, often fatal childhood illness characterized by swelling of the brain and toxic degeneration of the liver. It usually develops during recovery from a flu-like infection, measles, or chickenpox. Symptoms include fever, headache, delirium, loss of consciousness, and seizures. It is one of the 10 major causes of death in children aged 1 to 10 years. Evidence to date suggests that the syndrome may be due to the combined effects of viral infection and chemical toxins (possibly drugs) in a genetically predisposed child. Drugs that have been used just prior to the onset of symptoms include acetaminophen, aspirin, antibiotics, and antiemetics (drugs to control nausea and vomiting). Although it has not been definitely established that drugs actually cause Reye syndrome, it is thought that they may contribute to its development or adversely affect its course. Current recommendations are to avoid the use of aspirin in children with flu-like infections, chickenpox, or measles.

sedimentation rate The speed at which red blood cells in a sample of blood will settle to the bottom of a testing tube held in a vertical position. It is measured in millimeters of sediment within one hour. Normally the rate of sedimentation is slow: 0–20 mm/hr. In the presence of active inflammatory disease, the rate increases proportionately to the degree of inflammation and serves as an indicator of disease progression and response to treatment. It can be very useful in the management of diseases such as rheumatoid arthritis and systemic lupus erythematosus.

sensitivity The ability of a test to correctly identify a person who has a specific disorder. A sensitive test has few false-negative results.

side effect A normal, expected, and predictable response to a drug that accompanies the principal (intended) response sought in treatment. Side effects are part of a drug's pharmacological activity and thus are unavoidable. Most side effects are undesirable. The majority cause minor annoyance and inconvenience; some may cause serious problems in managing certain diseases; a few can be hazardous.

Example: The drug amitriptyline is often effective in treating depression and some kinds of pain. In addition to restoring normal mood and relieving pain (intended effects), it also causes blurred vision, dry mouth, constipation, and impaired urination; these are *side effects*.

specificity The ability of a test to correctly identify a person who does not have a specific disorder. A specific test has few false-positive results.

statistical significance The mathematical measure of the probability that the results of a study are attributable to chance rather than to the effect of the treatment being evaluated. If the probability is low enough, given the size of the study population and the nature of the findings, the results are considered to be "statistically significant."

tardive dyskinesia A late-developing, drug-induced disorder of the nervous system characterized by involuntary bizarre movements of the eyelids, jaws, lips, tongue, neck, and fingers. It occurs after long-term treatment with the more potent drugs used in the management of serious mental illness. Although it may occur in any age group, it is more common in the middle-aged and the elderly. Older, chronically ill women are particularly susceptible to this adverse drug effect. Once developed, the pattern of uncontrollable chewing, lip puckering, and repetitive tongue protruding (fly-catching movement) appears to be irreversible. No consistently satisfactory treatment or cure is available. To date there is no way of identifying beforehand the individual who may develop this distressing reaction to drug treatment, and there is no known prevention. Fortunately, the persistent dyskinesia (abnormal movement) is not accompanied by further impairment of mental function or deterioration of intelligence. It is ironic, however, that the patient who shows significant improvement in his mental illness but is unfortunate enough to develop tardive dyskinesia may have to remain hospitalized because of a reaction to a drug that was given to make it possible for him to leave the hospital.

tolerance An adaptation by the body that lessens responsiveness to a drug on continuous administration. Body tissues become accustomed to the drug's presence and react to it less vigorously. Tolerance can be beneficial or harmful in treatment.

Beneficial tolerance occurs when the hay fever sufferer finds that the side effect of drowsiness gradually disappears after four or five days of continuous use of antihistamines.

Harmful tolerance occurs when the patient with "shingles" (herpes zoster) finds that the usual dose of codeine is no longer sufficient to relieve pain and that the need for increasing dosage creates a risk of physical dependence.

toxicity The capacity of a drug to dangerously impair body functions or to damage body tissues. Most toxicity is related to total dosage: the larger the overdose, the greater the toxic effects. Some drugs, however, can produce toxic reactions when used in normal doses. Such adverse effects are not due to allergy or idiosyncrasy; in many instances their mechanisms of toxic action are not fully understood. Toxic effects due to overdosage are generally a harmful extension of the drug's normal pharmacological actions and—to some extent—are predictable and preventable. Toxic reactions that occur with normal dosage are unrelated to the drug's known pharmacology and for the most part are unpredictable and unexplainable.

WHO pain ladder A therapeutic scheme of utilizing increasing strengths of pain medications (analgesics) that include NSAIDs, opiates, and adjuvant drugs to control pain as specified by the World Health Organization.

withdrawal syndrome A pattern of symptoms that develops following the abrupt discontinuation of an addictive substance by an individual who has developed a physical (or chemical) dependence upon the substance. This is also referred to as an abstinence syndrome.

APPENDIXES

Health Care Practitioners/ Professionals/Providers

The numerous innovations in medical technology and the need for greater specialization have combined to spawn a remarkable proliferation of health care practitioners. The following is a list of the various types of health care providers practicing currently in the United States. The vast majority of these are required to be licensed by state or regional examining boards. Qualifying credentials of any practitioner can be verified by calling the appropriate licensing board in your state of residence.

Professional Degree Abbreviations

ALS	Advanced Life Support Technician
BS	Bachelor of Science
CNM	Certified Nurse-Midwife
CPN	Certified Nurse Practitioner
CRNA	Certified Registered Nurse Anesthetist
DC	Doctor of Chiropractic
DDS	Doctor of Dental Surgery
DMD	Doctor of Medical Dentistry or Doctor of Dental Medicine
DO	Doctor of Osteopathy
DPM	Doctor of Podiatric Medicine
EdD	Doctor of Education
LPN	Licensed Practical Nurse
LVN	Licensed Vocational Nurse
MD	Doctor of Medicine
MLS	Master of Library Science
MSW	Master of Social Work
NP	Nurse Practitioner
OD	Doctor of Optometry
OT	Occupational Therapist
PA	Physician Assistant

PharmD	Doctor of Pharmacy
PhD	Doctor of Philosophy
PsyD	Doctor of Psychology
PT	Physical Therapist
RD	Registered Dietitian
RN	Registered Nurse
RPh	Registered Pharmacist
RT	Radiologic Technician
RVT	Registered Vascular Technician

Health Care Providers

acupuncturist—MD, DO, or technician: one trained in the use of acupuncture to manage pain.

allergist—MD: a specialist in diagnosis and treatment of allergic disorders.

ALS technician—advanced life-support technician: one trained in life-saving and life-supporting techniques; utilized by ambulance teams and rescue squads.

anesthesiologist—MD or DO: a specialist in the use of anesthetic agents to facilitate surgical procedures.

anesthetist: same as ANESTHESIOLOGIST.

audiologist: one trained in the diagnostic evaluation and rehabilitation of the hearing-impaired.

bariatrician—MD or DO: a physician who specializes in the evaluation and management of obesity.

cardiac surgeon: see SURGEON, CARDIOVASCULAR.

cardiologist—MD or DO: an INTERNIST who specializes primarily in the diagnosis and treatment of heart diseases.

chest surgeon: see SURGEON, THORACIC.

chiropodist: see PODIATRIST.

chiropractor—DC: Doctor of Chiropractic, a treatment method based on the theory that all disease is due to irritation of the nervous system by mechanical, chemical, or psychic factors; therapy consists primarily of manual manipulation of spinal structures. Chiropractic literally means to practice (or do) with the hands.

colon/rectal surgeon: see SURGEON, COLON/RECTAL.

cosmetic/reconstructive surgeon: see SURGEON, PLASTIC/RECONSTRUCTIVE.

critical care physician: see SURGEON, CRITICAL CARE.

densitometrist, clinical—MD or PharmD: a practitioner who is specially trained in densitometry, the measurement of bone density and the interpretation of test results.

dental hygienist—BS or associate degree: practices under supervision of a DENTIST, cleans and polishes teeth, and detects dental problems; in some states, is permitted to administer local anesthetics.

dentist—DDS or DMD: Doctor of Dental Surgery or Doctor of Medical Dentistry; there is no significant difference in training, licensing, or practice between dentists that earn either degree. Dentists in general practice treat diseases of the teeth and gums, and examine for other disorders of the mouth and adjacent soft tissue structures.

dermatologist—MD or DO: a physician who specializes in diseases and disorders of the skin.

dietitian/nutritionist—RD: one who is qualified by formal training to advise and teach patients regarding food selection and preparation in accordance with health concerns.

endocrinologist—MD or DO: an INTERNIST who specializes in disorders of the endocrine (hormone-producing) glands, such as hypothyroidism, diabetes, Addison's disease, etc.

endodontist—DDS or DMD: a DENTIST who specializes in root canal surgery.

exodontist—DDS or DMD: see SURGEON, ORAL and SURGEON, MAXILLOFACIAL.

family physician—MD or DO: the modern version of the GENERAL PRACTITIONER, providing general medical care for all members of the family, with selective referral to specialists as appropriate. Family Practice is recognized as a specialty by the American Medical Association.

gastroenterologist—MD or DO: an INTERNIST who specializes in diseases and disorders of the digestive system—esophagus, stomach, intestine, colon, gallbladder, pancreas.

general practitioner—MD or DO: the FAMILY PHYSICIAN of earlier generations; General Practice is recognized as a specialty by the American Osteopathic Association.

geriatrician—MD or DO: an INTERNIST who specializes in medical care of the elderly—diseases and disorders associated with aging.

gynecologist—MD or DO: a physician who specializes in diseases and disorders of the female reproductive system.

hand surgeon: see SURGEON, HAND.

hematologist—MD or DO: an INTERNIST who specializes in diseases and disorders of the blood-forming organs.

hepatologist—MD or DO: an INTERNIST who specializes in diseases and disorders of the liver.

hospice physician: see PHYSICIAN, PALLIATIVE CARE.

hypnotherapist—MD or PhD or PsyD: Doctor of Medicine, Doctor of Philosophy in Psychology, Doctor of Psychology; a mental health professional who is skilled in the use of hypnosis as a therapeutic tool.

immunologist, clinical—MD: a physician who specializes in diseases and disorders of the immune system.

inhalation therapist: a MEDICAL TECHNICIAN who teaches and supervises the proper use of devices that facilitate breathing exercises and pulmonary therapy.

internist, general: see PHYSICIAN, INTERNIST.

maxillofacial surgeon: see SURGEON, ORAL and SURGEON, MAXILLOFACIAL.

medical librarian—MLS: Master of Library Science; one formally trained in library science who also has special knowledge and skills in the language and literature of the health sciences; invaluable aide to all health care professionals, patients, and families.

medical secretary: one trained in secretarial functions who also has a working knowledge of medical terminology.

medical social worker—MSW: Master of Social Work; one formally trained in social skills required to help patients adjust to chronic illness or disability.

medical technician: one formally trained in technical skills required to perform diagnostic or therapeutic procedures.

neonatologist—MD or DO: a PEDIATRICIAN who specializes in the management of disorders of newborn infants, including the premature.

nephrologist—MD or DO: an INTERNIST who specializes in diseases and disorders of the kidney.

neurological technician: one formally trained to perform diagnostic neurological procedures, such as electroencephalograms (EEG), electromyograms (EMG), etc.

neurologist—MD or DO: a physician who specializes in diseases and disorders of the nervous system.

neuropsychiatrist—MD or DO: a physician who specializes in disorders that share manifestations of organic brain disease and psychotic behavior.

neuroradiologist—MD or DO: a RADIOLOGIST who has expertise in the interpretation of nervous system imaging.

neurosurgeon: see SURGEON, NEUROLOGICAL.

nuclear medicine specialist: see PHYSICIAN, NUCLEAR MEDICINE.

nurse anesthetist—CRNA: Certified Registered Nurse Anesthetist; a registered nurse (RN) who is proficient in the use of inhalation anesthetic agents.

nurse, general duty—RN: Registered Nurse; one who has completed formal training in an accredited school of nursing and is registered to practice as a professional nurse in a wide variety of health care settings.

nurse-midwife—CNM: Certified Nurse-Midwife; a registered nurse (RN) who has taken advanced training and is certified by examination to monitor pregnancy and supervise birthing (delivery) in the absence of an obstetrician.

nurse, practical—LPN: Licensed Practical Nurse; one who has completed formal training in a vocational technical setting, community college, or hospital and is licensed to provide general care to patients, often under supervision of a registered nurse.

nurse practitioner—NP or CNP: a registered nurse (RN) who has taken additional training and is certified to perform some functions normally assumed by an MD or DO.

nurse's aide: one who assists hospital staff nurses by performing unspecialized tasks.

nurse, vocational—LVN: Licensed Vocational Nurse; same as Licensed Practical Nurse (see NURSE, PRACTICAL).

obstetrician—MD or DO: a physician who specializes in the management of pregnancy, prenatal care through delivery.

occupational therapist—OT: one who has completed formal training in the use of creative activities that help patients recover from illness, injury, or surgery.

oculist: same as OPHTHALMOLOGIST.

oncologist, medical—MD or DO: an INTERNIST who specializes in the diagnosis and treatment (chemotherapy) of all types of cancer.

oncologist, nurse—RN: a registered nurse who has received special training in the nursing aspects of oncology.

oncologist, radiation—MD or DO: a RADIOLOGIST who is skilled in the use of radiant energy and radioactive substances to treat cancer.

oncologist, surgical—MD or DO: a surgeon who is skilled in the surgical procedures that pertain to the diagnosis (biopsy) and treatment (surgical removal) of cancerous tissues.

ophthalmologist—MD or DO: a physician who specializes in the medical and surgical treatment of all disorders of the eye.

optician: an expert in the science of applied optics—the filling and adaptation of ophthalmic prescriptions for eyeglasses.

optometrist—OD: Doctor of Optometry; a professional formally trained and licensed to practice optometry, the primary care of the eye and vision, prescription of eyeglasses, and other diagnostic and therapeutic functions regulated by state law.

oral surgeon: see SURGEON, ORAL and SURGEON, MAXILLOFACIAL.

orthodontist—DDS or DMD: a DENTIST who specializes in the correction of malocclusion (improper positioning) of the teeth by the use of braces.

orthopedic surgeon: see SURGEON, ORTHOPEDIC.

osteopath: see PHYSICIAN, OSTEOPATHIC.

otolaryngologist—MD or DO: a surgeon specializing in diseases and disorders of the ear, nose, sinuses, and throat.

otologist—MD or DO: an OTOLARYNGOLOGIST who limits his practice to the diagnosis and treatment of disorders of the ear.

palliative care physician: see PHYSICIAN, PALLIATIVE CARE.

paramedic: a vernacular term applied to a MEDICAL TECHNICIAN who is trained and skilled in the provision of care in emergency situations.

pathologist—MD or DO: a Doctor of Medicine who specializes in the interpretation of laboratory test results of organs, tissues, body fluids, etc., to facilitate diagnosis during life (clinical pathology), or to establish the cause of death (autopsy pathology).

pediatrician, general—MD or DO: a physician who specializes in the diagnosis and treatment of diseases and disorders in infants and children.

pediatric neurologist—MD or DO: a PEDIATRICIAN who specializes in diseases and disorders of the nervous system.

pediatric oncologist—MD or DO: a PEDIATRICIAN who specializes in the diagnosis and treatment of cancer in children.

pediatric urologist—MD or DO: a PEDIATRICIAN who specializes in diseases and disorders of the urinary system in children.

pedodontist—DDS or DMD: a DENTIST who specializes in dental care of children.

pedorthist—DPM: a PODIATRIST who specializes in the use of orthotics (such as molded shoe inserts) for foot disorders.

periodontist—DDS or DMD: a DENTIST who specializes in the treatment of gums and the bones and supportive structures that hold the teeth.

pharmacist, clinical—PharmD: Doctor of Pharmacy; a specialist in pharmaceutical care: detailed knowledge of the availability and properties of medicinal drugs, their proper use in therapeutics, and appropriate counseling of patients regarding safe and effective drug use.

pharmacist, general—RPh: Registered Pharmacist; a graduate from an accredited school of pharmacy, proficient in the interpretation and filling of medical prescriptions and in counseling patients on the proper use of medicinal drugs.

pharmacologist, clinical—MD, DO, PhD, or PharmD: one who holds a doctorate degree and is highly skilled in all aspects of pharmacotherapy, the use of drugs in the treatment of disease or disorder.

physiatrist—MD or DO: a physician who specializes in physical medicine and rehabilitation—the evaluation, diagnosis, and treatment of patients with impairments or disabilities involving the neurological, musculoskeletal, cardiovascular, or other body systems.

physical therapist—PT: one who is formally trained and licensed to practice physical therapy, treatment procedures designed to rehabilitate from injuries, surgeries, and debilitating diseases; works under the direction of a physician.

physician, allopathic—MD: a Doctor of Medicine graduated from an accredited school of allopathic medicine—the dominant type of medical school in the United States; there are approximately 500,000 allopathic physicians practicing in this country. Allopathy is the modern theory of medicine firmly rooted in the basic medical sciences of anatomy, physiology, biochemistry, bacteriology, pathology, pharmacology, etc.; therapy is based upon the principle of producing a condition in the patient that is antagonistic to or incompatible with the disease or disorder to be cured or alleviated; it is represented in the United States by the American Medical Association.

physician, emergency medicine—MD or DO: a physician who is formally trained and specializes in the management of acutely ill and injured patients that require immediate and definitive treatment for survival; usually practices in hospital emergency rooms.

physician, hepatologist—MD or DO: an INTERNIST who specializes in diseases and disorders of the liver.

physician, homeopathic—MD or DO: an ALLOPATHIC or OSTEOPATHIC PHYSICIAN who has studied and adopted some of the principles of homeopathic medicine, an outdated therapeutic system that was based on the belief that diseases should be treated by drugs (in minute doses) that are capable of producing in healthy persons symptoms like those of the disease to be treated: the theory that "like cures like."

physician, infectious diseases—MD or DO: an INTERNIST who specializes in the diagnosis and treatment of life-threatening infectious diseases.

physician, internist—MD or DO: a physician who specializes in the diagnosis and treatment of diseases of the internal organs, primarily in adults; many internists practice general internal medicine, while others specialize in one organ or system: CARDIOLOGIST, GASTROENTEROLOGIST, NEPHROLOGIST, etc.

physician, nephrologist—MD or DO: an INTERNIST who specializes in diseases and disorders of the kidney.

physician, neurologist—MD or DO: a physician who specializes in the non-surgical management of diseases and disorders of the nervous system.

physician, nuclear medicine—MD or DO: a physician who specializes in the use of radioactive substances for diagnosis and treatment.

physician, occupational medicine—MD or DO: a physician certified in the specialty of preventive medicine who provides medical care for employee groups in industry.

physician, osteopathic—DO: a Doctor of Osteopathy graduated from an accredited school of osteopathic medicine; there are 15 osteopathic medical schools and over 28,000 osteopathic physicians in the United States, 52% of them practicing primary care medicine. Osteopathic physicians complete the same courses of medical education and pass the same licensure examinations as ALLOPATHIC PHYSICIANS; the fundamental difference between the two is a philosophical one: the osteopathic approach is a more holistic one—(1) the human body is a unified organism and the patient must be evaluated and managed as a whole person, (2) the musculoskeletal system is central to the patient's well-being and can influence the functional status of all other body systems, and (3) osteopathic manipulation of musculoskeletal structures can often provide effective and less intrusive therapy for many conditions. Osteopathy is represented in the United States by the American Osteopathic Association.

physician, palliative care—MD or DO: a physician qualified by training to provide comprehensive and compassionate hospice-type medical care for the terminally ill and dying patient.

physician, preventive medicine—MD or DO: a physician who specializes in the maintenance of individual health and well-being and the prevention of disease through immunization, healthful behavior, and avoidance of noxious environmental influences.

physician, pulmonologist—MD or DO: an INTERNIST who specializes in diseases and disorders of the pulmonary system—trachea, bronchial tubes, lungs.

physician, tropical medicine—MD or DO: an INTERNIST who specializes in the prevention, diagnosis, and treatment of tropical diseases.

physician assistant—PA: one formally trained in a medical setting to perform some of the functions normally done by the physician. Physician assistant programs have expanded to include many major specialties; PAs are usually trained to a higher level than NURSE PRACTITIONERS or MEDICAL TECHNICIANS—they work under the physician's supervision.

plastic surgeon: see SURGEON, PLASTIC/RECONSTRUCTIVE.

podiatrist—DPM: Doctor of Podiatric Medicine; a graduate of an accredited school of podiatry who is licensed to provide medical and surgical care of the feet (formerly known as a chiropodist).

practical nurse: see NURSE, PRACTICAL.

proctologist: see SURGEON, COLON/RECTAL.

prosthodontist—DDS or DMD: a DENTIST who specializes in the replacement of missing teeth with caps, bridges, and dentures; his services are usually recommended by a general dentist for patients with difficult problems of dental restoration.

psychiatrist—MD or DO: a physician who specializes in the prevention, diagnosis, and treatment of mental, emotional, and behavioral disorders; therapy may include the use of medicinal drugs (psychopharmacology), counseling (psychotherapy), or both.

psychologist—PhD, or PsyD or EdD: Doctor of Philosophy in psychology, Doctor of Psychology, Doctor of Education in psychology; a clinical psychologist is one formally trained to evaluate and treat patients with emotional problems; therapy is limited to counseling (psychotherapy); psychologists are not physicians and cannot legally prescribe drugs.

pulmonologist: see PHYSICIAN, PULMONOLOGIST.

radiologic technician—RT: one formally trained in the use of diagnostic X-ray equipment and the preparation of patients for radiation therapy; many states require licensure.

radiologist, diagnostic—MD or DO: a physician who specializes in the production and interpretation of diagnostic images: conventional X-ray films, computed axial tomography (CAT scans), magnetic resonance imaging (MRI) films, sonography (ultrasound).

radiologist, nuclear—MD or DO: a RADIOLOGIST trained in the use of radioactive materials for diagnostic and therapeutic procedures.

radiologist, therapeutic—MD or DO: a RADIOLOGIST trained in the use of all types of radiation for therapeutic purposes, especially the treatment of cancer (radiation ONCOLOGIST).

rheumatologist—MD or DO: an INTERNIST who specializes in arthritis and related musculoskeletal disorders.

roentgenologist: another name for RADIOLOGIST.

speech therapist: one trained in the evaluation and treatment of speech, language, and voice disorders that are not amenable to medical or surgical treatment.

surgeon, cardiovascular—MD: a surgeon who specializes in heart and great vessel surgery: coronary artery procedures, heart transplants, aorta repair, etc.

surgeon, colon/rectal—MD or DO: a surgeon who specializes in surgical procedures involving the colon or rectum. A surgeon who specializes in surgical procedures of only the rectum and anus is a proctologist.

surgeon, cosmetic—MD: a surgeon who specializes in reshaping structures of the body to improve appearance or enhance self-esteem.

surgeon, critical care—MD or DO: a surgeon who specializes in the management of trauma victims who require critical, life-saving care.

surgeon, general—MD or DO: a surgeon who performs common surgeries (such as appendectomies) that are not within the domain of more specific surgical specialties.

surgeon, hand—MD: a surgeon who limits his practice to all components of the hand and wrist.

surgeon, head and neck—MD or DO: an OTOLARYNGOLOGIST who specializes in surgical procedures of head and neck structures, excluding the brain and eyes.

surgeon, maxillofacial—DDS or DMD: a DENTIST who specializes in surgery of the mouth and jaw.

surgeon, neurological—MD: a surgeon who specializes in the evaluation and surgical treatment of disorders of the brain, spinal cord, and peripheral nerves—a neurosurgeon.

surgeon, oral—DDS or DMD: a DENTIST who specializes in the evaluation and diagnosis (by biopsy) of diseases of the mouth.

surgeon, orthopedic—MD or DO: a surgeon who specializes primarily in the management of bone fractures, repair and replacement of diseased joints, disorders of the spine, and reconstruction of bone deformities.

surgeon, plastic/reconstructive—MD: a surgeon who specializes in procedures designed to correct abnormalities due to congenital defects, flawed development, trauma, or disease; plastic surgery is usually performed to improve function or appearance.

surgeon, thoracic—MD: a surgeon who specializes in the evaluation and surgical management of diseases and disorders within the chest (thorax): coronary artery disease; defective heart valves; defects of the aorta; cancers of the lung, esophagus, or chest wall; chest wounds; etc.

surgeon, transplantation—MD: a surgeon who specializes in organ transplantation: kidney, bone marrow, liver, heart, pancreas.

surgeon, urological—MD: a UROLOGIST who specializes in surgical procedures involving the adrenal glands and the genitourinary system.

surgeon, vascular—MD: a surgeon who specializes in blood vessel surgery (other than brain, heart, or lung).

tropical disease physician: see PHYSICIAN, TROPICAL MEDICINE.

urologist, general—MD: a physician who specializes in diseases and disorders of the urinary system and the prostate gland.

vascular surgeon: see SURGEON, VASCULAR.

vascular technician—RVT: Registered Vascular Technician; one formally trained in diagnostic techniques used to detect and evaluate blood vessel disorders.

virologist, clinical—MD: an INFECTIOUS DISEASE PHYSICIAN with special expertise in the diagnosis and treatment of viral infections.

vocational nurse—LVN; same as licensed PRACTICAL NURSE (LPN).

X-ray technician: see RADIOLOGIC TECHNICIAN.

APPENDIX 2

The National Cancer Institute Designated Cancer Centers and Clinical Trials

Part One: The National Cancer Institute (NCI) Designated Cancer Centers

The following NCI Comprehensive Cancer Centers emphasize a multidisciplinary approach to cancer research, patient care, and community outreach. Information about referral procedures, treatment costs, and services available to patients can be obtained from the individual centers listed below.

ALABAMA
University of Alabama at Birmingham
Comprehensive Cancer Center
Basic Health Sciences Building, Room 108
1918 University Boulevard
Birmingham, AL 35294
Phone: (205) 934-5077

ARIZONA
University of Arizona Cancer Center
1501 North Campbell Avenue
Tucson, AZ 85724
Phone: (602) 626-6372

CALIFORNIA
USC/Norris Comprehensive Cancer Center
University of Southern California
1441 Eastlake Avenue

Los Angeles, CA 90033-0804
Phone: (213) 226-2370

Jonsson Comprehensive Cancer Center
University of California at Los Angeles
100 UCLA Medical Plaza, Suite 255
Los Angeles, CA 90024-1781
Phone: 1-800-825-2631

CONNECTICUT
Yale University Comprehensive Cancer Center
333 Cedar Street
New Haven, CT 06510
Phone: (203) 785-4095

DISTRICT OF COLUMBIA
Lombardi Cancer Research Center
Georgetown University Medical Center
3800 Reservoir Road, NW
Washington, DC 20007
Phone: (202) 687-2192

FLORIDA
Sylvester Comprehensive Cancer Center
University of Miami Medical School
1475 Northwest 12th Avenue
Miami, FL 33136
Phone: (305) 545-1000

MARYLAND
The Johns Hopkins Oncology Center
600 North Wolfe Street, Room B156
Baltimore, MD 21287-8915
Phone: (410) 955-8964

MASSACHUSETTS
Dana-Farber Cancer Institute
44 Binney Street
Boston, MA 02115
Phone: (617) 632-3476

MICHIGAN
Meyer L. Prentis Comprehensive Cancer Center of Metropolitan Detroit
110 East Warren Avenue
Detroit, MI 48201
Phone: (313) 745-4329

University of Michigan Comprehensive Cancer Center
101 Simpson Drive
Ann Arbor, MI 48109-0752
Phone: (313) 936-9583

MINNESOTA
Mayo Comprehensive Cancer Center
200 First Street Southwest
Rochester, MN 55902
Phone: (507) 284-3413

NEW HAMPSHIRE
Norris Cotton Cancer Center
Dartmouth-Hitchcock Medical Center
2 Maynard Street
Hanover, NH 03756
Phone: (603) 646-5505

NEW YORK
Memorial Sloan-Kettering Cancer Center
1275 York Avenue
New York, NY 10021
Phone: 1-800-525-2225

Roswell Park Cancer Institute
Elm and Carlton Streets
Buffalo, NY 14263
Phone: 1-800-ROSWELL (1-800-767-9355)

Kaplan Cancer Center
New York University Medical Center
462 First Avenue
New York, NY 10016-9103
Phone: (212) 263-6485

NORTH CAROLINA
Duke Comprehensive Cancer Center
Post Office Box 3814
Durham, NC 27710
Phone: (919) 684-2748

UNC Lineberger Comprehensive Cancer Center
University of North Carolina School of Medicine
Chapel Hill, NC 27599
Phone: (919) 966-4431

Cancer Center of Wake Forest University at Bowman Gray
    School of Medicine
300 South Hawthorne Road
Winston-Salem, NC 27103
Phone: (919) 748-4354

OHIO
Ohio State University Comprehensive Cancer Center
Arthur G. James Cancer Hospital
410 West 10th Avenue

Columbus, OH 43210
Phone: 1-800-638-6996

PENNSYLVANIA
Fox Chase Cancer Center
7701 Burholme Avenue
Philadelphia, PA 19111
Phone: (215) 728-2570

University of Pennsylvania Cancer Center
3400 Spruce Street
Philadelphia, PA 19104
Phone: (215) 662-6364

Pittsburgh Cancer Institute
200 Meyran Avenue
Pittsburgh, PA 15213-2592
Phone: 1-800-537-4063

TEXAS
The University of Texas M.D. Anderson Cancer Center
1515 Holcombe Boulevard
Houston, TX 77030
Phone: (713) 792-3245

VERMONT
Vermont Regional Cancer Center
University of Vermont
1 South Prospect Street
Burlington, VT 05401
Phone: (802) 656-4580

WASHINGTON
Fred Hutchinson Cancer Research Center
1124 Columbia Street
Seattle, WA 98104
Phone: (206) 667-5000
    Bone marrow transplantation is the primary treatment offered.

WISCONSIN
University of Wisconsin Comprehensive Cancer Center
600 Highland Avenue
Madison, WI 53792
Phone: (608) 263-8090

Part Two: Clinical Trials

What Are Clinical Trials?
    The National Cancer Institute (NCI) is the agency within our Public Health
Service that oversees all aspects of cancer research at the national level. It

brings together the very best minds and institutions in the country and supports a vast national network of basic and clinical research devoted to the understanding and management of malignant diseases. The ultimate goal is the incorporation of new knowledge gained through basic research into clinical practice that benefits people with cancer. This very lengthy and complex process culminates in the "clinical trial," a carefully designed study conducted with cancer patients. Most clinical trials are performed to determine if a new and promising treatment is both safe and effective. Many former cancer patients are alive and well today as a result of treatments developed and perfected in clinical trials.

Participating in a Clinical Trial

If you are interested in learning more about clinical trials, proceed as follows:

1. Obtain a copy of the following free publication:

What Are Clinical Trials All About?, A Booklet for Patients with Cancer, NIH Publication No. 92-2706, June 1992.

National Cancer Institute
Office of Cancer Communications
9000 Rockville Pike
Bethesda, MD 20892
Phone: 1-800-4-CANCER, or (301) 496-5583

This publication is also available by fax. If you have access to a fax machine, use it to dial the NCI CancerFAX Service at (301) 402-5874.

On voice prompt, enter the numbers 400109. The CancerFAX voice will confirm your selection and prompt you to press the START button on your machine and then hang up the hand set. Your fax machine will print out the 14-page booklet.

Read this completely.

2. If you decide that you want to explore the feasibility of participating in a clinical trial, ask your personal physician if this is in your best interest. Understanding you personally and knowing the nature and course of your disease, your physician is the logical and most appropriate advisor at this point.

3. If you and your physician agree that further consideration is reasonable, ask him to determine where an appropriate clinical trial is being conducted. Health professionals have access to the NCI clinical trial database known as PDQ—Physician's Data Query. This database provides information on (1) the latest treatments recommended for all forms of cancer, and (2) the institutions and principal investigators currently conducting clinical trials. Your physician will be able to determine if you are eligible for a clinical trial that is open to new patients. A copy of the study protocol can be obtained for you and your physician to review.

4. Another source of information available to cancer patients and their families is the Cancer Information Service (CIS), also sponsored by the National Cancer Institute (NCI). If you want information on clinical trials that may

be appropriate for you, call the toll-free number 1-800-4-CANCER (1-800-422-6237) and you will be connected to the CIS office serving your area. Because of the large number of callers who use this valuable service, you may encounter delays (on "hold" listening to music) before a cancer information specialist takes your call in turn. However, the information provided and the service rendered are well worth the wait—or the need to call again at a later time. In order to determine if there is an open clinical trial for you to consider, the information specialist will ask you to describe the kind of cancer you have, original site (breast, lung, ovary, etc.), the cell type, and the stage. The CIS information specialist has access to same PDQ database that serves health care professionals.

5. The PDQ database can be accessed also by personal computer and modem using the GratefulMed program sponsored by the National Library of Medicine (NLM). For more information call the MEDLARS Service Desk at the National Library of Medicine: 1-800-638-8480.

Cancer Pain Management

Approximately 70% of patients with terminal cancer will experience pain, most of it attributable to the disease, some occurring as a result of treatment procedures. It is well documented that cancer pain in both adults and children is greatly undertreated. This occurs in spite of the fact that we have ample means to control pain and relieve suffering in the majority of cases. It is imperative that the patient who is experiencing pain (or his advocate) make this known to caregivers, and that prompt and adequate relief is a demand, not a request. It is obligatory that caregivers honor the patient's assessment of pain and provide optimal relief.

If the severity of pain requires the use of opioid (narcotic) drugs, any consideration of their habit-forming potential is irrelevant in treating the terminally ill. Rarely, if ever, does true addiction occur.

The goal in cancer pain management is to *prevent pain if possible*. The optimal dose of analgesics should be determined and given on a regular schedule—by the clock—to prevent the recurrence of pain as the drug's analgesic action wears off. Numerous methods for relieving pain are available. The optimal *combination of treatments* should be determined and used fully. If possible, consultation with a pain specialist should be sought so that a full multidisciplinary approach can be made to individualize optimal therapy.

Analgesic Drugs

Three classes of drugs are effective in treating cancer pain:
- nonopioid (not morphinelike) drugs for mild to moderate pain
- opioid (morphinelike) drugs for mild to severe pain
- adjuvant drugs used concurrently with nonopioid and/or opioid drugs to enhance their analgesic effects

The current treatment of choice for managing cancer pain is the World Health Organization (WHO) three-step analgesic ladder:

Step 1: Begin treatment with nonopioid drugs, with or without an adjuvant drug (see drug lists below).

Step 2: If pain persists or increases, add an opioid drug for mild to moderate pain to those used in step 1.

Step 3: If pain continues or increases, change opioid drug to one for moderate to severe pain; continue nonopioid and adjuvant drugs as individual need requires.

Nonopioid Drugs

- aspirin
- acetaminophen (Tylenol, etc.)
- nonsteroidal anti-inflammatory drugs (NSAIDs):
  - ibuprofen (Advil, etc.)
  - indomethacin (Indocin)
  - ketoprofen (Orudis)
  - ketorolac (Toradol)
  - naproxen (Aleve, etc.)
  - others

Opioid Drugs for Mild to Moderate Pain

- codeine
- propoxyphene (Darvon, etc.)

Opioid Drugs for Moderate to Severe Pain

- fentanyl (Duragesic)
- hydrocodone (Lorcet, Vicodin, etc.)
- hydromorphone (Dilaudid)
- levorphanol (Levo-Dromoran)
- methadone (Dolophine)
- morphine (MS Contin, Oramorph) (the drug of choice)
- oxycodone (Roxicodone, Percocet, Percodan, etc.)

Adjuvant Drugs

- corticosteroids (cortisonelike drugs)
- anticonvulsants
- antidepressants (amitriptyline, the drug of choice)
- neuroleptics (antipsychotic drugs; methotrimeprazine is the drug of choice)
- hydroxyzine (Atarax, etc.)
- methylphenidate (Ritalin)

Nondrug Treatments

- Transcutaneous electrical nerve stimulation (TENS)
- Relaxation and imagery techniques
- Psychotherapy

- Support groups
- Pastoral counseling

Invasive Treatments for Pain Relief

- Nerve blocks
- Neurosurgical procedures
- Radiation (X-ray) therapy
- Surgical procedures (selective)

Recommended Additional Reading

Principles of Analgesic Use in the Treatment of Acute Pain and Cancer Pain, 3rd edition. Glenview, IL: American Pain Society, 1992.

Management of Cancer Pain, Clinical Practice Guideline, No. 9. U.S. Department of Health and Human Services, Public Health Service, Agency for Health Care Policy and Research, AHCPR Publication No. 94-0592, March 1994.

Questions and Answers About Pain Control: A Guide for People with Cancer and Their Families, American Cancer Society and The National Cancer Institute. Call 1-800-4-CANCER.

Cancer Pain Relief and Palliative Care. Report of a WHO Expert Committee, Technical Report Series No. 804, World Health Organization, Geneva, 1990.

You Don't Have to Suffer: A Complete Guide to Relieving Cancer Pain for Patients and Their Families, Susan S. Lang and Richard B. Patt. Oxford University Press, 1994.

Management of Nausea and Vomiting Associated with Cancer Chemotherapy

Chemotherapy (the use of anticancer drugs) is one of the major treatments utilized today to manage malignant diseases, along with surgery and radiation. Some forms of cancer, such as Hodgkin's lymphoma and some acute leukemias, are actually being cured by appropriate chemotherapy. Other cancers, though not curable, can be significantly suppressed (palliative treatment), thus relieving symptoms and improving the patient's quality of life. One feature of chemotherapy that seriously limits its usefulness is the frequency of nausea and vomiting that follows the use of some highly effective drugs. Fortunately, we now have medications that can significantly reduce the frequency and severity of these side effects and allow patients to receive the potential benefits of chemotherapy.

At the very beginning of chemotherapy it is most important that *nausea and vomiting be prevented*. If nausea and vomiting are allowed to occur and are not properly controlled, some patients will develop a conditioned response known as "anticipatory nausea and vomiting" when chemotherapy is recommended in the future. Uncontrolled nausea and vomiting is a major cause of noncompliance with chemotherapy, causing many patients to discontinue treatment before an adequate course of treatment is completed.

Good management requires follow-up evaluation for several days after each dose of chemotherapy. Over 80% of patients will experience delayed nausea and vomiting that begins from 24 to 72 hours after treatment and lasts for five to seven days. Adjustments in drug selection and dosage schedules are made at this time to provide better control. Antiemetic (anti-vomiting) drugs are most effective when used in combination. Different mechanisms responsible for drug-induced nausea and vomiting require a selection of drugs with differing actions.

CHEMOTHERAPEUTIC DRUGS THAT CAUSE NAUSEA AND VOMITING

Drugs	Incidence of Nausea and Vomiting
cisplatin (Platinol)	>90%
mechlorethamine (Mustargen)	>90%
streptozocin (Zanosar)	>90%
dacarbazine (DTIC-Dome)	>90%
dactinomycin (Cosmegen)	30–90%
cyclophosphamide (Cytoxan, Neosar)	30–90%
carmustine (BiCNU)	30–90%
procarbazine (Matulane)	30–90%
daunorubicin (Cerubidine)	30–90%
doxorubicin (Adriamycin RDF, Rubex)	30–90%
asparaginase (Elspar)	30–90%
cytarabine (Cytosar-U)	30–90%
fluorouracil (Adrucil)	30–90%
mitomycin (Mutamycin)	30–90%
bleomycin (Blenoxane)	<30%
hydroxyurea (Hydrea)	<30%
melphalan (Alkeran)	<30%
etoposide (VePesid)	<30%
ifosfamide (Ifex)	<30%
methotrexate (Folex)	<30%
busulfan (Myleran)	<30%
chlorambucil (Leukeran)	<30%
vinca alkaloids	<30%

Note: Drug selections and dosage schedules are determined by the medical oncologist for each patient individually.

The above information was adapted from "Chemotherapy-Induced Nausea and Vomiting," Syed Bilgrami, M.D., and Barbara G. Fallon, M.D. *Postgraduate Medicine*, Vol. 94, No. 5, October 1993.

ANTIEMETIC DRUGS THAT PREVENT OR RELIEVE NAUSEA AND VOMITING

Drugs	Route of Administration
diphenhydramine (Benadryl)	By mouth or injection
scopolamine (Transderm-Scop)	Skin patch
prochlorperazine (Compazine)	By mouth, injection, or suppository
haloperidol (Haldol)	By mouth or injection
droperidol (Inapsine)	By injection
methylprednisolone (Solu-Medrol)	By injection
dexamethasone (Decadron, etc.)	By mouth or injection
lorazepam (Ativan)	By injection
metoclopramide (Reglan)	By mouth or injection
ondansetron (Zofran)	By mouth or injection
granisetron (Kytril)	By mouth or injection

Note: Drug selections and dosage schedules are determined by the medical oncologist for each patient individually.

The above information was adapted from "Chemotherapy-Induced Nausea and Vomiting," Syed Bilgrami, M.D., and Barbara G. Fallon, M.D. *Postgraduate Medicine*, Vol. 94, No. 5, October 1993.

ANTIEMETIC DRUG COMBINATIONS AND THEIR EFFECTIVENESS

Drug Combinations	Effective Response
dexamethasone ondansetron	91%

dexamethasone
   diphenhydramine
   droperidol
   metoclopramide
	76%

dexamethasone
   lorazepam
   metoclopramide
	63%

dexamethasone
   diphenhydramine
   metoclopramide
	60%

Note: Drug selections and dosage schedules are determined by the medical oncologist for each patient individually.

The above information was adapted from "Chemotherapy-Induced Nausea and Vomiting," Syed Bilgrami, M.D., and Barbara G. Fallon, M.D. *Postgraduate Medicine*, Vol. 94, No. 5, October 1993.

The Immune System

The immune system is an integrated, collaborative network of organs, tissues, blood cells, and chemical substances that have evolved together to provide effective mechanisms designed to protect our bodies against invasion by pathogenic (disease-producing) microorganisms. It has the innate ability to recognize "self"—all of the normal components of our bodies. It can also recognize foreign life forms—that are "not self"—which it can seek out and destroy. Hence the immune system is a vital unit of the body's total biology that contributes to the maintenance of a healthy state.

What It Is

The Bone Marrow

This is the tissue that produces all types of blood cells and is the first "master organ" of the immune system—the principal site for the formation and development of all types of blood cells: red blood cells (erythrocytes), white blood cells (leukocytes), and blood platelets (thrombocytes).

Lymphocytes

Among the five types of leukocytes (white blood cells) are the lymphocytes, major elements in the immune system. The two principal lymphocytes are the B lymphocyte (or B cell) and the T lymphocytes (or T cells). The B cells produce antibodies. The T cells are of two kinds: (1) CD4 T cells, also called "helper" T cells because they help B cells produce antibodies; and (2) CD8 T cells, also called "killer" T cells because they destroy cells infected by viruses and bacteria, as well as cells undergoing cancerous change. The CD8 T cells provide *cellular immunity*.

The Thymus Gland

This small gland located in the upper chest above the heart is the second "master organ" of the immune system. It receives young lymphocytes from the bone marrow and matures them into functional T cells. During maturation, the T cells differentiate into either "helper" T cells or "killer" T cells. In addition, the T cells learn to distinguish "self" tissues from "nonself" materials, an extremely important function (see organ rejection and autoimmune disorders below).

Lymph Nodes

These small glands of lymphoid tissue are strategically located along the network of lymphatic vessels that are spread throughout the body. Their primary purpose is to produce concentrations of lymphocytes that serve as filters for detecting and destroying infectious organisms and toxins as lymph flows through the nodes. The resultant debris of foreign matter is engulfed and digested by large scavenger white blood cells known as macrophages.

The Spleen

This is the largest organ of the lymphoid system; it sits in the upper left abdominal cavity. Its primary function is to serve as a reservoir for blood. In addition, it produces lymphocytes and plasma cells, the latter being fully differentiated B cells that produce antibodies.

Antibodies

Specifically configured protein molecules (immunoglobulins) that are designed to bind and neutralize foreign substances: bacteria, fungi, viruses, parasites, toxins, etc. The immunoglobulins are divided into five classes: IgA, IgD, IgE, IgG, and IgM. The IgE antibody is unique in that it causes allergic (hypersensitivity) reactions when it reacts with certain allergens: allergic rhinitis (hay fever) is due to histamine that is released when pollens (allergens) and IgE antibodies interact. Antibodies provide *humoral immunity*—proteins dissolved in the blood as opposed to cells.

Specialized Chemical Messengers

The following chemical substances are produced by components of the immune system; they convey messages and signals that organize and regulate the intricate interactions that control immune functions:

  Interleukins: a group of 11 distinct chemical messengers produced by various cells of the immune system that orchestrate specific interactions among them.

  Lymphokines: a type of interleukin produced by CD4 "helper" T cells; they assist B cells in production of antibodies and assist maturation of CD8 "killer" T cells.

  Interferons: a subset of lymphokines that are produced by lymphocytes when they have been activated by viral invasion; interferons mobilize other immune cells and enhance antiviral defense.

  Neurotransmitters: chemicals that facilitate the transmission of nerve impulses across junction points in the network of nerves throughout the body, a process called innervation.

Neurohormones: chemical substances (hormones) that are produced by the brain, released into the bloodstream, and circulated throughout the body; they exert specific effects on "target" organs and tissues of the immune system.

The Brain/Mind Connection

It is now well established that the brain/mind and the immune system share an ongoing two-way system of communication—each is aware of and understands the language of the other. This dialogue is evident in a number of ways:

1. All immune tissues (thymus, lymph nodes, spleen, etc.) are extensively connected with the brain by (1) nerve fibers and neurotransmitters and (2) neurohormones produced by the hypothalamus and the pituitary gland in the brain.
2. B cells and T cells of the immune system have receptors for both neurotransmitters and neurohormones, providing them with a mechanism to receive messages from the brain.
3. The brain has receptors for interleukins that can monitor lymphokine messages exchanged between lymphocytes.
4. Lymphocytes make and release into the bloodstream the exact same ACTH molecule made and released by the brain's pituitary gland. (Adrenocorticotropic hormone—ACTH—stimulates the adrenal gland to produce cortisone; psychological stress may cause excessive production of ACTH and cortisone which can impair immunity, probably by inhibiting T-cell functions.)
5. The immune system is able to make over 20 neurohormones also made by the brain.
6. The brain can make interleukins similar to those produced by lymphocytes.
7. It is well known that intense grief and bereavement can initiate or aggravate such immune disorders as cancer, rheumatoid arthritis, and ulcerative colitis.
8. The brain—through the five senses of sight, sound, touch, taste, and smell—monitors the outside world for the body. The immune system—functioning somewhat like a sixth sense—monitors the inside world of the body and keeps the brain informed.

When the Immune System Is in Control: Normal Functions

Natural Immunity

When all elements of the immune system are present and functioning normally, we enjoy reasonably complete protection from infection by environmental pathogens. Sometimes we acquire a natural immunity to some infections through repeated exposures to small doses of pathogens that do not result in illness, but do induce the formation of protective antibodies.

Induced Immunity

By the process of active immunization—the administration of vaccines in appropriate doses—immunity to specific pathogens can be established. Immunization programs have greatly reduced the frequency and severity of many infectious diseases. Smallpox has been completely eliminated through a program of worldwide vaccination.

Tumor Surveillance

It is now quite evident that the immune system continually monitors body tissues for cells that are undergoing malignant change that transforms them into "nonself" structures, to destroy them; thus the immune system is an instrument of primary cancer prevention.

Organ Rejection Following Transplantation

Except in cases of identical twin donor and recipient, any attempt to transplant an organ (kidney, liver, heart, etc.) from one individual to another is met with automatic rejection by the immune system—refusal to tolerate "nonself" tissue. This reaction is based upon the fact that every individual possesses a unique pattern of proteins (antigens) on the surface of all cells in the body, which provide a very specific marker of "self." These antigens are called HLA (human leukocyte antigens); they are the cell markers that are used in the process of typing and matching of organ donor and recipient to determine the degree of tissue compatibility, hence the designation "histocompatibility antigens." The closer the match, the greater the likelihood that the transplant will "take" (not be rejected) if appropriate immunosuppressant drugs are given to prevent rejection.

The actual rejection of donor tissue by the immune system is due to the action of CD8 "killer" T cells (also called cytotoxic T lymphocytes or CTLs). Doing the job that nature programmed them to do—functioning normally—CD8 T cells will destroy the "nonself" donor tissue within two weeks, if not prevented by immunosuppressant drugs.

When the Immune System Is Out of Control: Immune Disorders

The marked complexity of the immune system makes it vulnerable to malfunction. A deficiency of one element or an excess of another can result in serious illness. The following summary of immune disorders illustrates the magnitude of the system's impact on our health.

Primary Immune Deficiency Disorders

There are more than 70 well-defined primary immune deficiency diseases that occur in humans. All of these are genetic in origin—the inheritance of a faulty gene from a parent. About 400 new cases occur annually, the majority becoming apparent within the first few years of life. The following examples illustrate the nature of some of these childhood immune disorders.

- Bruton's agammaglobulinemia (also known as XLA, for X-linked agamma-globulinemia—the defective gene is located on the X chromosome): this disorder occurs almost exclusively in young boys (only one X chromosome). This gene controls the development of B cells that make antibodies; the defective gene fails to produce functional B cells, hence the absence of antibodies (gammaglobulins); the result is the lack of immunity to bacterial infections.
- DiGeorge syndrome: children who have normal levels of antibodies in their blood but are unusually susceptible to infections caused by viruses and fungi; this is due to genetically defective development of the thymus gland and the resultant absence of functional T cells.
- severe combined immunodeficiency disease (SCID): children with genetic defects that impair both B-cell and T-cell production; they are unable to produce antibodies or to develop immunity to viral and fungal pathogens. The complete lack of immune response results in overwhelming infections by all pathogens—bacteria, viruses, fungi, and parasites; attempts to vaccinate these children can be fatal.

Secondary Immune Deficiency Disorders

These disorders are not due to defective genes, but are acquired later in life from a variety of causes. The principal causes include:
- immunosuppressant drugs used to treat cancer and to prevent rejection of organ transplants
- stress, burns, malnutrition
- autoimmune disorders (see below)
- AIDS—the acquired immune deficiency syndrome—due to infection with HIV-1 or HIV-2, the human immunodeficiency viruses. These specifically target the CD4 "helper" T lymphocytes, the key cell that prompts the B cells to make antibodies and promotes maturation of CD8 "killer" T cells. As the number of CD4 T cells gradually declines, both humoral and cellular immunity fade, permitting the development of numerous opportunistic infections.

Allergy and Hypersensitivity

These terms are often used interchangeably; strictly speaking, allergy refers to *immediate type hypersensitivity*—the condition of being sensitized (overly sensitive and overly reactive) to small amounts of allergens (pollens, foods, drugs, etc.) that cause allergic rhinitis (hay fever), asthma, hives, dermatitis (skin rash), and anaphylactic shock. Allergic reactions occur very promptly following contact with the allergen; they are caused by IgE antibodies that are produced on the first exposure to the antigen (sensitization). Why the immune system of some individuals produces IgE antibodies—and renders them allergic—is not understood.

Delayed-type hypersensitivity (DTH) develops from 12 to 48 hours after exposure to an antigen and is due to activation of CD8 T lymphocytes, not antibodies. Examples of delayed hypersensitivity are the skin reactions to poison ivy, oak, and sumac leaves, and the tuberculin skin test that is positive (red and swollen) in those previously infected by the tuberculosis germ. More drastic examples of DTH are the progressive destruction of lung tissue in tuberculosis and of liver tissue in chronic hepatitis B by T lymphocytes and macrophages, the killers and scavengers of the immune system. Lung tissue cells infected by tubercle bacilli and liver tissue cells infected by hepatitis B virus are so altered that the T cells of the immune system judge them to be "nonself" and proceed to destroy them.

Autoimmune Disorders

Approximately 5% of Americans suffer from an autoimmune disorder. Our present understanding of the immune system does not clearly explain why, without apparent provocation, it attacks normal tissues of the body of which it is a part—why it fails to recognize and honor "self." There appears to be no single answer, but several explanations have been offered.

1. By the time of birth, the immune system has acquired the ability to recognize that all body constituents are "self;" B and T lymphocytes are so imprinted. B and T cells live only a few weeks; every succeeding generation must be imprinted with the same instructions—flawlessly. It is conceivable that biological variability could result in erroneous imprinting and impair the ability to distinguish "self" from "nonself."

2. Genetic flaws can predispose some individuals to the development of autoimmune disorders. Many of them are known to "run in families."

3. Environmental factors can initiate autoimmune disorders in susceptible individuals. Very low grade infections with small numbers of viruses or bacteria (clinically undetectable) can cause a delayed type hypersensitivity reaction. An invading microorganism can contain a molecular segment that mimics a normal "self" tissue structure and thus delude the immune system to attack—destroying foreign and native elements alike.

4. Sex hormones can influence the potential for developing autoimmune disorders. Many such diseases are significantly more common in women than men, with the highest incidence during reproductive years.

5. The brain/mind, via psychological stress, anxiety, depression, etc., can initiate or intensify immune dysfunction. This is a common clinical observation in patients with autoimmune disease.

The following disorders are now considered to be autoimmune diseases:

    Addison's disease
    autoimmune hemolytic anemia
    autoimmune hepatitis
    autoimmune nephritis
    Crohn's disease
    diabetes, type I, insulin-dependent
    Graves' disease
    Hashimoto's thyroiditis
    lupus erythematosus
    multiple sclerosis

myasthenia gravis
pemphigus
rheumatic carditis
rheumatoid arthritis
scleroderma
Sjögren's syndrome

Recommended Additional Reading

At War Within: The Double-Edged Sword of Immunity, William R. Clark. New York: Oxford University Press, 1995.

A comprehensive and beautifully written summary of the history and present understanding of immunology.

"The End of the Self," Sarah Richardson. *Discover Magazine,* Vol. 17, No. 4, pages 80–87, April 1996.

An insightful and clearly presented review of the work of Polly Matzinger, immunologist at the National Institutes of Health, who postulates an alternate interpretation of how the immune system works.

APPENDIX 6

Long-Term Corticosteroid (Cortisone) Therapy

Corticosteroid (cortisonelike) drugs are most commonly used for short periods of time—several days to a few weeks. However, there are numerous chronic conditions that require corticosteroid therapy (usually prednisone or prednisolone) for periods of several months to several years, intermittently or continuously. Long-term use requires very careful dosage adjustment and close monitoring for adverse effects. Optimal treatment schedules can be very beneficial in managing the following disorders:
- alcoholic hepatitis
- asthma
- celiac sprue
- chronic active hepatitis (with negative hepatitis B test)
- Crohn's disease
- hemolytic anemia
- idiopathic thrombocytopenia
- mixed connective tissue disease
- nephrosis
- nonalcoholic cirrhosis in women
- organ transplantation
- pemphigus
- polyarteritis nodosa
- polymyalgia rheumatica
- polymyositis
- rheumatoid arthritis
- sarcoidosis
- subacute hepatic necrosis
- systemic lupus erythematosus
- temporal arteritis
- ulcerative colitis
- Wegener's granulomatosis

General Principles of Corticosteroid Therapy

- Corticosteroid drugs are not curative for any of the above disorders. They may be beneficial because of their anti-inflammatory and immunosuppressive effects.
- The optimal dose is the smallest one that will achieve the desired results; it must be determined by trial and error.
- The maintenance dose must be monitored closely and adjusted according to the course of the illness and the patient's response to treatment.
- The goal of long-term therapy should not be the complete relief of symptoms, but reduction of symptoms to a tolerable level.
- After the disease process has been stabilized and the smallest effective dose determined, attempts should be made to reduce the dose to every other day.
- Prednisone and prednisolone, when prescribed once daily, should be given before 9 A.M. to minimize suppression of pituitary gland function (secretion of ACTH, the pituitary hormone that regulates cortisone production by the adrenal gland).
- Prolonged therapy with high doses should be used only for life-threatening disease. The longer the course of treatment and the higher the dose, the greater is the risk of suppressing function of the pituitary and adrenal glands.
- Following long-term use, corticosteroid drugs must be discontinued gradually to prevent acute deficiency of the adrenal glands; rapid withdrawal can also result in a prompt return of symptoms of the disorder being treated—asthma, arthritis, sarcoidosis, etc.
- Prolonged use of corticosteroid drugs usually causes some suppression of adrenal gland function that can require from 9 to 12 months for recovery following discontinuation. During this period and for an additional one to two years, the patient may require prompt administration of corticosteroids in the event of acute illness, injury, or surgery.

Possible Adverse Effects of Long-Term Corticosteroid Therapy

Abnormal thinning and bruising of the skin

Acne

Aseptic necrosis of bone (bone death not due to infection); most commonly occurs in the head of the humerus (upper arm) or femur (thigh bone)

Cataracts

Cushing's syndrome fat deposits: "moon face," "buffalo hump," "central obesity"

Excessive hair growth

Hypertension (high blood pressure)

Impaired immunity, increased susceptibility to infection

Impairment of calcium absorption

Increased blood sugar

Increased internal eye pressure (glaucoma)

Menstrual irregularities

Mental and emotional disturbances (nervousness, insomnia, mood changes, manic-depression, schizophrenia)

Myopathy (muscle weakness of arms and legs)

Osteoporosis (with rib and vertebra fractures)

Pancreatitis

Peptic ulcer (with risk of bleeding or perforation)

Reactivation of latent tuberculosis

Retarded growth in children

Salt and water retention

Pain Management Centers

Many patients living with a chronic disorder find that coping with chronic pain is one of the more difficult aspects of disease management. While other features of their illness may have responded well to treatment, a chronic pain syndrome (CPS) continues to mar their quality of life. After long periods of unrelieved suffering, some patients seek evaluation and treatment at a pain center as a last resort.

By its very nature, chronic pain is seldom curable. Due to disappointing treatment outcomes in spite of elaborate and costly procedures offered by some pain centers, many consumer groups have become confused and suspicious. Within the past 10 years, several organizations have developed practice guidelines and accreditation procedures for the management of pain by health care providers and facilities. The most noteworthy are the International Association for the Study of Pain (IASP), The American Pain Society (APS), and the Commission on Accreditation of Rehabilitation Facilities (CARF). The American Academy of Pain Medicine now offers a comprehensive examination for physicians interested in board certification in pain medicine.

Characteristics of Patients with Chronic Pain Syndrome

There are four basic groups of individuals who experience chronic pain as a feature of their disorder.

1. Those with mild to moderate pain that is associated with a known condition under treatment and who are functioning (coping) reasonably well, but pain is persistent in spite of treatment. Patients in this group are not truly pain-disabled and can usually be managed satisfactorily by their primary care physician.

2. Those with mild to moderate pain that is associated with a known condition under treatment but who are not coping well and are basically pain-disabled. Patients in this group may benefit from evaluation and treatment by a limited specialty pain facility, such as a tension-headache clinic.

3. Those with moderate to severe pain that is a known feature of their disorder and who are coping poorly with their total illness. Patients in this group are truly pain-disabled and may benefit from evaluation and treatment by an interdisciplinary pain management program.
4. Those who report chronic persistent pain in the absence of a known physical disorder that could cause the pain. Patients in this group are reported to be pain-disabled, but the underlying cause is a psychological disturbance or a psychiatric disorder; appropriate treatment should be sought in a mental health facility.

Currently Available Pain Treatment Facilities

Among facilities that offer evaluation and management of chronic pain, there are four basic types:
1. Multidisciplinary pain centers: large, complex components of medical universities or teaching hospitals that are well staffed with medical specialists of numerous disciplines and provide research, teaching, and medical care. These centers accept patients with acute or chronic pain, and usually provide both inpatient and outpatient services. A collaborative, integrated, multidisciplinary approach to assessment and management of pain is stressed.
2. Multidisciplinary pain clinics: medical care facilities that are organized and staffed like pain centers but do not provide research or teaching. The principal focus is the interdisciplinary diagnosis and management of patients with chronic pain. Services may be provided for inpatient or outpatient care or both.
3. Pain clinics: relatively smaller health care facilities devoted to the diagnosis and management of patients with particular types of chronic pain. Pain clinics specialize in specific pain syndromes, such as headaches, back pain, hand pain, etc. Pain clinics are generally staffed by single-discipline health professionals.
4. Modality-oriented clinics: health care facilities that offer specific types of treatment that may be helpful in the management of chronic pain syndromes. They do not provide comprehensive evaluation or management of the pain problem. Examples of such clinics include facilities that provide acupuncture, biofeedback, nerve blocks, etc.

Desirable Features of a Pain Management Facility

Consult your personal physician regarding the advisability of seeking help in a pain management facility. Being familiar with your medical condition and your psychological status, he is the best one to provide advice and guidance. If you decide to consider this further, select a facility with the following features:
- Provides outpatient services
- Provides a multidisciplinary approach capable of evaluating and treating both physical and psychological aspects of chronic pain

- Utilizes conservative therapy; minimal use of such therapeutic agents as diathermy, electrical nerve stimulation, ultrasound, etc., for pain relief
- Utilizes individualized, goal-oriented treatment plans with the following objectives:
  - Reduction of pain intensity
  - Reduction of dependence on pain medications
  - Improved ability to manage pain and related problems
  - Increased capacity for productive activity

Resources

Recommended Reading

Patient or Person: Living with Chronic Pain, P. Cowan. New York: Gardner Press, 1992.

Additional Information and Services

American Pain Society (APS)
A National Chapter of the International Association for the Study of Pain (IASP)
4700 West Lake Avenue
Glenview, IL 60025-1485
Phone: (847) 375-4715; Fax: (847) 375-4777

Maintains a current Pain Facilities Directory for the entire United States and Canada. Will provide a listing of all Pain Facilities within caller's state.

Commission on Accreditation of Rehabilitation Facilities (CARF)
4891 East Grant Road
Tucson, AZ 85712
Phone: (520) 325-1044; Fax: (520) 318-1129

Maintains a current file of Accredited Pain Management Facilities in the United States and Canada. Will provide names, addresses, and phone numbers of facilities within caller's area.

American Chronic Pain Association
P.O. Box 850
Rocklin, CA 95677
Phone: (916) 632-0922

National Chronic Pain Outreach Association
7979 Old Georgetown Road, Suite 100
Bethesda, MD 20814-2429
Phone: (301) 652-4948

Nonsteroidal Anti-Inflammatory Drugs (NSAIDs): A Guide to Selection for Therapy

Musculoskeletal disorders are currently the second most common reason for seeking medical attention in the United States. Nonsteroidal anti-inflammatory drugs (NSAIDs) are the most frequently used medications for treating these conditions. It is now generally recognized that the NSAIDs class is the most frequently used class of drugs throughout the world, an indication of the drugs' relative effectiveness and safety. In addition to their dominant role in treating rheumatic disorders, NSAIDs are now widely used to manage headache, menstrual discomfort, postoperative pain, cancer-associated pain, and the prevention of unwanted blood clotting (thrombosis).

The established ability of NSAIDs to relieve pain and inflammation clearly accounts for their universal acceptance and enormous consumption. They all share a common mechanism of action: the inhibition of prostaglandin production in affected tissues. Because of the widespread presence of prostaglandins throughout the body and their very significant roles in numerous body functions, the suppression of prostaglandin production can have both beneficial and harmful consequences.

While all NSAIDs inhibit prostaglandin production and thereby relieve pain and inflammation, there is great variation among individuals as to relief of symptoms (benefits) and the occurrence of adverse drug effects (risks). Unfortunately, in most instances it is not possible to know in advance which NSAID will prove to be beneficial—or harmful—for any one person. A trial-and-error approach is usually unavoidable. At this time, prescribing NSAIDs is more of an art than a science.

Pain relief provided by NSAIDs is due more to their analgesic actions than to their anti-inflammatory effects. There is evidence that suggests other mechanisms (in addition to prostaglandin suppression) are involved in relieving pain. When pain relief is the goal, the smallest effective dose of an NSAID should be used.

The greatest frequency and severity of adverse effects from NSAIDs occur in the elderly, who are also among the heaviest users. Elderly women appear to be the most likely to experience adverse drug reactions due to NSAIDs. If possible, it is advisable to avoid using the following long-acting NSAIDs in the elderly: diflunisal, nabumetone, naproxen, piroxicam, sulindac.

There is no evidence that NSAIDs are superior to acetaminophen (Tylenol, etc.) in relieving pain due to osteoarthritis.

There is no evidence that using NSAIDs in combination with each other increases their effectiveness in relieving pain. The use of NSAIDs in combination is not recommended.

If an adequate trial of an NSAID fails to provide satisfactory pain relief, a trial of an NSAID from another chemical class is recommended (see below).

There is no evidence that NSAIDs used alone are protective of joint cartilage. On the contrary, there is evidence that indicates some NSAIDs may contribute to the deterioration of cartilage in osteoarthritic joints in dogs and humans.

It is advisable to avoid the use of NSAIDs during the last three months of pregnancy. Some NSAIDs can cause premature closure of the ductus arteriosus in the fetus and alter the normal circulation of blood between the heart and lungs.

Compliance with dosage instructions is usually best when taking one or two doses daily. However, long-acting dosage forms are best avoided by anyone with impaired kidney function.

NSAIDs are used solely to provide relief of symptoms. They do not alter the underlying nature of the disorder or favorably influence its course.

It is advisable to use NSAIDs only as needed to relieve significant pain, adjusting the dosage appropriately. When possible, they should be used intermittently and not continuously without interruption. The chronic, long-term use of NSAIDs increases the risk of damage to the gastrointestinal tract, kidneys, and joint cartilage.

Patients requiring chronic use of NSAIDs (over three months) should be followed closely by their physician; periodic blood counts and kidney and liver function tests should be monitored.

NSAIDs Currently Available

Salicylates
aspirin (ASA, Bufferin, Ecotrin, Empirin, others)

Nonacetylated Salicylates
choline magnesium salicylate (Trilisate)
choline salicylate (Arthropan)
magnesium salicylate (Doan's, Magan, Mobidin)

salsalate (Amigesic, Disalcid, Salsitab)
sodium salicylate (Dodd's Pills)

Acetic Acids
diclofenac potassium (Cataflam)
diclofenac sodium (Voltaren, Voltaren XR)
etodolac (Lodine)
indomethacin (Indochron E-R, Indocin, Indocin SR)
ketorolac (Toradol)
nabumetone (Relafen)
sulindac (Clinoril)
tolmetin (Tolectin, Tolectin DS)

Fenamates
meclofenamate (Meclomen)
mefenamic acid (Ponstel)

Oxicams
piroxicam (Feldene)

Propionic Acids
diflunisal (Dolobid)
fenoprofen (Nalfon)
flurbiprofen (Ansaid)
ibuprofen (Advil, Medipren, Motrin, Motrin IB, Nuprin, Rufen)
ketoprofen (Orudis, Orudis KT, Orvail)
naproxen (Naprelan, Naprosyn, Naprosyn EC)
naproxen sodium (Aleve, Anaprox, Anaprox DS)
oxaprozin (Daypro)
suprofen (Profenal)

Pyrazolones
phenylbutazone (Azolid, Butazolidin)

Major Disorders Treated with NSAIDs

Rheumatoid Arthritis
- Preferred NSAIDs: aspirin, nonacetylated salicylates, ibuprofen, naproxen, oxaprozin, others
- NSAIDs not recommended: indomethacin (highest toxicity scores); avoid concurrent use of all NSAIDs, especially salicylates, and methotrexate if possible

Juvenile Rheumatoid Arthritis
- Preferred NSAIDs: ibuprofen, naproxen, tolmetin
- NSAIDs not recommended: aspirin (causes elevated liver enzymes in 40% of patients)

Osteoarthritis
- Preferred NSAIDs: ibuprofen, naproxen, nonacetylated salicylates
- NSAIDs not recommended: indomethacin, ketorolac (not appropriate for chronic use)
- *Note:* The long-term use of NSAIDs is not preferred in this condition.

Ankylosing Spondylitis
- Preferred NSAIDs: indomethacin, naproxen, diclofenac, piroxicam, keto-profen, others
- NSAIDs not recommended: salicylates (increased gastrointestinal toxicity)

Psoriatic Arthritis
- Preferred NSAIDs: diclofenac, indomethacin, ketoprofen, meclofenamate, naproxen, piroxicam
- NSAIDs not recommended: salicylates

Acute Gout
- Preferred NSAIDs: indomethacin, ketoprofen, ketorolac, naproxen
- NSAIDs not recommended: nonacetylated salicylates, tolmetin (ineffective in relieving pain)

Systemic Lupus Erythematosus
- Preferred NSAIDs: diclofenac, ketoprofen, naproxen, sulindac, others
- NSAIDs not recommended: aspirin (causes elevated liver enzymes in 44% of patients), ibuprofen (may induce aseptic meningitis)

Bursitis, Tendinitis, etc.
- Preferred NSAIDs: diclofenac, ibuprofen, naproxen, others
- NSAIDs not recommended: nonacetylated salicylates

Principal Adverse Effects Due to NSAIDs

Gastrointestinal Effects
- All NSAIDs may cause stomach irritation and indigestion.
- Some NSAIDs may cause diarrhea; others may cause constipation.
- Most NSAIDs can cause peptic ulcer disease in susceptible individuals; complications of ulcer bleeding and perforation cause significant morbidity and mortality.
- Some NSAIDs can activate latent Crohn's disease or ulcerative colitis or aggravate existing disease.
- Long-term use of NSAIDs can initiate lower-bowel damage.
- Studies of relative risks among NSAIDs for causing peptic ulcer disease in the elderly (the most vulnerable patients) report the following:

ibuprofen	2.3 (lowest risk)
naproxen	4.3
indomethacin	4.7

piroxicam   6.4
tolmetin   8.5
meclofenamate   8.6
piroxicam   11.1 (highest risk)

- It is estimated that NSAIDs are the direct cause of 20–30% of all cases of peptic ulcer complications.
- Continued use of NSAIDs may slow healing of ulcers or slow eradication of *Helicobacter pylori* infections.

Effects on Kidney Function

- NSAIDs do not adversely affect functions of the normal kidney.
- Chronically diseased kidneys with impaired function are vulnerable to adverse effects induced by some NSAIDs. Prostaglandins produced within the kidney are often able to compensate for some impaired functions. By suppressing the production of prostaglandins, NSAIDs eliminate their compensatory influence and precipitate kidney failure.
- The following conditions predispose to NSAID-induced kidney failure: age-related kidney deterioration (nephrosclerosis), congestive heart failure, cirrhosis of the liver, abnormally low blood volume and low blood protein levels.
- Sulindac and nonacetylated salicylates are probably the safest NSAIDs to use in the presence of impaired kidney function.
- Another kind of NSAID-induced kidney disorder is interstitial nephritis. This very rare drug reaction is due to individual idiosyncrasy (see Glossary). Although eight commonly used NSAIDs are known to have caused interstitial nephritis, fenoprofen accounted for 60% of the cases.
- Binge drinking and concomitant use of NSAIDs can cause kidney toxicity even in young, healthy individuals.

Effects on Liver Function

- All NSAIDs can cause drug-induced hepatitis. However, this is a very rare adverse reaction—1 in 100,000 to 1 in 500,000 NSAID users.
- Diclofenac and sulindac have been associated with the highest incidence of hepatitis.
- Ibuprofen, indomethacin, ketoprofen, and naproxen have been associated with the lowest incidence of hepatitis.
- Nonacetylated salicylates have not been associated with drug-induced hepatitis.
- It is advisable for anyone with a history of significant drug-induced liver reaction or with active liver disease to avoid the use of NSAIDs.

Effects on Blood Clotting

- All NSAIDs, except sodium salicylate, inhibit the aggregation of blood platelets and thus impair blood clotting; this prolongs the bleeding time and increases the risk of serious hemorrhage.

- Aspirin renders blood platelets ineffective for clotting during their life span of 7–12 days; aspirin should be avoided during this period prior to elective surgery.
- Other NSAIDs inhibit platelet activity only during the time the drug is present in the bloodstream and in contact with platelets; the bleeding time will return to normal within one to six days after the last dose, depending upon the NSAID taken.
- Those NSAIDs that increase the anticoagulant effects of warfarin may also increase the risk of significant bleeding.

Effects on Blood Cell Production
- The two most dangerous and threatening adverse reactions to NSAIDs are agranulocytosis and aplastic anemia. They are the result of suppression of bone marrow production of vital blood cells, a potentially fatal condition. Fortunately, these reactions are extremely rare. In a study population of over 22 million people, only 221 cases of agranulocytosis and 113 cases of aplastic anemia were found. See bone marrow depression in Glossary.
- Indomethacin and phenylbutazone were the only two NSAIDs significantly associated with these blood disorders.
- There are no tests that can identify individuals who may be at risk for this type of drug reaction. Judicious use of this class of drugs is mandatory.

Effects on the Central Nervous System
- Indomethacin may cause headaches and mental depression.
- Ibuprofen used during active systemic lupus erythematosus may cause aseptic meningitis.
- Sulindac and tolmetin may cause aseptic meningitis (rarely).
- Some NSAIDs can impair mental functions in the elderly, causing drowsiness, inability to think clearly or concentrate, memory loss, and apathy—symptoms that may be misdiagnosed as senile dementia.

Effects on the Skin
- All NSAIDs are capable of causing some type of skin reaction. A wide variety of reactions are possible, from mild rash and itching to sun sensitivity to toxic epidermal necrolysis—a life-threatening skin destruction with infection. The vast majority of skin reactions consist of mild rash and itching; serious skin reactions are quite rare but are associated with all classes of NSAIDs.
- Any given NSAID can produce a variety of skin reactions; no type of reaction is peculiar to a specific NSAID.
- Aspirin is thought to be responsible for 5–10% of cases of acute and chronic hives.

Effects on Joint Cartilage
- Living joint cartilage is a dynamic tissue that undergoes continuous renewal and maintenance—a balance of tissue loss (degeneration) and tissue replacement (synthesis). Recent experimental studies of normal and

osteoarthritic human cartilage suggest that some NSAIDs can inhibit the synthesis of new (replacement) cartilage, thus preventing the repair of damaged cartilage. This implies that long-term NSAID therapy may cause chronic, low-grade inhibition of cartilage repair, ultimately leading to joint deterioration. The studies revealed significant variations in the effects produced by different NSAIDs. Aspirin and diclofenac caused minimal inhibition of repair in osteoarthritic cartilage. Ibuprofen, indomethacin, and naproxen were shown to cause significant inhibition in the renewal (synthesis) phase of cartilage maintenance.

- Further studies and observations are needed to translate these findings into clinical practice. However, the potential value of the information for NSAID selection deserves consideration.

Precautions

Possible Contraindications for NSAID Therapy
- Known hypersensitivity (allergy) to aspirin or other NSAIDs
- Active peptic ulcer disease; history of recurrent peptic ulcer disease
- Active Crohn's disease or ulcerative colitis
- Active liver disease
- Active bleeding disorder
- Chronic kidney disease with impaired function
- Untreated congestive heart failure
- Cirrhosis of the liver with ascites
- Pregnancy, especially in third trimester or near term

Indomethacin
- The total daily dose should not exceed 200 mg; dosage above this level increases the frequency of adverse reactions.
- Studies demonstrate that indomethacin significantly increases systolic blood pressure in patients with mild hypertension.
- Indomethacin (to a greater degree than other NSAIDs) is reported to interfere with drug therapy of hypertension and heart failure in patients receiving angiotensin-converting enzyme (ACE) inhibitors, beta-blockers, and diuretics (see Appendix 16, Drug Classes).
- Clinical observations suggest that indomethacin may accelerate joint destruction—"analgesic arthropathy." It is not clear whether this finding is due to drug-induced cartilage damage or to excessive joint wear-and-tear following pain relief provided by indomethacin therapy.

Impaired Kidney Function
- It is advisable to initiate NSAIDs at half the usual dose.
- Kidney function should be monitored periodically; NSAID dosage should be adjusted accordingly.
- Concurrent use of an NSAID and a diuretic increases the risk of acute kidney failure.

Drug Interactions of Significance

- NSAIDs may *increase* the anticoagulant effects of *warfarin*; prothrombin times should be monitored carefully.
- Most NSAIDs *increase* the effects of *lithium*; to avoid toxicity, lithium blood levels should be monitored periodically. Sulindac may be an exception to this potential interaction.
- NSAIDs may *increase* the effects of *digoxin*; heart rate and rhythm should be monitored closely.
- Salicylates may *increase* the effects of *sulfonylurea drugs* and cause hypoglycemia (see Appendix 16, Drug Classes).
- Aspirin may *increase* the effects of *phenytoin* and *valproic acid* and cause toxicity.
- Most NSAIDs can *decrease* the effectiveness of antihypertensive drugs: *hydralazine, prazosin, diuretics, beta-blockers,* and *angiotensin-converting enzyme (ACE) inhibitors* (see Appendix 16, Drug Classes).
- NSAIDs taken concurrently with *cortisonelike drugs* (corticosteroids) may increase the risk of gastrointestinal bleeding.
- NSAIDs taken concurrently with *cyclosporine* may increase the risk of impaired kidney function.
- NSAIDs taken concurrently with *methotrexate* may *increase* methotrexate levels by slowing its elimination (kidney clearance).
- Indomethacin taken concurrently with *triamterene* may impair the kidneys' ability to clear creatinine by 60–72%.
- Piroxicam taken concurrently with *cimetidine* may *increase* blood levels of piroxicam.
- Probenecid may *increase* the blood levels of certain NSAIDs by 50%. This does not apply to diclofenac, ibuprofen, or tolmetin.
- Aluminum hydroxide antacids *decrease* the effects of *diflunisal* and *naproxen*.

Chronotherapeutics

- It is helpful to observe the patient's "symptom rhythm" and to individualize the timing of medications accordingly.
- Rheumatoid arthritis: joint stiffness, pain, swelling, and decreased grip strength are usually more pronounced in the morning; NSAIDs are best taken at bedtime and on arising.
- Osteoarthritis: joint pain and swelling are usually worse in the late afternoon, evening, or early morning; sustained-release NSAIDs are best taken in the evening. For those with early afternoon pain, NSAIDs should be taken in the morning.

Conclusions

- Systematic comparisons of numerous studies have been unable to identify the "best NSAID" among those currently available. This is attributed to the

fact that all NSAIDs share (in varying degrees) the same therapeutic benefits and risks.

- The selection of an NSAID for each patient should be a highly individualized procedure. As with all drug therapy, the optimal choice is the NSAID
  that is judged to provide the greatest benefit with the least risk in light of
  the characteristics of the individual who is to use it.
- Treatment outcomes that involve the use of NSAIDs will be determined by
  the match of the drug and the patient. Unfortunately, quite often decisions
  must be made in the absence of complete information in advance. The
  experimental nature of much NSAID therapy is unavoidable. The patient
  should understand this and work closely with the physician to monitor
  response to treatment and make adjustments as necessary.
- Based upon information provided above, the patient should inform the
  physician of any conditions that must be considered with regard to the use
  of NSAIDs. Such conditions include:
  - known allergies, especially allergy to aspirin and other NSAIDs
  - history of prior adverse reactions to medications
  - medications taken currently; medical conditions under treatment
  - history of peptic ulcer disease, Crohn's disease, or ulcerative colitis
  - history of high blood pressure (hypertension), or disorders of the heart,
    liver, or kidneys
  - excessive use of alcohol or tobacco
  - pregnancy, current or planned
  - scheduled surgical or dental procedures

APPENDIX 9

Tyramine-Free Diet

Tyramine is a chemical present in many foods and beverages that causes no difficulties under normal circumstances. The principal pharmacological action of tyramine is to raise blood pressure. Normally this action of tyramine (in quantities found in the average diet) is neutralized by enzymes present in many body tissues. The principal enzyme responsible for neutralizing tyramine (and chemicals with similar action) is monoamine oxidase (MAO) type A. This enzyme provides important regulatory functions in body chemistry, including stabilization of blood pressure. If this action of MAO type A is blocked, chemicals like tyramine can cause dangerous elevations of blood pressure.

Several drugs in use today are capable of blocking the actions of MAO type A; these drugs are referred to as MAO type A inhibitors (see Appendix 16, Drug Classes). If an individual is taking one of these drugs and his diet includes foods or beverages that contain significant amounts of tyramine, he may experience a sudden increase in blood pressure and be at risk for having a stroke (brain hemorrhage).

Any protein-containing food that has undergone partial decomposition may present a hazard because of its increased tyramine content. The following foods and beverages have been reported to contain varying amounts of tyramine (or chemicals with similar action). Unless their tyramine content is known to be insignificant, they should be avoided completely while taking an MAO inhibitor drug. If you are taking such a drug, discuss this possible drug–food interaction with your physician.

Foods and Beverages Likely to Contain Tyramine

Avoid the following if you are taking a monoamine oxidase (MAO) type A inhibitor drug:

Foods
Aged cheeses of all kinds
Avocados

Bananas
Bean curd
Bologna
"Bovril" extract
Broad bean pods
Buttermilk
Caviar
Chicken liver (unless fresh and used at once)
Chocolate
Fava beans
Figs, canned
Fish, canned
Fish, dried and salted
Herring, pickled
Liver, if not very fresh
"Marmite" extract
Meat extracts
Mincemeat pie
Monosodium glutamate, in excessive amounts
Papaya
Passion fruit
Peanuts
Pepperoni
Plums, red
Raisins
Raspberries
Salami
Shrimp paste
Sour cream
Sourdough bread or doughnuts
Soy sauce
Summer sausage
Yeast bread or coffee cake, hot and fresh
Yeast extracts
Yogurt

Beverages
Beer (unpasteurized)
Chianti wine
Sherry wine
Vermouth

High-Potassium Foods

Diuretic drugs that cause loss of potassium from the body are often used to treat conditions that also require a reduced intake of sodium. The high-potassium foods listed below have been selected for their compatibility with a sodium-restricted diet (500 to 1000 mg of sodium daily).

Beverages
Orange juice
Prune juice
Skim milk
Tea
Tomato juice
Whole milk

Breads and Cereals
Brown rice
Cornbread
Griddle cakes
Muffins
Oatmeal
Shredded wheat
Waffles

Fruits
Apricots
Avocados
Bananas
Figs
Honeydew melons
Mangos
Oranges

Papaya
Prunes

Meats
Beef
Chicken
Codfish
Flounder
Haddock
Halibut
Liver
Pork
Rockfish
Salmon
Turkey
Veal

Vegetables
Baked beans
Lima beans
Mushrooms
Navy beans
Parsnips
Radishes
Squash
Sweet potatoes
Tomatoes
White potatoes

Genetic Disorders and Gene Therapy

All of the tissues that constitute our bodies (skin, muscle, organs, etc.) consist of microscopic units called cells. All cells (except fully developed red blood cells) contain a nucleus—a central control point. Within the nucleus are 23 pairs of chromosomes, one-half of each pair derived from the mother, the other half from the father. Each chromosome is a rod-shaped structure that contains a compressed double-ribbon of deoxyribonucleic acid (DNA). The ribbons (or strands) are divided into segments that are called genes. Each gene occupies a specific location on its chromosome, and the components of each gene are arranged in a specific sequential order; genes are capable of undergoing DNA rearrangements to perform specific tasks. Genes are the biological units of heredity, controlling all of the mechanisms that govern how we develop, grow, and function. They largely determine the course of our lives—the features of the infant at birth, the developing body and mind of childhood, the maturing of adulthood, and the aging and ultimate demise of the elderly. The total collection of genes within an individual is known as the genome. The human genome consists of approximately 100,000 genes, of which an estimated 6,300 are considered to be relevant to human diseases and disorders. Today 1 American in 100 is born with a serious genetic defect.

Unfortunately, DNA segments that constitute genes are somewhat unstable chemical structures and are subject to both minor and major alterations. A wide variety of influences can affect the processes involved when genes are copied to provide for sexual reproduction and new generations of cells during development and growth. Physical or chemical alteration of gene structure (from whatever cause) is known as mutation. Mutant genes are responsible for a wide range of deleterious effects that may manifest throughout an individual lifetime. Given the number of genes at risk for alteration and the inherent instability of DNA, it is not surprising that mankind displays such marked diversity and is vulnerable to a significant array of genetic (inherited) defects and disorders.

Genetic Disorders

Geneticists now believe that genes largely determine the nature and timing of the majority of diseases and disorders we experience during our lifetime. Some genetic disorders are present and detectable at birth, such as cretinism (thyroid hormone deficiency) and sickle cell disease. Some manifest during childhood, such as acute lymphoblastic leukemia; others during adolescence, such as epilepsy and schizophrenia. Some become apparent during midlife, such as hypertension, coronary artery disease, and Huntington's disease; and some in late life, such as Alzheimer's disease. It is now thought that genes determine our predisposition and susceptibility to disorders we usually think of as due to environmental factors—autoimmune disorders, cancer, or Parkinson's disease. We apparently inherit the potential to develop these if and when we encounter an environmental stimulus that can trigger their development, such as excessive sun exposure that causes skin cancer.

More than 4,300 disorders that are clearly of genetic origin are now recognized. Notable examples include the following:

- ADA—serious combined immune deficiency (early childhood)
- breast cancer (some types)
- Bruton's X-linked agammaglobulinemia (early childhood)
- cystic fibrosis
- diabetes type II (noninsulin-dependent)
- familial colon polyposis/colon cancer
- hemophilia
- Huntington's disease
- muscular dystrophy
- pancreatic cancer
- polycystic kidney disease
- progressive myoclonus epilepsy
- X-linked serious combined immune deficiency (early childhood)

Genetic Testing

Within the next few years, genetic tests for a variety of diseases and disorders will be widely available. Such tests will be able to demonstrate that (1) a person has a genetic potential for developing a given disorder in the future, (2) an individual is a carrier of a potentially harmful gene that can be transmitted to children, or (3) a developing fetus has a defective gene that is known to cause a genetic disorder.

Knowledge of genetic predisposition for significant illness can be a combination of blessing and curse. Early detection of incipient disease could motivate one to modify known risk factors and so deter the onset of disease or limit its manifestations. On the other hand, such knowledge could adversely affect employment, insurance eligibility, family relationships, and emotional health.

ALERT!

Patients and families who are considering genetic testing should first seek the wisdom and guidance of experienced counselors in genetic testing centers.

The following would be reasonable candidates for genetic testing:

- individuals who have reason to think they may have a genetic disorder or are at risk for developing one
- women who are pregnant after age 34
- couples with a child who has a genetic disorder, mental retardation, or a birth defect
- women who have had two or more miscarriages (spontaneous abortions) or whose babies died in infancy
- couples concerned about the risk of congenital defects that occur frequently in their ethnic group
- couples who are first cousins or other blood relatives

Genetic testing is currently targeted to a specific disease. Examples of available tests include those for the following disorders:

- ADA-SCID—serious combined immune deficiency
- Alzheimer's disease (uncommon type in young adults)
- breast and ovarian cancer (hereditary type)
- colon cancer (hereditary type)
- cystic fibrosis
- Down syndrome
- Duchenne muscular dystrophy
- fragile X syndrome
- hemophilia
- Huntington's disease
- Marfan's syndrome
- sickle cell disease
- Tay-Sachs disease

Genetic Counseling

Medical genetics is a family-oriented specialty. The clinical geneticist serves as a coordinator between the family unit and those medical specialists who have relevance to the genetic disorder of concern. Consideration must be given to the psychological and financial costs for the patient with genetic disease, the possible carrier status of other family members, and the potential for transmission of genetic disease to children.

The role of the fully qualified genetic counselor is indispensable to the successful practice of medical genetics. The counselor is properly trained in gathering and interpreting pertinent information, explaining genetic disorders to patients and families, and coordinating the selection and timing of diagnostic tests and therapeutic procedures. The goals of counseling include the following:

- evaluation of test results and the degree of certainty of the diagnosis
- estimation of the implied burden of the diagnosis in terms of physical, emotional, and financial costs
- assessment of risk for genetic disease in other family members, living children, currently developing fetuses, and future children
- consideration of individualized management options as appropriate for each situation

The National Society of Genetic Counselors will accept *written* requests for referral to certified counselors located in the geographic area of the requester. Write to:

National Society of Genetic Counselors
233 Canterbury Drive
Wallingford, PA 19086-6617

Gene Therapy

The first successful attempt to use gene therapy occurred in 1990. It involved a four-year-old girl with a form of SCID—serious combined immune deficiency disease, a fatal disorder caused by a defective gene. Both of her parents carried one defective copy of the gene that enables the production of the enzyme ADA, adenosine deaminase. This enzyme in T lymphocytes enables the cell to mature normally and to assist the production of antibodies by B lymphocytes (see Appendix 5, The Immune System). Young Ashanti had inherited two defective genes, one from each parent; her immune system was unable to protect her from deadly bacterial and viral infections. The gene therapy designed to correct Ashanti's immune deficiency involved drawing samples of her blood and isolating her defective T cells. A copy of a normal human gene for ADA production was first incorporated into a harmless virus that had been rendered unable to reproduce itself. The newly engineered virus was then allowed to "infect" the sample of Ashanti's T cells; it delivered the normal ADA gene to the nucleus of the T cells, where it was incorporated into the cell's DNA, instructing the cell to henceforth produce normal ADA. Following a period of incubation, the newly constituted T cells were injected back into Ashanti's bloodstream. After six repetitions of this procedure, Ashanti's immune system was performing normally. A few months later, a second child with ADA-SCID was treated using the same procedure and with equal success.

Gene therapy is designed to treat a specific genetic disorder by replacing or modifying the defective gene that is responsible for the disorder. It is not intended to be used for the enhancement of desirable traits. Gene therapy does not involve alteration of sperm or egg cells and cannot affect a patient's offspring.

Currently there are 149 ongoing research projects in this country designed to evaluate various methods of gene therapy for a variety of diseases. The principal procedures under investigation utilize the following approaches:

- the use of altered (harmless) viruses as vectors for the delivery of replacement genes into mature blood cells
- the introduction of corrective genes into bone marrow "stem cells," the primary source for the development of all types of blood cells
- the insertion of corrective genes directly into afflicted tissues, often using a virus vector. Example: the insertion of normal genes into the bronchial tubes of a patient with cystic fibrosis.
- the injection of a "killer" gene into cancerous tumors to make them more susceptible to chemotherapy

Current genetic research clearly indicates that within the next 10 years gene therapy will not be limited to correction of genetic diseases, but will also be used to treat various forms of cancer and disorders of the immune system.

Resource for Additional Information and Referral

March of Dimes Birth Defects Foundation
National Office
1275 Mamaroneck Avenue
White Plains, NY 10605
Phone: (914) 428-7100

APPENDIX 12

Drug Enforcement Administration (DEA) Schedules of Controlled Substances

The controlled substances that come under the jurisdiction of the Controlled Substances Act of 1970 are divided into five schedules.

Schedule I

Nonmedicinal substances with high abuse potential and dependence liability. Used for research purposes only. Not legally available for medicinal use by prescription. Examples are dihydromorphine, heroin, LSD, marijuana, and others.

Schedule II

Medicinal drugs in current use that have the highest abuse potential and dependence liability. A written prescription is required. Telephoned prescribing is prohibited. No refills are allowed. Examples are opium derivatives (morphine, codeine, oxycodone, etc.); opioids (meperidine, methadone, etc.); amphetamines (Dexedrine) and methylphenidate (Ritalin); short-acting barbiturates (Amytal, Nembutal, Seconal).

Schedule III

Medicinal drugs with abuse potential and dependence liability less than Schedule II drugs but greater than Schedule IV or V drugs. A telephoned prescription is permitted, to be converted to written form by the dispensing pharmacist. Prescriptions must be renewed every six months. Refills are limited to five. Examples are codeine, hydrocodone, and paregoric in combination with one or more non-narcotic drugs; some sedative/hypnotics (butabarbital, methyprylon); some appetite suppressants (Didrex, Sanorex, Tenuate).

Schedule IV

Medicinal drugs with less abuse potential and dependence liability than Schedule III drugs. Prescription requirements are the same as for Schedule III drugs. Examples include pentazocine (Talwin), propoxyphene (Darvon), and all benzodiazepines (Librium, Valium, etc.).

Schedule V

Medicinal drugs with the lowest abuse potential and dependence liability. Examples are diphenoxylate (Lomotil) and loperimide (Imodium). Drugs requiring a prescription are handled the same as any nonscheduled prescription drug. Some nonprescription drugs can be sold only with approval of the pharmacist; the buyer is required to sign a log of purchase at the time the drug is dispensed. Examples include codeine and hydrocodone in combination with other active, non-narcotic drugs sold in preparations that contain limited quantities for control of cough or diarrhea.

APPENDIX 13

Arthritis and Musculoskeletal Disease Centers

The National Institute of Arthritis and Musculoskeletal and Skin Diseases, one of the National Institutes of Health, has designated the following institutions as Multipurpose Arthritis and Musculoskeletal Disease Centers. As "centers of excellence," these 12 institutions offer the expertise needed by those with difficult-to-diagnose or difficult-to-treat conditions.

ALABAMA
William J. Koopman, M.D.
University of Alabama at Birmingham
UAB Station/THT 429A
Birmingham, AL 35294
Phone: (205) 934-5306; Fax: (205) 934-1564

CALIFORNIA
Dennis A. Carson, M.D.
University of California, San Diego
9500 Gilman Drive, 0664
La Jolla, CA 92093-0664
Phone: (619) 534-5408; Fax: (619) 534-5399

Bevra H. Hahn, M.D.
University of California, Los Angeles
1000 Veterans Avenue
Los Angeles, CA 90024-1670
Phone: (310) 825-7991; Fax: (310) 206-8606

Halsted R. Holman, M.D.
Stanford University Medical Center
1000 Welch Road, Suite 203
Palo Alto, CA 94304
Phone: (415) 723-5907; Fax: (415) 723-9656

ILLINOIS

Richard M. Pope, M.D.
Northwestern University Medical School
303 East Chicago Avenue
Chicago, IL 60611
Phone: (312) 503-8003; Fax: (312) 503-0994

INDIANA

Kenneth Brandt, M.D.
Indiana University School of Medicine
542 Clinical Drive, Room 492
Indianapolis, IN 46202-5103
Phone: (317) 274-4225; Fax: (317) 274-7792

MASSACHUSETTS

Mathew H. Liang, M.D., M.P.H.
Brigham and Women's Hospital
75 Francis Street
Boston, MA 02115
Phone: (617) 732-5356; Fax: (617) 732-5505

David Felson, M.D., M.P.H.
Boston University School of Medicine
71 East Concord Street, K-5
Boston, MA 02118
Phone: (617) 638-5180; Fax: (617) 638-5239

MICHIGAN

David A. Fox, M.D.
University of Michigan Medical School
1500 East Medical Center Drive
Ann Arbor, MI 48109-0358
Phone: (313) 936-5566; Fax: (313) 763-1253

NEW YORK

Robert P. Kimberly, M.D.
The Hospital for Special Surgery
535 East 70th Street
New York, NY 10021
Phone: (212) 606-1189; Fax: (212) 439-1857

OHIO

David N. Glass, M.D.
Children's Hospital Research Foundation
Elland and Bethesda Avenues
Cincinnati, OH 45229-2899
Phone: (513) 559-8854; Fax: (513) 559-4615

Roland W. Moskowitz, M.D.
Case Western Reserve University
2074 Abington Road
Cleveland, OH 44106
Phone: (216) 844-3168; Fax: (216) 844-5172

APPENDIX 14

Monosodium Glutamate (MSG) Syndrome

Despite the common association with Chinese food, monosodium glutamate (MSG) is a chemical compound normally present in various forms of animal and plant life. Mushrooms, carrots, and some seaweeds are rich sources of MSG. It is one of the most abundant chemical messengers (neurotransmitters) in the human central nervous system (brain and spinal cord). MSG exerts a stimulant (excitatory) effect on the transmission of nerve impulses throughout the brain.

The Medical Significance of MSG

The brain produces MSG from sugar in quantities necessary for normal function. Should some disturbance cause higher than normal concentrations of MSG, the resulting excessive stimulation may have deleterious effects on brain tissues. Most individuals tolerate the usual fluctuations of MSG levels very well and experience no symptoms from transient elevations due to large intakes with food. However, some individuals are quite sensitive to MSG levels above the normal range. For them, symptoms develop within a few hours after eating foods that contain liberal amounts of MSG. The following patterns illustrate the more common manifestations of sensitivity to this food additive.

"The Chinese Restaurant Syndrome"
- Headache, often of a throbbing nature
- Lightheadedness or faintness
- Flushing and burning sensation of the face and neck
- Facial swelling, pressure, numbness around mouth
- Tightness in the jaw, neck, shoulders, chest, or back
- Nervous twitching, tremors

ALERT!
This can be mistaken for a heart attack.

Vascular Headaches
- Onset of headache within 20 minutes to 5 hours after eating
- Headache may have a pulsating or throbbing quality
- May begin with facial flushing, fatigue, or nausea
- May be accompanied by tingling of the tongue, hands, or feet
- Headache may resemble migraine or cluster headache
- Headache may be true migraine triggered by MSG

Sleep Disorders
MSG eaten during the later half of the day can cause:
- Difficulty falling asleep or staying asleep
- Active, bizarre dreaming
- Restless leg syndrome

These disorders are more common in the elderly.

MSG and Labels

MSG is generally known to be a flavor enhancer, hence its wide use by the food industry. It can be found in a wide variety of packaged foods and seasonings: canned soups, processed meats, frozen dinners, soy sauce, meat tenderizer, etc. The Food and Drug Administration designates MSG as "Generally Recognized as Safe" (GRAS). However, in consideration of those who are truly sensitive to MSG, the FDA requires that all food containing MSG disclose its presence on the label. Unfortunately, the average consumer will not recognize that MSG is a component of some of the items listed, some of which are 20% MSG. Those who read labels to determine if MSG is present should learn to recognize the following items that "hide" the MSG within:
- autolyzed yeast
- flavoring
- hydrolyzed corn gluten
- hydrolyzed plant protein
- hydrolyzed soy protein
- hydrolyzed vegetable protein
- kombu extract
- natural flavor
- seasoning
- sodium caseinate

Food and Drug Administration (FDA) Pregnancy Categories

ALERT!

Regardless of the designated Pregnancy Category or its implied safety, no drug should be taken during any period of pregnancy, or if you believe you might be pregnant, unless it is definitely needed and the anticipated benefits clearly outweigh possible risks.

Category A

Adequate and well-controlled studies in pregnant women are *negative* for fetal abnormalities. Risk to the fetus is deemed remote.

Category B

Animal reproduction studies are *negative* for fetal abnormalities. Information from adequate and well-controlled studies in pregnant women is not available.

OR

Animal reproduction studies are *positive* for fetal abnormalities. Adequate and well-controlled studies in pregnant women are *negative* for fetal abnormalities. Risk to the fetus is deemed to be relatively unlikely.

Category C

Animal reproduction studies are *positive* for fetal abnormalities. Information from adequate and well-controlled studies in pregnant women is not available.

OR

Information from animal reproduction studies *and* from adequate and well-controlled studies in pregnant women is not available. Possible benefits of the drug may justify potential risks to the fetus.

Category D

Studies in pregnant women and/or premarketing (investigational) or postmarketing experience demonstrate *positive* evidence of human fetal risk. The drug is needed to treat serious disease or in life-threatening situations where safer drugs are ineffective or cannot be used.

Category X

Animal reproduction studies and/or human pregnancy studies are *positive* for fetal abnormalities.

OR

Studies in pregnant women and/or premarketing (investigational) or postmarketing experience demonstrate *positive* evidence of human fetal risk.

AND

Potential risks to the fetus outweigh possible benefits of the drug. Use of the drug is *contraindicated* in women who are or may become pregnant.

Drugs Designated as Category D

acetohexamide
alfentanil—if prolonged use, or high doses at term
alphaprodine—if prolonged use, or high doses at term
alprazolam
amitriptyline
amobarbital
anileridine—if prolonged use, or high doses at term
anisindione
aspirin—if full dose used in third trimester
atenolol
azathioprine
benazepril
bendroflumethiazide
benzthiazide
bleomycin
bromides
bumetanide
busulfan
butalbital—if prolonged use, or high doses at term
butorphanol—if prolonged use, or high doses at term

calcifediol—if doses exceed recommended daily allowances
calcitriol—if doses exceed recommended daily allowances
captopril
carbarsone
carbimazole
chlorambucil
chlordiazepoxide
chlorothiazide
chlorpropamide
chlortetracycline
cholecalciferol—if doses exceed recommended daily allowances
cisplatin
clorazepate
codeine—if prolonged use, or high doses at term
colchicine
cortisone
cyclophosphamide
cytarabine
daunorubicin
demeclocycline
diazepam
dihydrocodeine—if prolonged use, or high doses at term
dihydrotachysterol—if doses exceed recommended daily allowances
doxorubicin
doxycycline
enalapril
ergocalciferol—if doses exceed recommended daily allowances
ergotamine
ethacrynic acid
fentanyl—if prolonged use, or high doses at term
fluorouracil
glyburide
hydrochlorothiazide
hydrocodone—if prolonged use, or high doses at term
hydroflumethiazide
hydromorphone—if prolonged use, or high doses at term
hydroxyurea
ibuprofen—if used in third trimester or near term
imipramine
indapamide
indomethacin—if used for more than 48 hours, or after 34 weeks of preg-
    nancy
iodine
kanamycin
ketoprofen—if used in third trimester or near term
levorphanol—if prolonged use, or high doses at term

lisinopril
lithium
lorazepam
meclofenamate—if used in third trimester or near term
medroxyprogesterone
melphalan
meperidine—if prolonged use, or high doses at term
meprobamate
mercaptopurine
metaraminol
methadone—if prolonged use, or high doses at term
methimazole
methotrexate
methyclothiazide
metolazone
metrizamide
midazolam
minocycline
morphine—if prolonged use, or high doses at term
naproxen—if used in third trimester or near term
nortriptyline
oxazepam
oxycodone— if prolonged use, or high doses at term
paregoric—if prolonged use, or high doses at term
penicillamine
pentazocine—if prolonged use, or high doses at term
pentobarbital
phenobarbital
phenylbutazone—if used in third trimester or near term
phenytoin
piroxicam—if used in third trimester or near term
plicamycin
polythiazide
potassium iodide
povidone-iodine
primidone
procarbazine
propoxyphene—if prolonged use
propylthiouracil
quinapril
ramipril
secobarbital
spironolactone
streptomycin
"sulfa" drugs—if taken near term
sulindac—if used in third trimester or near term

teniposide
tetracycline
thiotepa
tobramycin
tolazamide
tolbutamide
tolmetin—if used in third trimester or near term
triamterene
trichlormethiazide
trimethadione
vaccine, yellow fever
vinblastine
vitamin D—if doses exceed recommended daily allowances

Drugs Designated as Category X

alcohol—if prolonged use or large amounts
aminopterin
chenodiol
chlorotrianisene
clomiphene
coumarin derivatives
danazol
dicumarol
dienestrol
diethylstilbestrol
estradiol
estrogens, conjugated
estrone
ethinyl estradiol
etretinate
flurazepam
hormonal pregnancy test tablets
iodinated glycerol
isotretinoin
leuprolide
lovastatin
mestranol
mifepristone (RU 486)
misoprostol
norethindrone
norethynodrel
norgestrel
oral contraceptives
phencyclidine (PCP)
quinine

ribavirin
sodium iodide (I^{125})
sodium iodide (I^{131})
temazepam
triazolam
vaccine, measles
vaccine, mumps
vaccine, rubella
vaccine, smallpox
vitamin A—if doses exceed recommended daily allowances
warfarin

Drug Classes

List of Drug Classes

Adrenocortical steroids
Alpha-adrenergic-blocking drugs (alpha-blockers)
Aminoglycosides
Amphetaminelike drugs
Analgesics, mild
Analgesics, strong (see Opioid drugs)
Androgens
Angiotensin-converting enzyme (ACE) inhibitor drugs
Angiotensin II receptor antagonist drugs
Anorexiants
Anti-AIDS drugs
Anti-anginal drugs
Antianxiety drugs
Antiarrhythmic drugs
Antiasthmatic drugs (bronchodilators)
Antibiotics
Anticholinergic drugs
Anticoagulant drugs
Anticonvulsant drugs
Antidepressant drugs
Antidiabetic drugs, oral (see Sulfonylureas)
Antiemetic drugs
Antiepileptic drugs (see Anticonvulsants)
Antifungal drugs
Anti-glaucoma drugs
Anti-gout drugs
Antihistamines

Antihypertensive drugs
Anti-infective drugs
Antileprosy drugs
Antimalarial drugs
Anti-migraine drugs
Anti-motion sickness/antinausea drugs (see Antiemetics)
Antiparkinsonism drugs
Antiplatelet drugs
Antipsychotic drugs (neuroleptics)
Antispasmodics, synthetic
Antituberculosis drugs
Antitussive drugs
Antiviral drugs
Appetite suppressants (see Anorexiants)
Atropinelike drugs (see Anticholinergic drugs)
Barbiturates
Benzodiazepines
Beta-adrenergic-blocking drugs (beta-blockers)
Bronchodilators (see Antiasthmatic drugs)
Calcium channel-blocking drugs (calcium blockers)
Cephalosporins
Cholesterol-reducing drugs
Cortisonelike drugs (see Adrenocortical steroids)
Cough suppressants (see Antitussives)
Decongestants
Digitalis preparations
Diuretics
Estrogens
Female sex hormones (see Estrogens and Progestins)
Fluoroquinolones
Heart rhythm regulators (see Antiarrhythmic drugs)
Histamine-blocking drugs
Hypnotic drugs
Male sex hormones (see Androgens)
Macrolide antibiotics
Monoamine oxidase (MAO) inhibitor drugs
Muscle relaxants
Narcotic drugs (see Opioid drugs)
Nitrates
Nonsteroidal anti-inflammatory drugs (NSAIDs)
Opioid drugs (narcotics)
Penicillins
Phenothiazines
Progestins
Salicylates

Sedatives/sleep inducers (see Hypnotic drugs)
Sulfonamides ("sulfa" drugs)
Sulfonylureas
Tetracyclines
Thiazide diuretics
Tranquilizers, minor (see Antianxiety drugs)
Tranquilizers, major (see Antipsychotic drugs)
Vasodilators
Xanthines

Adrenocortical Steroids

Cortisonelike Drugs
beclomethasone (Beclovent, Vanceril)
betamethasone (Celestone)
cortisone (Cortone)
dexamethasone (Decadron)
flunisolide (AeroBib)
fluticasone (Flonase)
hydrocortisone (Cortef)
methylpredisolone (Medrol)
prednisolone (Delta-Cortef)
prednisone (Deltasone)
triamcinolone (Aristocort, Azmacort)

Alpha-adrenergic-blocking drugs

Alpha-Blockers
doxazosin (Cardura)
prazosin (Minipress)
terazosin (Hytrin)

Aminoglycosides

Anti-infectives
kanamycin (Kantrex)
neomycin (Mycifradin, Neobiotic)
paromomycin (Humatin)

Amphetaminelike Drugs

amphetamine (no brand name)
benzphetamine (Didrex)
dextroamphetamine (Dexedrine)
diethylpropion (Tenuate, Tepanil)
methamphetamine (Desoxyn)

methylphenidate (Ritalin)
phendimetrazine (Anorex, Plegine)
phenmetrazine (Preludin)
phentermine (Fastin, Ionamin)
phenylpropanolamine (Dexatrim)

Analgesics, Mild

acetaminophen (Datril, Tylenol)
aspirin
lidocaine/prilocaine cream (EMLA)
   See Nonsteroidal Anti-Inflammatory Drugs (NSAIDs) below.

Androgens

Male Sex Hormones
fluoxymesterone (Halotestin)
methyltestosterone (Android, Metandren, Oreton)
testosterone (Depotest, Testone)

Angiotensin-Converting Enzyme (ACE) Inhibitors

benazepril (Lotensin)
captopril (Capoten)
enalapril (Vasotec)
fosinopril (Monopril)
lisinopril (Prinivil, Zestril)
quinapril (Accupril)
ramipril (Altace)

Angiotensin II Receptor Antagonist

losartan (Cozaar)

Anorexiants

Appetite Suppressants
dexfenfluramine (Redux)
fenfluramine (Pondimin)
mazindol (Mazanor, Sanorex)
   See also Amphetaminelike Drugs.

Anti-AIDS Drugs

didanosine (DDI, Videx)
lamivudine (3TC)

stavudine (Zerit)
zalcitabine (dideoxycytidine, DDC, Hivid)
zidovudine (AZT, Retrovir)
  See Disorder Profile of AIDS in Section Three for drugs used to treat the
"indicator diseases" of AIDS.

Antianginal Drugs

See Disorder Profile of coronary artery disease in Section Three for detailed
list.
Beta-adrenergic-blocking class (see below)
bepridil (Vascor)
diltiazem (Cardizem)
nicardipine (Cardene)
nifedipine (Adalat, Procardia)
Nitrates (see below)
verapamil (Calan, Isoptin)

Antianxiety Drugs

Minor Tranquilizers
See Benzodiazepine class below.
buspirone (Buspar)
chlormezanone (Trancopal)
hydroxyzine (Atarax, Vistaril)
meprobamate (Equanil, Miltown)

Antiarrhythmic Drugs

Heart Rhythm Regulators
acebutolol (Sectral)
amiodarone (Cordarone)
digitoxin (Crystodigin)
digoxin (Lanoxin)
disopyramide (Norpace)
flecainide (Tambocor)
mexiletine (Mexitil)
moricizine (Ethmozine)
procainamide (Procan SR, Pronestyl)
propafenone (Rythmol)
propranolol (Inderal)
quinidine (Quinaglute, Quinidex, Quinora)
tocainide (Tonocard)
verapamil (Calan, Isoptin)

Antiasthmatic Drugs

Bronchodilators

albuterol (Proventil, Ventolin)
aminophylline (Phyllocontin)
bitolterol (Tornalate)
dyphylline (Lufyllin)
ephedrine (Efed II)
epinephrine (Adrenalin, Bronkaid Mist, Primatene Mist)
isoetharine (Bronkosol, Dey-Lute)
isoproterenol (Isuprel)
metaproterenol (Alupent, Metaprel)
oxtriphylline (Choledyl)
pirbuterol (Maxair)
salmeterol (Serevent)
terbutaline (Brethaire, Brethine, Bricanyl)
theophylline (Bronkodyl, Elixophyllin, Slo-Phyllin, others)

Mast Cell-Stabilizing Drugs

cromolyn sodium (Gastrocrom, Intal)
nedocromil (Tilade)

Antibiotics

See specific antibiotic class (Cephalosporins, Erythromycins, Penicillins, etc.).

Anticholinergic Drugs

Atropinelike Drugs

atropine
belladonna
hyoscyamine
scopolamine
Antidepressants, tricyclic (see class below)
Antihistamines, some (see class below)
Antiparkinsonism drugs, some (see class below)
Antispasmodics, synthetic, some (see class below)
Muscle Relaxants, some (see class below)

Anticoagulant Drugs

anisindione (Miradon)
dicumarol (no brand name)
warfarin (Coumadin, Panwarfin)

Anticonvulsant Drugs

Antiepileptic Drugs
acetazolamide (Diamox)
carbamazepine (Tegretol)
clonazepam (Klonopin)
clorazepate (Tranxene)
diazepam (Valium)
ethosuximide (Zarontin)
ethotoin (Peganone)
felbamate (Felbatol)
gabapentin (Neurontin)
lamotrigine (Lamictal)
mephenytoin (Mesantoin)
methsuximide (Celontin)
paramethadione (Paradione)
phenacemide (Phenurone)
phenobarbital (Luminal)
phensuximide (Milontin)
phenytoin (Dilantin)
primidone (Mysoline)
trimethadione (Tridione)
valproic acid (Depakene)

Antidepressant Drugs

Bicyclic Antidepressants
fluoxetine (Prozac)
venlafaxine (Effexor)

Tricyclic Antidepressants
amitriptyline (Elavil, Endep)
amoxapine (Asendin)
clomipramine (Anafranil)
desipramine (Norpramin, Pertofrane)
doxepin (Adapin, Sinequan)
imipramine (Janimine, Tofranil)
nortriptyline (Aventyl, Pamelor)
protriptyline (Vivactil)
trimipramine (Surmontil)

Tetracyclic Antidepressant
maprotiline (Ludiomil)

Other Antidepressants
bupropion (Wellbutrin)
fluvoxamine (Luvox)
nefazodone (Serzone)
paroxetine (Paxil)
sertraline (Zoloft)
trazodone (Desyrel)

Monoamine Oxidase (MAO) Inhibitors
See class below.

Antiemetic Drugs

Anti-Motion Sickness, Antinausea Drugs
chlorpromazine (Thorazine)
cyclizine (Marezine)
dimenhydrinate (Dramamine)
diphenhydramine (Benadryl)
granisetron (Kytril)
hydroxyzine (Atarax, Vistaril)
meclizine (Antivert, Bonine)
ondansetron (Zofran)
prochlorperazine (Compazine)
promethazine (Phenergan)
scopolamine (Transderm Scop)
trimethobenzamide (Tigan)

Antifungal Drugs

Anti-Infectives
amphotericin B (Fungizone)
fluconazole (Diflucan)
flucytosine (Ancobon)
griseofulvin (Fulvicin, Grifulvin, Grisactin)
itraconazole (Sporanox)
ketoconazole (Nizoral)
miconazole (Monistat)
nystatin (Mycostatin)

Anti-Glaucoma Drugs

acetazolamide (Diamox)
betaxolol (Betoptic)
epinephrine (Glaucon)
pilocarpine (Isopto-carpine)
timolol (Timoptic)

Anti-Gout Drugs

allopurinol (Zyloprim)
colchicine (no brand name)
diclofenac (Cataflam, Voltaren)
fenoprofen (Nalfon)
ibuprofen (Advil, Motrin, Nuprin, Rufin)
indomethacin (Indocin)
ketoprofen (Orudis)
mefenamic acid (Ponstel)
naproxen (Anaprox, Naprosyn)
oxaprozin (Daypro)
phenylbutazone (Azolid, Butazolidin)
piroxicam (Feldene)
probenecid (Benemid)
sulfinpyrazone (Anturane)
sulindac (Clinoril)

Antihistamines

astemizole (Hismanal)
azatadine (Optimine)
brompheniramine (Dimetane, others)
carbinoxamine (Clistin, Rondec)
chlorpheniramine (Chlor-Trimeton, Teldrin)
clemastine (Tavist)
cyclizine (Marezine)
cyproheptadine (Periactin)
dimenhydrinate (Dramamine)
diphenhydramine (Benadryl)
doxylamine (Unisom)
loratadine (Claritin, Claritin Extra)
meclizine (Antivert, Bonine)
orphenadrine (Norflex)
pheniramine (component of Triaminic)
promethazine (Phenergan, others)
pyrilamine (component of Triaminic)
terfenadine (Seldane)
tripelennamine (Pyribenzamine, PBZ)
triprolidine (component of Actifed and Sudahist)

Antihypertensive Drugs

See the Disorder Profile of hypertension in Section Three for a detailed list.
clonidine (Catapres)
doxazosin (Cardura)

guanabenz (Wytensin)
guanadrel (Hylorel)
guanethidine (Ismelin)
guanfacine (Tenex)
hydralazine (Apresoline)
methyldopa (Aldomet)
minoxidil (Loniten)
prazosin (Minipres)
reserpine (Serpasil)
terazosin (Hytrin)
    See also the following Drug Classes:
Angiotensin-converting enzyme (ACE) inhibitors
Angiotensin II receptor antagonist
Beta-adrenergic-blocking drugs
Calcium channel-blocking drugs
Diuretics

Anti-Infective Drugs

See specific anti-infective Drug Class:
Aminoglycosides
Antifungal drugs
Antileprosy drugs
Antimalarial drugs
Antituberculosis drugs
Antiviral drugs
Cephalosporins
Fluoroquinolones
Macrolides
Penicillins
Sulfonamides
Tetracyclines

Miscellaneous Anti-Infective Drugs
atovaquone (Mepron)
chloramphenicol (Chloromycetin)
clindamycin (Cleocin)
colistin (Coly-Mycin S)
furazolidone (Furoxone)
lincomycin (Lincocin)
nalidixic acid (NegGram)
nitrofurantoin (Furadantin, Macrodantin)
novobiocin (Albamycin)
pentamidine (Pentam-300)
trimethoprim (Proloprim, Trimpex)
vancomycin (Vancocin)

Antileprosy Drugs

Anti-Infectives
clofazimine (Lamprene)
dapsone (no brand name)

Antimalarial Drugs

Anti-Infectives
chloroquine (Aralen)
doxycycline (Vibramycin)
hydroxychloraquine (Plaquenil)
mefloquine (Lariam)
primaquine (no brand name)
pyrimethamine (Daraprim)
quinacrine (Atabrine)
quinine (no brand name)
sulfadoxine/pyrimethamine (Fansidar)

Anti-Migraine Drugs

See the Disorder Profile of migraine headache in Section Three for a detailed
list.
atenolol (Tenormin)
ergotamine (Ergostat)
methysergide (Sansert)
metoprolol (Lopressor)
nadolol (Corgard)
nifedipine (Procardia)
propranolol (Inderal)
sumatriptan (Imitrex)
timolol (Blocadren)
verapamil (Calan, Isoptin)

Antiparkinsonism Drugs

amantadine (Symmetrel)
benztropine (Cogentin)
bromocriptine (Parlodel)
diphenhydramine (Benadryl)
levodopa (Dopar, Larodopa)
levodopa/bensarazide (Prolopa)
levodopa/carbidopa (Sinemet, Sinemet CR)
pergolide (Permax)
selegiline (Eldepryl)
trihexyphenidyl (Artane)

Antiplatelet Drugs

Platelet Aggregation Inhibitors
aspirin (Bufferin, Ecotrin, others)
dipyridamole (Persantine)
sulfinpyrazone (Anturane)
ticlopidine (Ticlid)

Antipsychotic Drugs

Neuroleptics, Major Tranquilizers
See Phenothiazine class below.
chlorprothixene (Taractan)
clozapine (Clozaril)
haloperidol (Haldol)
loxapine (Loxitane)
molindone (Moban)
pimozide (Orap)
risperidone (Risperdol)
thiothixene (Navane)

Antispasmodics, Synthetic

anisotropine (Valpin)
clidinium (Quarzan)
glycopyrrolate (Robinul)
hexocyclium (Tral)
isopropamide (Darbid)
mepenzolate (Cantil)
methantheline (Banthine)
methscopolamine (Pamine)
propantheline (Pro-Banthine)
tridihexethyl (Pathilon)

Antituberculosis Drugs

aminosalicylate sodium (Sodium P.A.S.)
capreomycin (Capastat)
cycloserine (Seromycin)
ethambutol (Myambutol)
ethionamide (Trecator-SC)
isoniazid (Laniazid, Nidrazid)
pyrazinamide (no brand name)
rifabutin (Mycobutin)
rifampin (Rifadin, Rimactane)
streptomycin (no brand name)

Antitussive Drugs

Cough Suppressants
benzonatate (Tessalon)
codeine (no brand name)
dextromethorphan (Hold DM, Suppress)
diphenhydramine (Benylin)
hydrocodone (Hycodan)
hydromorphone (Dilaudid)
promethazine (Phenergan)

Antiviral Drugs

Anti-Infectives
acyclovir (Zovirax)
amantadine (Symmetrel)
didanosine (Videx)
famciclovir (Famvir)
foscarnet (Foscavir)
ganciclovir (Cytovene)
ribavirin (Virazole)
rimantadine (no brand name)
stavudine (Zerit)
vidarabine (Vira A)
zalcitabine (Hivid)
zidovudine (Retrovir)

Barbiturates

amobarbital (Amytal)
aprobarbital (Alurate)
butabarbital (Butisol)
mephobarbital (Mebaral)
metharbital (Gemonil)
pentobarbital (Nembutal)
phenobarbital (Luminal, Solfoton)
secobarbital (Seconal)
talbutal (Lotusate)

Benzodiazepines

alprazolam (Xanax)
bromazepam (Lectopam)
chlordiazepoxide (Libritabs, Librium)
clonazepam (Klonopin)
clorazepate (Tranxene)

diazepam (Valium, Vazepam)
flurazepam (Dalmane)
halazepam (Paxipam)
ketazolam (Loftran)
lorazepam (Ativan)
midazolam (Versed)
nitrazepam (Mogadon)
oxazepam (Serax)
prazepam (Centrax)
quazepam (Doral)
temazepam (Restoril)
triazolam (Halcion)

Beta-Adrenergic-Blocking Drugs

Beta-Blockers
acebutolol (Sectral)
atenolol (Tenormin)
betaxolol (Kerlone)
bisoprolol (Zebta)
bisoprolol/hydrochlorothiazide (Ziac)
carteolol (Cartrol)
labetalol (Normodyne, Trandate)
metoprolol (Lopressor)
nadolol (Corgard)
penbutolol (Levatol)
pindolol (Visken)
propranolol (Inderal)
timolol (Blocadren)

Calcium Channel-Blocking Drugs

Calcium Blockers
bepridil (Vascor)
diltiazem (Cardizem)
felodipine (Plendil)
isradipine (DynaCirc)
nicardipine (Cardene)
nifedipine (Adalat, Procardia)
nimodipine (Nimotop)
verapamil (Calan, Isoptin)

Cephalosporins

Anti-Infectives
cefaclor (Ceclor)
cefadroxil (Duricef, Ultracef)

cefamandole (Mandol)
cefazolin (Ancef, Kefzol, Zolicef)
cefixime (Suprax)
cefmetazole (Zefazone)
cefonicid (Monocid)
cefoperazone (Cefobid)
ceforanide (Precef)
cefotaxime (Claforan)
cefotetan (Cefotan)
cefoxitin (Mefoxin)
cefprozil (Cefzil)
ceftazidime (Fortaz, Tazidime, Tazicef)
ceftizoxime (Cefizox)
ceftriaxone (Rocephin)
cefuroxime (Ceftin, Kefurox, Zinacef)
cephalexin (Keflex, Keftab)
cephalothin (Keflin)
cephapirin (Cefadyl)
cephradine (Anspor, Velosef)
moxalactam (Moxam)

Cholesterol-Reducing Drugs

cholestyramine (Cholybar, Questran)
clofibrate (Atromid-S)
colestipol (Colestid)
dextrothyroxine (Choloxin)
fenofibrate (Lipidil)
gemfibrozil (Lopid)
lovastatin (Mevacor)
niacin (Nicobid, Slo-Niacin, others)
pravastatin (Pravachol)
probucol (Lorelco)
simvastatin (Zocor)

Decongestants

ephedrine (Efedron, Ephedsol)
naphazoline (Naphcon, Vasocon)
oxymetazoline (Afrin, Duration, others)
phenylephrine (Neo-Synephrine, others)
phenylpropanolamine (Propadrine, Propagest, others)
pseudoephedrine (Afrinol, Sudafed, others)
tetrahydrozoline (Tyzine, Visine, others)
xylometazoline (Otrivin)

Digitalis Preparations

deslanoside (Cedilanid-D)
digitoxin (Crystodigin)
digoxin (Lanoxicaps, Lanoxin)

Diuretics

acetazolamide (Diamox)
amiloride (Midamor)
bumetanide (Bumex)
chlorthalidone (Hygroton)
ethacrynic acid (Edecrin)
furosemide (Lasix)
indapamide (Lozol)
metolazone (Diulo, Zaroxolyn)
spironolactone (Aldactone)
thiazide diuretics (see Class below)
triamterene (Dyrenium)

Estrogens

Female Sex Hormones
chlorotrianisene (Tace)
diethylstilbestrol (DES, Stilphostrol)
estradiol (Estrace, Estraderm, others)
estrogens, conjugated (Premarin)
estrogens, esterified (Estratab, Menest)
estrone (Theelin, others)
estropipate (Ogen)
ethinyl estradiol (Estinyl)
quinestrol (Estrovis)

Fluoroquinolones

Anti-Infectives
ciprofloxacin (Cipro)
lomefloxacin (Maxaquin)
norfloxacin (Noroxin)
ofloxacin (Floxin)

Histamine-Blocking Drugs

Histamine H-2 Blockers
cimetidine (Tagamet)
famotidine (Pepcid)

nizatidine (Axid)
ranitidine (Zantac)

Hypnotic Drugs

Sedatives/Sleep Inducers
acetylcarbromal (Paxarel)
chloral hydrate (Aquachloral, Noctec)
estazolam (ProSom)
ethchlorvynol (Placidyl)
ethinamate (Valmid)
flurazepam (Dalmane)
glutethimide (Doriden)
methyprylon (Noludar)
paraldehyde (Paral)
propiomazine (Largon)
quazepam (Doral)
temazepam (Restoril)
triazolam (Halcion)
zolpidem (Ambien)
    See also Barbiturate class.

Macrolide Antibiotics

Anti-Infectives
azithromycin (Zithromax)
clarithromycin (Biaxin)
erythromycin (E-Mycin, Ilosone, Erythrocin, E.E.S.)
troleandomycin (Tao)

Monoamine Oxidase (MAO) Inhibitor Drugs

Type A: Antidepressants
isocarboxazid (Marplan)
phenelzine (Nardil)
tranylcypromine (Parnate)

Muscle Relaxants

Skeletal Muscle Relaxants
baclofen (Lioresal)
carisoprodol (Rela, Soma, others)
chlorphenesin carbamate (Maolate)
chlorzoxazone (Paraflex, Parafon Forte)
cyclobenzaprine (Flexeril)
dantrolene (Dantrium)
diazepam (Valium)

meprobamate (Equanil, Miltown, others)
metaxalone (Skelaxin)
methocarbamol (Robaxin, others)
orphenadrine (Norflex, others)

Nitrates

amyl nitrate (Amyl Nitrate Vaporole, others)
erythrityl tetranitrate (Cardilate)
isosorbide dinitrate (Isordil, Sorbitrate, others)
isosorbide mononitrate (Ismo)
nitroglycerin (Nitrostat, Nitrolingual, Nitrogard, Nitrong, others)
pentaerythritol tetranitrate (Duotrate, Peritrate)

Nonsteroidal Anti-Inflammatory Drugs (NSAIDs)

Aspirin Substitutes

diclofenac (Cataflam, Voltaren)
diflunisal (Dolobid)
etodolac (Lodine)
fenoprofen (Nalfon)
flurbiprofen (Ansaid)
ibuprofen (Advil, Haltran, Motrin, Nuprin, others)
indomethacin (Indocin, others)
ketoprofen (Orudis)
ketorolac (Toradol)
meclofenamate (Meclomen)
mefenamic acid (Ponstel)
nabumetone (Relafen)
naproxen (Aleve, Anaprox, Naprosyn)
oxaprozin (Daypro)
phenylbutazone (Azolid, Butazolidin)
piroxicam (Feldene)
sulindac (Clinoril)
suprofen (Profenal)
tolmetin (Tolectin)

Opioid Drugs

Narcotics

alfentanil (Alfenta)
codeine (no brand name)
fentanyl (Sublimaze, Duragesic)
hydrocodone (Hycodan)
hydromorphone (Dilaudid)
levorphanol (Levo-Dromoran)
meperidine (Demerol)

methadone (Dolophine)
morphine (Astramorph, Duramorph, MS Contin, Roxanol)
oxycodone (Roxicodone)
oxymorphone (Numorphan)
propoxyphene (Darvon)
sufentanil (Sufenta)

Penicillins

Anti-Infectives
amoxicillin (Amoxil, Larotid, Polymox, Trimox, others)
amoxicillin/clavulanate (Augmentin)
ampicillin (Omnipen, Polycillin, Principen, Totacillin)
ampicillin/sulbactam (Unasyn)
bacampicillin (Spectrobid)
carbenicillin (Geocillin, Geopen, Pyopen)
cloxacillin (Cloxapen, Tegopen)
dicloxacillin (Dynapen, Pathocil, Veracillin)
methicillin (Staphcillin)
mezlocillin (Mezlin)
nafcillin (Nafcil, Unipen)
oxacillin (Prostaphlin)
penicillin G (Pentids, others)
penicillin V (Pen Vee K, V-Cillin K, Veetids, others)
piperacillin (Pipracil)
ticarcillin (Ticar)
ticarcillin/clavulanate (Timentin)

Phenothiazines

Antipsychotic Drugs
acetophenazine (Tindal)
chlorpromazine (Thorazine)
fluphenazine (Permitil, Prolixin)
mesoridazine (Serentil)
perphenazine (Trilafon)
prochlorperazine (Compazine)
promazine (Sparine)
thioridazine (Mellaril)
trifluoperazine (Stelazine)
triflupromazine (Vesprin)

Progestins

Female Sex Hormones
ethynodiol (no brand name)
hydroxyprogesterone (Duralutin, Gesterol L.A., others)

medroxyprogesterone (Amen, Curretab, Provera)
megestrol (Megace)
norethindrone (Micronor, Norlutate, Norlutin)
norgestrel (Ovrette)
progesterone (Gesterol 50, Progestaject)

Salicylates

aspirin (ASA, Bufferin, Ecotrin, Empirin, others)
choline salicylate (Arthropan)
magnesium salicylate (Doan's, Magan, Mobidin)
salsalate (Amigesic, Disalcid, Salsitab)
sodium salicylate (no brand name)
sodium thiosalicylate (Rexolate, Tusal)

Sulfonamides

Anti-Infectives
multiple sulfonamides (Triple Sulfa No. 2)
sulfacytine (Renoquid)
sulfadiazine (no brand name)
sulfamethizole (Thiosulfil)
sulfamethoxazole (Gantanol)
sulfasalazine (Azulfidine)
sulfisoxazole (Gantrisin)

Sulfonylureas

Oral Antidiabetic Drugs
acetohexamide (Dymelor)
chlorpropamide (Diabinese)
glipizide (Glucotrol)
glyburide (DiaBeta, Micronase)
tolazamide (Ronase, Tolamide, Tolinase)
tolbutamide (Orinase)

Tetracyclines

Anti-Infectives
demeclocycline (Declomycin)
doxycycline (Doryx, Doxychel, Vibramycin)
methacycline (Rondomycin)
minocycline (Minocin)
oxytetracycline (Terramycin)
tetracycline (Achromycin V, Panmycin, Sumycin)

Thiazide Diuretics

bendroflumethiazide (Naturetin)
benzthiazide (Aquatag, Exna, Marazide)
chlorothiazide (Diuril)
cyclothiazide (Anhydron)
hydrochlorothiazide (Esidrix, Hydrodiuril, Oretic)
hydroflumethiazide (Diucardin, Saluron)
methyclothiazide (Enduron, Aquatensen)
polythiazide (Renese)
trichlormethiazide (Metahydrin, Naqua)

Vasodilators

Peripheral Vasodilators
cyclandelate (Cyclospasmol)
ethaverine (Ethaquin, Isovex)
isoxsuprine (Vasodilan)
nylidrin (Arlidin)
papaverine (Cerespan, Pavabid)

Xanthines

Bronchodilators
aminophylline (Phyllocontin, Truphylline)
dyphylline (Dilor, Lufyllin)
oxtriphylline (Choledyl)
theophylline (Bronkodyl, Slo-Phyllin, Theolair, others)

APPENDIX 17

Drug Information Sources

Within each Disorder Profile in Section Three you will find information categories that review drug therapies currently available for the disorder. Names of the drugs most commonly prescribed are listed, and some general principles regarding their use are presented. Space limitations do not allow the in-depth coverage of drug information that all patients need to use their medications effectively and safely. However, such information is readily available from a variety of sources. The following reference books provide appropriate drug information in detail. It is advisable to use one of these in conjunction with this book to further enhance your ability to be an active participant in the management of your health care. They can be found in community libraries, purchased at local bookstores, or obtained directly from the publisher. Prices are current at this writing but are subject to change.

References Written Primarily for the Patient

The Essential Guide to Prescription Drugs 1997, James J. Rybacki, Pharm.D., and James W. Long, M.D. New York: HarperCollins, 1997. Order Dept.: 1-800-242-7737. $20.00

USP DI Volume II, Advice for the Patient: Drug Information in Lay Language 1997. Rockville, MD: The United States Pharmacopeia, 1997. Order Dept.: 1-800-877-6733. $61.00

Worst Pills, Best Pills II: The Older Adult's Guide to Avoiding Drug-Induced Death or Illness, Sidney Wolfe, M.D. Washington, DC: Public Citizen. Order Dept.: (202) 588-1000. $15.00

References Written Primarily for Health Care Professionals

USP DI Volume I, Drug Information for the Health Care Professional 1997. Rockville, MD: The United States Pharmacopeia. Order Dept.: 1-800-877-6733. $117.00

Physicians' GenRx 1997: The Complete Drug Reference, Denniston Publishing Inc. St. Louis, MO: Mosby-Year Book. Order Dept.: 1-800-426-4545. $63.00

AHFS Drug Information 97. Bethesda, MD: The American Society of Health-System Pharmacists. Order Dept.: (301) 657-4383. $130.00

Drug Facts and Comparisons 1997, annual hardbound edition. St. Louis, MO: Facts and Comparisons. Order Dept.: 1-800-223-0554. $120.00

General Health Information Sources

It is well documented that patients who actively participate in the diagnostic and therapeutic aspects of their health care are more satisfied with their physicians and attain better treatment outcomes. To be successful, active participation requires involvement in two ways: (1) research—learning as much as possible about your condition; and (2) communication—discussing your problems openly with your health care professionals and getting the answers you need.

Patient education is a growing industry. There are numerous sources of useful information readily available to health care consumers. Many publications are free for the asking; others can be purchased at modest cost. The following sources are recommended.

Government Publications and Services

• The National Institutes of Health: 1-800-644-6627
Call to ask for the listing of Consensus Statements on more than 60 disorders. These are the conclusions reached by experts during the three-day Consensus Developing Conferences sponsored by NIH.
• The Public Health Service's Agency for Health Care Policy and Research: 1-800-358-9295
Call to ask for the current listing of Clinical Practice Guidelines developed by experts.
• The Office of Disease Prevention and Health Promotion
National Health Information Center
P.O. Box 1133
Washington, DC 20013-1133
Phone: 1-800-336-4979
This agency provides a referral service to specific health information organizations that are pertinent to the caller's disorder.

Private Organization Publications and Services

The last information category of the Disorder Profiles in Section Three is labeled "Resources." All appropriate nonprofit organizations that raise funds for education and research (for a particular disorder) are listed there; they are a most valuable source of information. Most of them provide substantive written information; some of them also provide a referral service to appropriate specialists in the caller's area.

Libraries

- Most public libraries have a well-stocked section devoted to health and medical matters. The collection usually includes books that provide information on a single disorder—heart disease, hypertension, prostate disorders, etc. Ask the librarian to help you find the specific reference you need. Many community libraries participate in an interlibrary loan service and can obtain books not available in their collection.
- Medical libraries are usually found in hospitals, medical schools, and some government agencies; their services may be limited to the medical staff of the institution. Call the National Network of Libraries of Medicine—1-800-338-7657—to find a medical library that is open to the public.
- Some public libraries may also subscribe to computer services provided by the National Library of Medicine (NLM) in Bethesda, Maryland, the largest medical library in the world. Using the interactive computer program "Grateful Med," the librarian can assist you in conducting a search for specific information in the NLM MEDLINE database.

Commercial Publications

Books

- *The Consumer's Medical Desk Reference: Everything You Need to Know for the Best in Health Care.* The People's Medical Society, 462 Walnut Street, Lower Level, Allentown, PA 18102. Phone: 1-800-624-8773. Also provides a Health Library Catalog that describes numerous books on common disorders.
- *Mayo Clinic Family Health Book,* David E. Larson, M.D., ed. New York: William Marrow, 1990.
- *The Johns Hopkins Medical Handbook: The 100 Major Medical Disorders of People over the Age of 50,* Simeon Margolis, M.D., Ph.D., ed. New York: Rebus, 1995.
- *Johns Hopkins Symptoms and Remedies: The Complete Home Medical Reference,* Simeon Margolis, M.D., Ph.D., ed. New York: Rebus, 1995.
- *All About Eve: The Complete Guide to Women's Health and Well-being,* Tracy Chutorian Semler. New York: HarperCollins Publishers, 1995.
- *Caring for the Mind: The Comprehensive Guide to Mental Health,* Dianne Hales and Robert E. Hales, M.D. New York: Bantam Books, 1995.

- *The American Geriatrics Society's Complete Guide to Aging and Health,* Mark E. Williams, M.D. New York: Harmony Books, Crown Publishers, 1995.

Electronic Media

Dr. Schueler's Health Information, Inc.
P.O. Drawer 410129
Melbourne, FL 32941-0129
Phone: 1-800-788-2099
 CD-ROMs: *Dr. Schueler's Home Medical Advisor Pro V 5.0; Dr. Schueler's Corner Drug Store; Dr. Schueler's Self-Health*

Alpha Media
P.O. Box 1719
Maryland Heights, MO 63043-1719
Phone: 1-800-832-1000
 CD-ROM: *Mayo Clinic Family Health Book,* Interactive Edition
 CD-ROM: *The Merck Manual, 16th Edition*
 Access to *US HealthLink* On-Line

Sources

The following sources were consulted in the creation of this book:

Abrams, W.B., and Berkow, R., eds. *The Merck Manual of Geriatrics.* Rahway, NJ: Merck, 1990.

Acute Pain Management: Operative or Medical Procedures and Trauma. Clinical Practice Guideline. AHCPR Pub. No. 92-0032. Rockville, MD: Public Health Service, February 1992.

Adverse Drug Reaction Bulletin. D.M. Davies, ed. Weybridge, Surrey, United Kingdom: Meditext, 1995.

AMA Department of Drugs, *AMA Drug Evaluations.* Chicago: American Medical Association, 1995.

Anderson, J., and Deskins, B., *The Nutrition Bible.* New York: William Morrow, 1995.

Andriole, G.L., and Catalona, W.J., eds. "Advanced Prostatic Carcinoma." *The Urologic Clinics of North America,* Vol. 18, No. 1, February 1991. Philadelphia: W.B. Saunders.

Andreoli, T.E., Carpenter, C.C.J., Plum, F., and Smith, L.H., eds. *Cecil Essentials of Medicine.* Philadelphia: W.B. Saunders, 1986.

Arndt, K.A., *Manual of Dermatologic Therapeutics,* 4th edition. Boston: Little, Brown and Co., 1989.

Atkinson, A.J., Ambre, J.J., *Kalman and Clark's Drug Assay, The Strategy of Therapeutic Drug Monitoring,* 2nd edition. New York: Masson Publishing USA, 1985.

Ayd, F.J., *Lexicon of Psychiatry, Neurology, and the Neurosciences.* Baltimore: Williams and Wilkins, 1995.

Bartlett, J., *Medical Management of HIV Infection.* Glenview, IL: Physicians and Scientists Publishing, 1994.

Berkow, R., ed., *The Merck Manual,* 16th edition. Rahway, NJ: Merck Sharp and Dohme Research Laboratories, 1992.

Bone, R.C., and Rosen, R.L., *Quick Reference to Internal Medicine: Outline Format.* New York: Igaku-Shoin, 1994.

Borda, I.T., and Koff, R.S., *NSAIDs: A Profile of Adverse Effects.* St. Louis: Mosby-Year Book, 1992.

Braddom, R.L., *Physical Medicine & Rehabilitation.* Philadelphia: W.B. Saunders, 1996.

Branch, W.T., *Office Practice of Medicine,* 3rd edition. Philadelphia: W.B. Saunders, 1994.

Briggs, G.G., Freeman, R.K., and Yaffee, S.J., *Drugs in Pregnancy and Lactation.* Baltimore: Williams and Wilkins, 1994.

Brooke, M.H., *A Clinician's View of Neuromuscular Diseases,* 2nd edition. Baltimore: Williams and Wilkins, 1986.

Cancer Facts. PDQ Search Service, National Cancer Institute, National Institutes of Health, 1996.

Carr, P.L., Freund, K.M., and Somani, S., *The Medical Care of Women.* Philadelphia: W.B. Saunders, 1995.

Centers for Disease Control and Prevention, *HIV/AIDS Surveillance Report,* Vol. 7, December 1995.

Clark, W.R., *At War Within: The Double-Edged Sword of Immunity.* New York: Oxford University Press, 1995.

Clin-Alert. Medford, NJ: Clin-Alert, 1989–1996.

Clinical Abstracts/Current Therapeutic Findings. D.J. Thordsen and P.G. Jaworski, eds. Cincinnati: Harvey Whitney Books, 1995.

Collier, J.A.B., Longmore, J.M., and Hodgetts, T.J., *Oxford Handbook of Clinical Specialties.* New York: Oxford University Press, 1995.

Coyle, P.K., *Lyme Disease.* St. Louis: Mosby-Year Book, 1993.

Davies, D.M., ed., *Textbook of Adverse Drug Reactions,* 4th edition. New York: Oxford University Press, 1991.

DeGregorio, M.W., and Wiebe, V.J., *Tamoxifen and Breast Cancer.* New Haven: Yale University Press, 1994.

Diamond, S., and Dalessio, D.J., eds., *The Practicing Physician's Approach to Headache,* 4th edition. Baltimore: Williams and Wilkins, 1986.

Dorland's Medical Dictionary, 28th edition. Philadelphia: W.B. Saunders, 1994.

Drug Interaction Facts. D.S. Tatro, ed. St. Louis: Facts and Comparisons, 1996.

Drug Newsletter. B.R. Olin, ed. St. Louis: Facts and Comparisons, 1996.

Drug Therapy, Physicians Prescribing Update. Lawrenceville, NJ: Excerpta Medica, 1996.

Drugs of Choice. New Rochelle, NY: The Medical Letter, 1996.

Dukes, M.N.G., ed., *Meyler's Side Effects of Drugs,* 11th edition. Amsterdam: Excerpta Medica, 1988.

Dunner, D.L., *Current Psychiatric Therapy.* Philadelphia: W.B. Saunders, 1993.

Encyclopedia of Associations, 30th edition. Vol. 1, Part 2, Section 8. Detroit: Gale Research, 1996.

Facts and Comparisons. B.R. Olin, ed. St. Louis: Facts and Comparisons, 1995.

F.D.A. Drug Bulletin. Rockville, MD: Department of Health and Human Services, Food and Drug Administration.

Foley, J.F., Vose, J.M., and Armitage, J.O., *Current Therapy in Cancer.* Philadelphia: W.B. Saunders, 1994.

Fraunfelder, F.T., *Drug-Induced Ocular Side Effects and Drug Interactions,* 3rd edition. Philadelphia: Lea and Febiger, 1989.

Goodman, L.S., and Gilman, A., eds., *The Pharmacological Basis of Therapeutics,* 8th edition. New York: Macmillan, 1990.

Greenberger, N.J., Arvanitakis, C., and Hurwitz, A., *Drug Treatment of Gastrointestinal Disorders.* New York: Churchill Livingstone, 1978.

Guide to Clinical Preventive Services, Report of the U.S. Preventive Services Task Force, 2nd edition. Baltimore: Williams and Wilkins, 1996.

Hales, D., and Hales, R.E., *Caring for the Mind: The Comprehensive Guide to Mental Health.* New York: Bantam Books, 1995.

Hallowell, E.M., and Ratey, J.J., *Answers to Distraction.* New York: Pantheon Books, 1994.

Hazzard, W.R., et al., eds., *Principles of Geriatric Medicine and Gerontology.* New York: McGraw-Hill, 1994.

Heinonen, O.P., Slone, D., and Shapiro, S., *Birth Defects and Drugs in Pregnancy.* Littleton, MA: PSG Publishing Co., 1977.

Hollister, L.E., *Clinical Pharmacology of Psychotherapeutic Drugs,* 2nd edition. New York: Churchill Livingstone, 1983.

Hurst, J.W., ed., *Medicine for the Practicing Physician,* 2nd edition. Boston: Butterworths, 1988.

Inlander, C.B., *The Consumer's Medical Desk Reference.* New York: Hyperion, 1995.

International Drug Therapy Newsletter. F.J. Ayd, ed. Baltimore: Ayd Medical Communications, 1996.

Jefferson, J.W., and Greist, J.H., *Primer of Lithium Therapy.* Baltimore: Williams and Wilkins, 1977.

Journal of the American Medical Association. G.D. Lundberg, ed. Chicago: American Medical Association, 1996.

Kelley, W.N., et al., *Textbook of Rheumatology,* 4th edition. Vol. 1. Philadelphia: W.B. Saunders, 1993.

Kirby, R.S., and Christmas, T.J., *Benign Prostatic Hyperplasia.* London: Gower Medical Publishing, 1993.

Klippel, J.H., ed., "Systemic Lupus Erythematosus." *Rheumatic Disease Clinics of North America*, Vol. 14, No. 1, April 1988. Philadelphia: W.B. Saunders.

Koller, W.C., ed., *Handbook of Parkinson's Disease.* New York: Marcel Dekker, 1987.

Lawrence, R.A., *Breast-Feeding.* St. Louis: Mosby, 1980.

Lepor, H., and Walsh, P.C., eds. "Benign Prostatic Hyperplasia." *The Urologic Clinics of North America,* Vol. 17, No. 3, August 1990. Philadelphia: W.B. Saunders.

Matthay, R.A., ed., "Lung Cancer." *Clinics in Chest Medicine*, Vol. 14, No. 1, March 1993. Philadelphia: W.B. Saunders.

McEvoy, G.K., ed., *American Hospital Formulary Service, Drug Information 1993.* Bethesda, MD: American Society of Hospital Pharmacists, 1996.

The Medical Letter on Drugs and Therapeutics. H. Aaron, ed. New Rochelle, NY: The Medical Letter, 1996.

Messerli, F.H., ed., *Current Clinical Practice.* Philadelphia: W.B. Saunders, 1987.

The New England Journal of Medicine. J.P. Kassirer, ed. Boston: The Massachusetts Medical Society, 1996.

Noble, J., ed., *Textbook of Primary Care Medicine,* 2nd edition. St. Louis: Mosby-Year Book, 1996.

Nuland, S.B., *How We Die: Reflections on Life's Final Chapter.* New York: Alfred A. Knopf, 1994.

Nyhus, L.M., and Baker, R.J., eds., *Mastery of Surgery,* 2nd edition. Vol. 1. Boston: Little, Brown and Co., 1992.

Patient Drug Facts. B.R. Olin, ed. St. Louis: Facts and Comparisons, 1996.

Postgraduate Medicine, The Journal of Applied Medicine for the Primary Care Physician. Minneapolis: McGraw-Hill, 1996.

Raj, P.P., *Practical Management of Pain,* 2nd edition. St. Louis: Mosby-Year Book, 1992.

Rakel, R.E., ed., *Conn's Current Therapy 1996.* Philadelphia: W.B. Saunders, 1996.

Rakel, R.E., ed., *Saunders Manual of Medical Practice.* Philadelphia: W.B. Saunders, 1996.

Reynolds, J.E.F., ed. *Martindale, The Extra Pharmacopoeia,* 30th edition. London: The Pharmaceutical Press, 1993.

Rogers, C.S., and McCue, J.D., eds., *Managing Chronic Disease.* Oradell, NJ: Medical Economics Books, 1987.

Rous, S.N., *The Prostate Book*. New York: W.W. Norton, 1988.

Ruoff, M., *Helicobacter Pylori and the Stomach*. Mediguide to Infectious Diseases, 1993.

Rybacki, J.J., and Long, J.W., *The Essential Guide to Prescription Drugs 1996*. New York: HarperCollins Publishers, 1996.

Sauer, G.C., *Manual of Skin Diseases,* 5th edition. Philadelphia: J.B. Lippincott, 1985.

Semla, T.P., Beizer, J.L., and Higbee, M.D., *Geriatric Dosage Handbook*. Hudson, OH: Lexi-Comp, 1993.

Sickle Cell Disease: Screening, Diagnosis, Management, and Counseling in Newborns and Infants. Clinical Practice Guideline No. 6, Public Health Service, Agency for Health Care Policy and Research, Rockville, MD. AHCPR Publication No. 93-0562.

Sleisenger, M.H., and Fordtran, J.S., eds., *Gastrointestinal Disease: Pathophysiology/Diagnosis/Management,* 5th edition. Philadelphia: W.B. Saunders, 1993.

Smith, J.A., ed., "Early Detection and Treatment of Localized Carcinoma of the Prostate." *The Urologic Clinics of North America,* Vol. 17, No. 4, November 1990. Philadelphia: W.B. Saunders.

Smith, L.H., and Thier, S.O., *Pathophysiology, The Biological Principles of Disease,* 2nd edition. Philadelphia: W.B. Saunders, 1985.

Snider, D.E., ed., "Mycobacterial Diseases." *Clinics in Chest Medicine,* Vol. 10, No. 3, September 1989. Philadelphia: W.B. Saunders.

Speight, T.M., ed., *Avery's Drug Treatment,* 3rd edition. Auckland: ADIS Press, 1987.

Stein, J.H., ed., *Internal Medicine,* 4th edition. St. Louis: Mosby-Year Book, 1994.

Swash, M., and Schwartz, M.S., *Neuromuscular Diseases,* 2nd edition. Berlin: Springer-Verlag, 1988.

USP Dispensing Information 1996, 16th edition. Vol. 1: Drug Information for the Health Care Professional. Rockville, MD: United States Pharmacopeial Convention, 1996.

Utian, W.H., *Menopause in Modern Perspective*. New York: Appleton-Century-Crofts, 1980.

Wallace, R.J., ed., "Lower Respiratory Tract Infections." *Infectious Disease Clinics of North America,* Vol. 5, No. 3, September 1991. Philadelphia: W.B. Saunders.

Wallach, J., *Interpretation of Diagnostic Tests,* 5th edition. Boston: Little, Brown and Co., 1992.

Williams, M.E., *Complete Guide to Aging and Health*. New York: Harmony Books, 1995.

Young, D.S., *Effects of Drugs on Clinical Laboratory Tests, 1991 Supplement*. Washington: AACC Press, 1991.

Index

ABOUT THE AUTHOR

James W. Long, M.D., was born in Allentown, Pennsylvania. He received his premedical education from the University of Maryland and his medical degree from the George Washington University School of Medicine in Washington, D.C. Following residency training in internal medicine, he served two years in the U.S. Army Medical Corps during World War II. His tour of duty on the infectious disease service at the George G. Meade Regional Hospital provided the opportunity to witness the earliest uses of penicillin and the birth of the antibiotic era. After a teaching fellowship at Johns Hopkins School of Medicine, he engaged in the private practice of internal medicine for 20 years in the Washington metropolitan area. For 25 years he served on the faculty of the George Washington University School of Medicine.

The second 20 years of Dr. Long's medical career included service in several pivotal settings within the federal government that allowed him to acquire a generalist's view of this most revolutionary period in American medicine. He held positions in the Food and Drug Administration, the National Library of Medicine, and the Bureau of Health Manpower at the National Institutes of Health. During the last 15 years of federal service, Dr. Long was director of Health Services for the National Science Foundation in Washington. It was in this setting that he discovered the alarming dearth of useful drug information available to the general public. In direct opposition to the official position of the American Medical Association at that time, he published *The Essential Guide to Prescription Drugs* in 1977, the first book of organized, detailed drug information written specifically for the consumer.

Now living in retirement and experiencing firsthand the serious infirmities of aging, the author is forced to accept an unavoidable and somewhat traumatic reversal of roles—the physician is now the patient. And once again he finds much of the general medical literature written primarily for the patient and family to be relatively superficial and of little practical value. With the advent of managed medical care and its attendant shifts of time, attention, and responsibility for monitoring the course of care, patients are finding it increasingly necessary to educate themselves regarding the accuracy of diagnosis and the management of therapy. This book is an attempt to provide some useful information for those who may need it.